Thank you for all you are doing to build a culture of health!

Claudia Fernandez

Your commitment to Engagement & Equity are inspiring

~ Giselle Corbie

Leading Community Based Changes in the Culture of Health in the US - Experiences in Developing the Team and Impacting the Community

Edited by Claudia S. P. Fernandez and Giselle Corbie-Smith

Published in London, United Kingdom

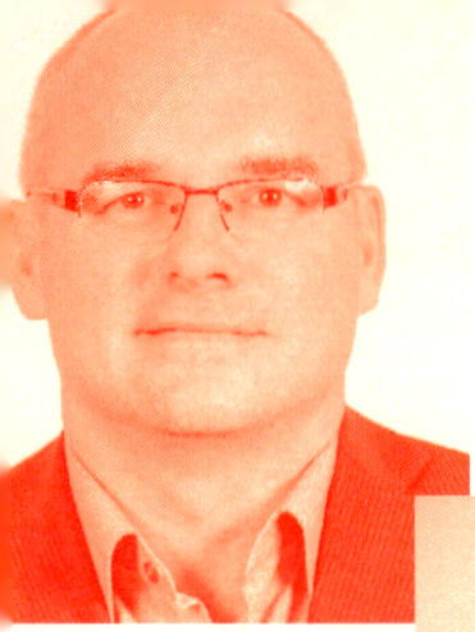
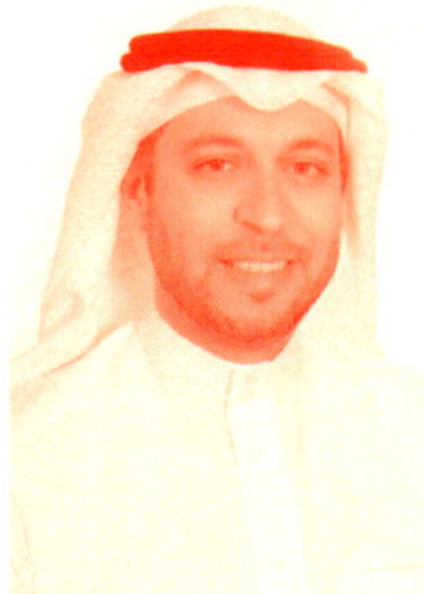
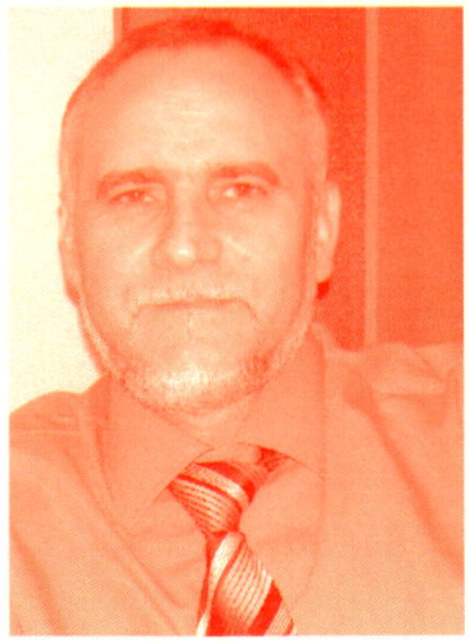
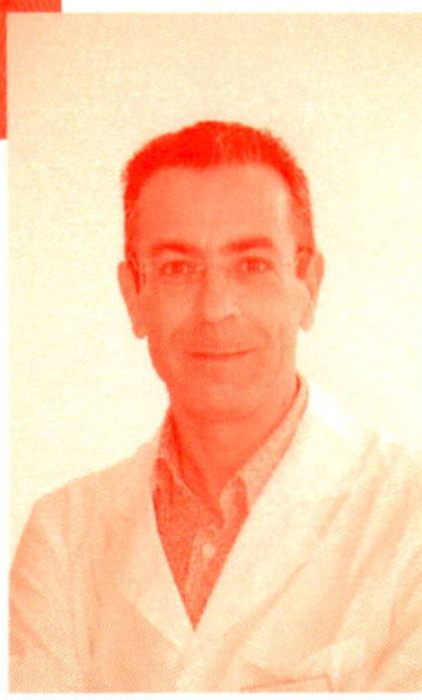
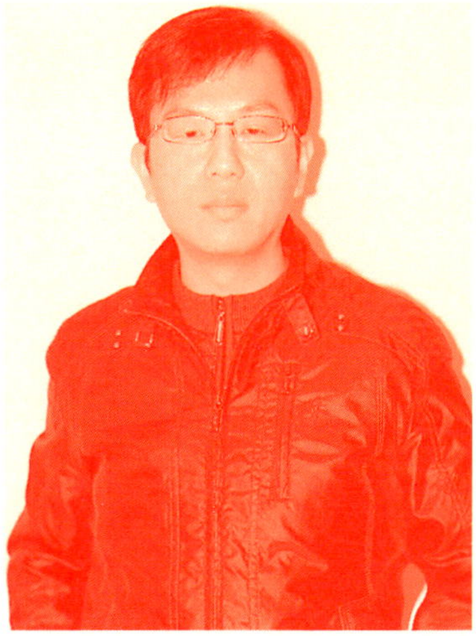
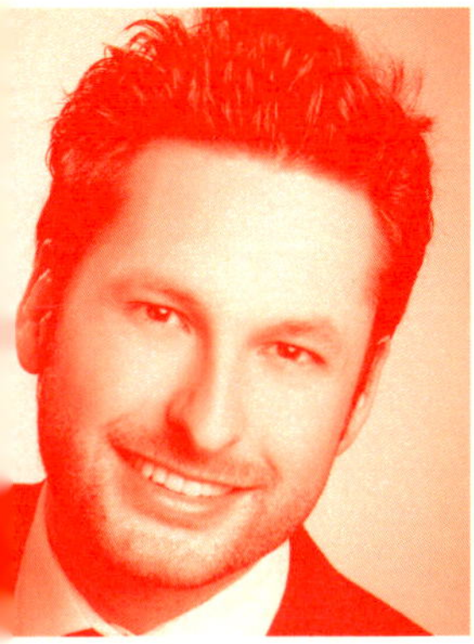
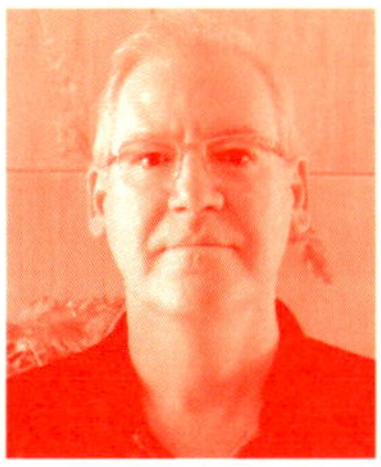

IntechOpen

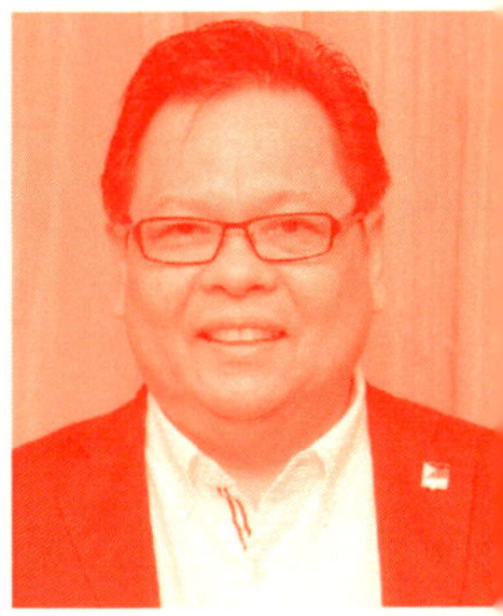
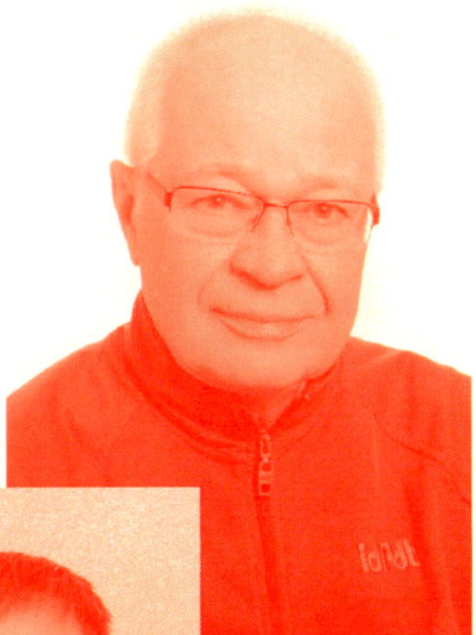
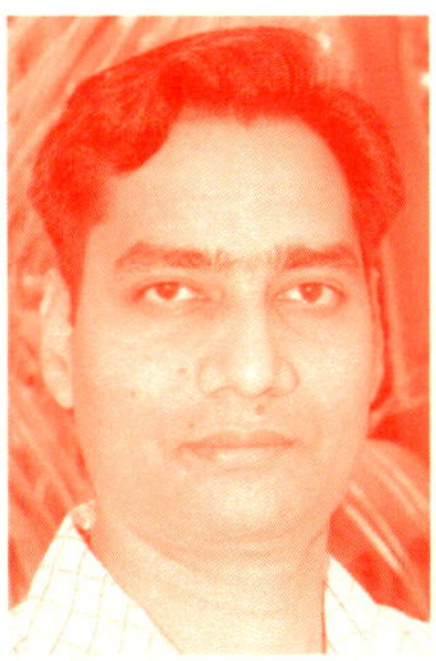
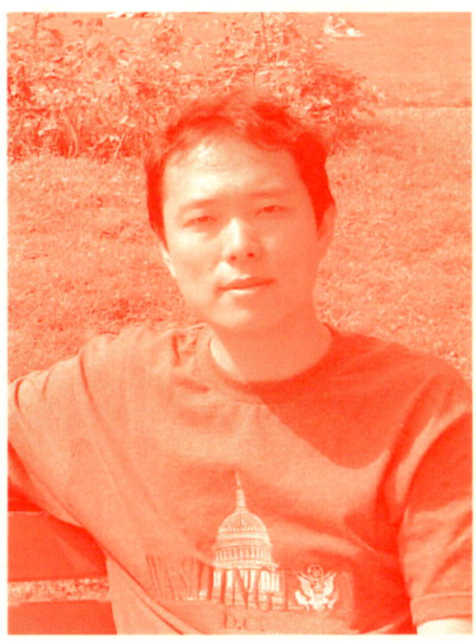
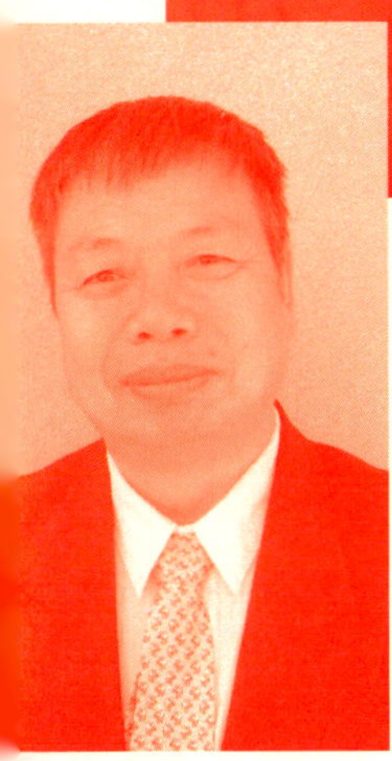
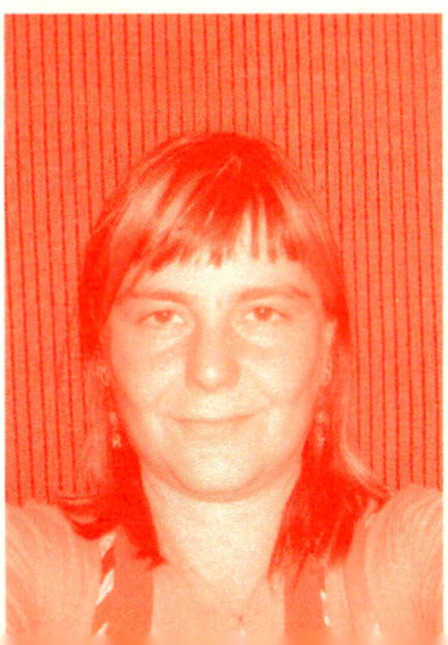

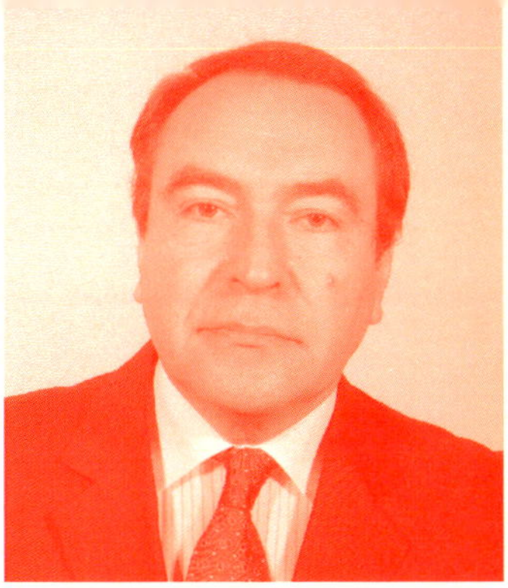
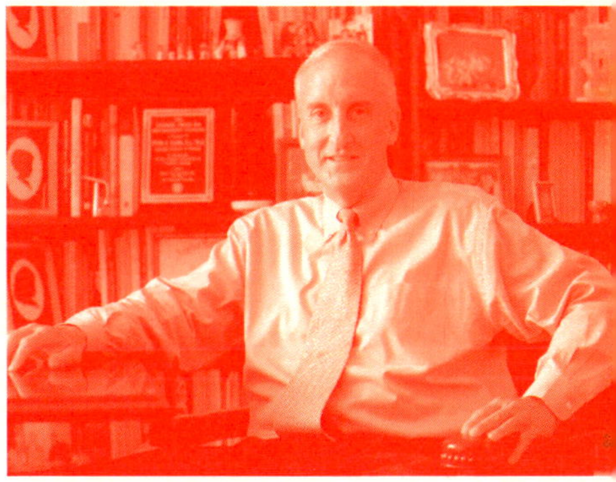
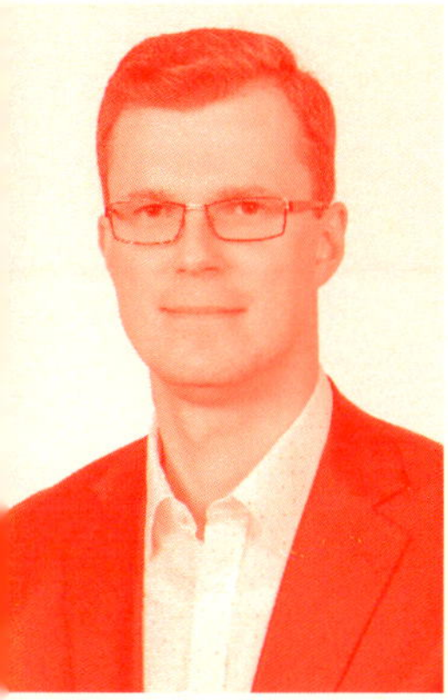
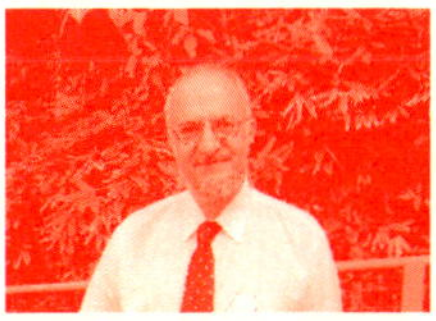
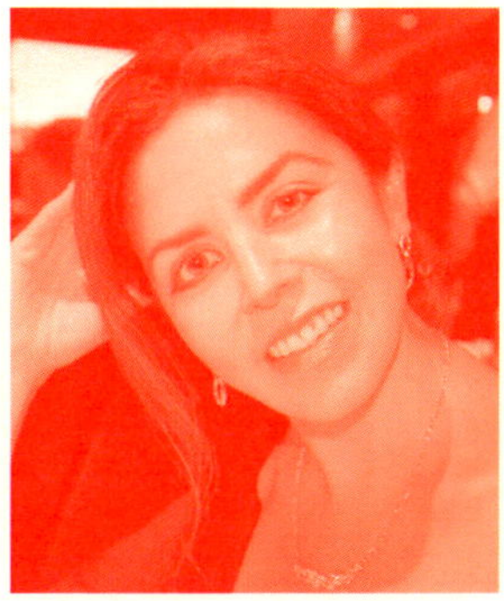

Supporting open minds since 2005

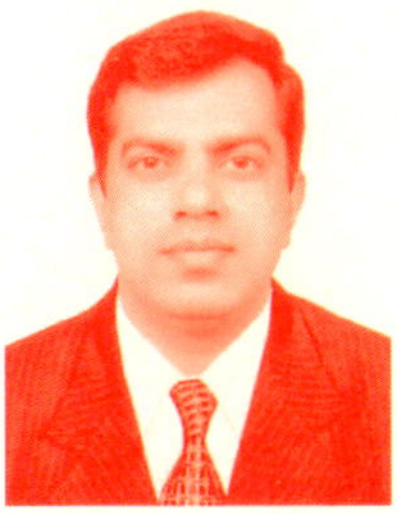
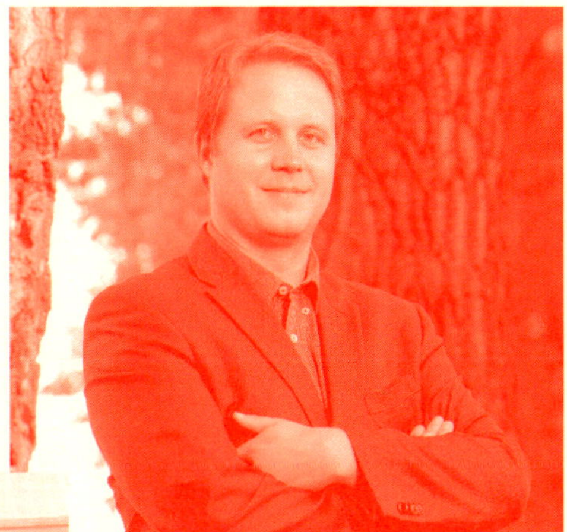
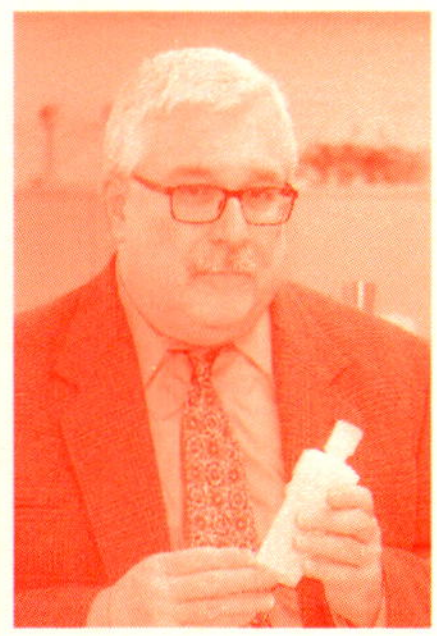
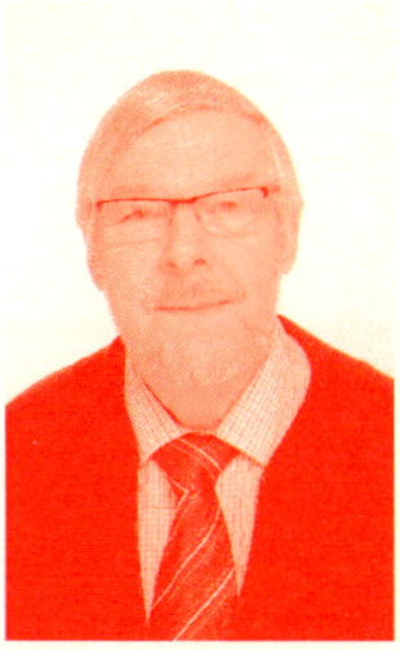
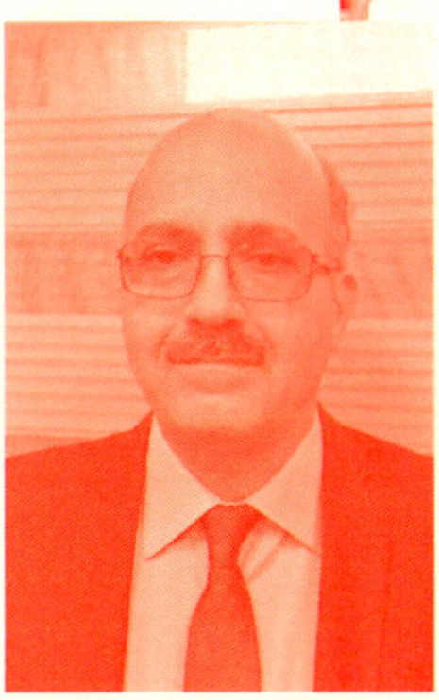
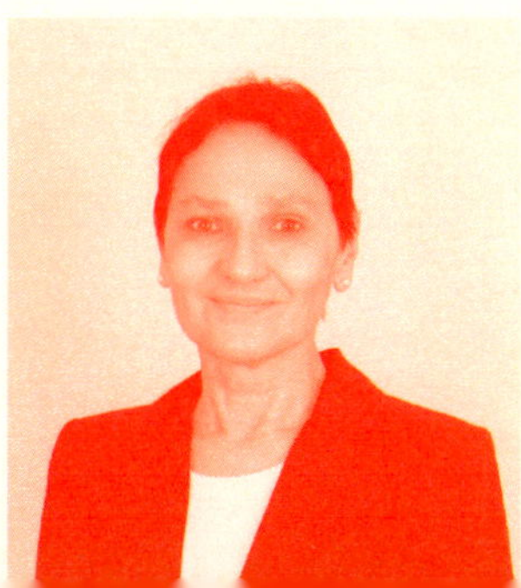
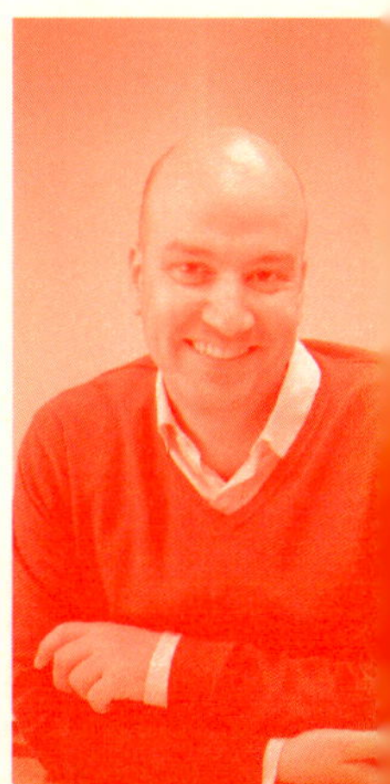

Leading Community Based Changes in the Culture of Health in the US - Experiences in Developing the Team and Impacting the Community
http://dx.doi.org/10.5772/intechopen.80243
Edited by Claudia S. P. Fernandez and Giselle Corbie-Smith

Contributors
Claudia S.P. Fernandez, Giselle Corbie-Smith, Melissa Green, Kathleen Brandert, Cheryl Noble, Gaurav Dave, Rachel Berthiaume, Caroline Chandler, Natalie S. Burke, Gail C. Christopher, Tara S. Hacker, Jeffrey Moy, Andrea Williams, Carolyn Wolf-Gould, Mark DeRuiter, Jeffrey Karp, Peter Scal, Charles E. Moore, Hope Bussenius, David Reznik, Annette Bell, Slyving Bordeau, Asha Davis, Amanda Stanec, Derrick Stephens, Aviril Sepulveda, Dean M. Coffey, Jed David, Horacio Lopez, Joyce R. Javier, Kamil Bantol, Kent Key, Tonita Smith, Edith Amponsah, Lia Garman, Seth Himelhoch, Marion Currens, Jewell Benford, Eric Weintraub, Laurel Berman, Nnemdi Kamanu Elias, Alfred Larbi, Kevin Washington, Erin Athey, Anjali Taneja, William Wagner

First published in London, United Kingdom, 2021 by IntechOpen
IntechOpen is the global imprint of INTECHOPEN LIMITED, registered in England and Wales, registration number: 11086078, 5 Princes Gate Court, London, SW7 2QJ, United Kingdom
Printed in Croatia

British Library Cataloguing-in-Publication Data
A catalogue record for this book is available from the British Library

Additional hard and PDF copies can be obtained from orders@intechopen.com

Leading Community Based Changes in the Culture of Health in the US - Experiences in Developing the Team and Impacting the Community
Edited by Claudia S. P. Fernandez and Giselle Corbie-Smith
p. cm.
Print ISBN 978-1-80355-155-5
Online ISBN 978-1-80355-153-1
eBook (PDF) ISBN 978-1-80355-154-8

Meet the editors

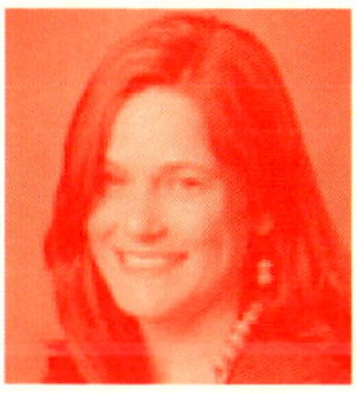

Claudia S. Plaisted Fernandez, DrPH, MS, RD, LDN, is an associate professor in the Gillings School of Global Public Health, University of North Carolina at Chapel Hill. She is the co-author of It-Factor Leadership: Become a Better Leader in 13 Steps. Dr. Fernandez has extensive experience developing custom executive education programs that focus on personal leadership development, innovation, and business skills for senior, middle, and frontline managers and leaders. As a licensed and registered dietitian, she has a particular interest in leadership in healthcare systems and high-performing healthcare and public health teams. Since 2006, she has directed the American College of Obstetricians and Gynecologists Robert C. Cefalo ACOG National Leadership Institute. Since 2005 she has served as the director of the Leadership Core of the Food Systems Leadership Institute, which was ranked number 2 in the country for open enrollment/continuing education in leadership by Leadership Excellence in 2016. In 2015 she was named the Co-Principal Investigator of the Clinical Scholars Fellowship for the Robert Wood Johnson Foundation's Advancing Change Leadership initiative. She has co-created and/or led several other leadership institutes, including the Managing in Turbulent Times: The Kellogg Fellowship for Emerging Leaders in Public Health Program (a minority leadership development program), the Southeast Public Health Leadership Institute, and Leadership Novant for the Novant Healthcare system. As an executive coach, Dr. Fernandez incorporates a wide array of leadership and psychological assessment tools and simulations and she is a trained hypnotherapist and stress management specialist with twenty years of experience counseling clients. Her programs offer values-based coaching, appreciative inquiry, and engaged learning. Dr. Fernandez earned her BS from Miami University of Ohio in 1986 and her MS from Boston University in 1988. She then pursued further education in psychology and counseling at the Harvard University Extension School and at the University of North Carolina at Chapel Hill, where she earned her doctorate in leadership studies in 2003 through the Public Health Leadership Department and Health Policy and Administration. Dr. Fernandez worked in the Harvard Medical School-affiliated hospital system for more than five years before joining the Duke Center for Living in 1992. In 1997 she accepted a faculty position with UNC and subsequently worked at the North Carolina Institute for Public Health. In 2007 she joined the faculty in the Department of Maternal and Child Health at the renowned UNC Gillings School of Global Public Health.

Giselle Corbie-Smith, MD, MSc, is Kenan Distinguished Professor, Departments of Social Medicine and Medicine, Director of the UNC Center for Health Equity Research at the University of North Carolina at Chapel Hill, and Associate Provost for UNC Rural. Internationally recognized for her scholarly work and expertise in community-engaged and patient-oriented research, Dr. Corbie-Smith has empirically studied methodological, ethical, and practical issues relating to studying racial disparities in health. Dr. Corbie-Smith has served as the Principal Investigator of several community-based participatory research projects focused on disease risk reduction among rural racial and ethnic minorities. These projects have included funding through the National

Heart Lung and Blood Institute, the Robert Wood Johnson Foundation (RWJF), the National Center for Minority Health and Health Disparities, the National Institute of Nursing Research, Greenwall Foundation, and the National Human Genome Research Institute. Dr. Corbie-Smith is accomplished in drawing communities, faculty, and healthcare providers into working partnerships in clinical and translational research. This engagement ultimately transforms the way that academic investigators and community members interact while boosting public trust in research. She has also shown a deep commitment to working in North Carolina by bringing research to communities, involving community members as partners in research, and improving the health of minority populations and underserved areas. In 2013 she established the UNC Center for Health Equity Research (CHER) to bring together collaborative multidisciplinary teams of scholars, trainees, and community members to improve North Carolina communities' health through a shared commitment to innovation, collaboration, and health equity. Dr. Corbie-Smith is also the Co-Principal Investigator for RWJF's Advancing Change Leadership Clinical Scholars Program, which provides intensive learning, collaboration, networking, and leadership development to seasoned clinicians to create a community of practitioners promoting health equity across the country. She served as President of the Society of General Internal Medicine (SGIM) in 2018–2019. In 2018 she was elected to the National Academy of Medicine. In 2019 Dr. Corbie-Smith created and is the current host of A Different Kind of Leader, a podcast that captures insights from diverse leaders so that organizations are in a stronger position to grow, innovate, and meet the challenges of our day. Dr. Corbie-Smith earned her MD from the Albert Einstein College of Medicine, NY, and MSc in Clinical Research from Emory University, Georgia.

Meet the authors

Erin Athey, DNP, FNP, BSN, is faculty at the George Washington University School of Nursing (GW Nursing) and a family nurse practitioner specializing in HIV/AIDS in Washington, DC. For almost a decade, Dr. Athey has worked in Ward 8 of Washington, DC, as a clinician, educator, and community-engaged scholar in an effort to bring quality care and innovation to a population most in need of healthcare. Dr. Athey has a keen understanding of social determinants of health (SDoH) and applies a holistic approach to the care of patients. She has strong connections to both the Rodham Institute and the Nashman Center for Civic Engagement, both GW-based institutions that are committed to using university resources to address health disparities and inequities in Washington, DC. Dr. Athey is also a member of the Ward 8 Health Council and co-created its first subcommittee on mental health and wellness. Through this community-engaged work, she was selected as a fellow into the inaugural Robert Wood Johnson Foundation Clinical Scholars Change Leadership program in 2016. She and her colleague developed the Mental Health Improvement through Studying, Teaching, Rebranding, Embedded Education and Technology (MHI-STREET) initiative, using barbershops in Southeast DC to promote mental health literacy in African American men. Recently, Dr. Athey was awarded the Hillman Emergent Innovation Award to expand the reach of the program by training DC youth to use storytelling to improve mental health literacy to other youth in other non-traditional spaces. In addition to being an educator at GW Nursing, Dr. Athey is also engaged in community education as a speaker for the Mid-Atlantic AIDS Education Training Center and is on the local and national board of directors for the Association of Nurses in AIDS Care. In 2017 she was awarded the Rising Star Award from the National Organization of Nurse Practitioner Faculties and in 2018 she was named an NP to Admire: 10 Role Models Improving the Lives of Vulnerable Populations by the Nurse Practitioner Education Blog.

Edith Amponsah, MPH, IBCLC, is a first-year medical student at Tulane University School of Medicine, Louisiana. She earned her Master's of Public Health in Maternal and Child Health at the University of North Carolina (UNC) Gillings School of Global Public Health. While at UNC, she completed a Pathway 2 Lactation Consultant program through the Mary Rose Tully Training Initiative (MRTTI) at the Carolina Global Breastfeeding Institute (CGBI). She also trained and volunteered as a birth doula with the UNC Birth Partners Program. Ms. Amponsah's research interests include disparities in pregnancy outcomes, MCH program evaluation, and effects of childhood trauma over the life course. Ms. Amponsah earned her Bachelor of Science in Global and International Health Development from the College of William and Mary, Virginia.

Kamil Evy Bantol, BS, previously served as a research assistant at Children's Hospital Los Angeles (CHLA). There she worked alongside Dr. Joyce Javier and Team Kapwa to promote Filipino American youth mental health and wellness in Los Angeles. Ms. Bantol obtained her bachelor's degree in Health Promotion and Disease Prevention from the University of Southern California. She is currently a second-year medical student at Drexel University College of Medicine, Pennsylvania, and hopes to address health disparities in the Filipino community as a future physician.

Annette Bell, MD, is a board-certified family physician who earned a Bachelor of Science (First Class Honours) from St. Francis Xavier University, Antigonish, Nova Scotia, and a Doctor of Medicine from Dalhousie University, Halifax, Nova Scotia. She completed her family medicine residency at the University of Alberta, Edmonton before relocating to Florida. She is certified with the College of Family Physicians of Canada and a fellow of the American Academy of Family Physicians. Dr. Bell currently practices as an emergency room physician in the Baptist Health System in Northeast Florida. In addition to providing direct patient care in the ER, she has worked with organizations in her community to impact the lives of patients with physical and mental health disorders by breaking down barriers to treatment. She is an alumnus with the Robert Wood Johnson Foundation Clinical Scholars Program and the recipient of the Baptist Medical Center Nassau Spirit of Magnet Evidence-based Quality Practice Award. She currently serves as chair of the McArthur Family YMCA Advisory Board and is a proud wife and mom of three wonderful children.

Jewell Benford, LCSW-C, is Program Director for the University of Maryland Drug Treatment Center administered by the University of Maryland Department of Psychiatry's Division of Alcohol and Drug Abuse. He also serves as Director of Compliance for the University of Maryland Medical Center Community Substance Abuse Programs. He also is a treating clinician for the National Football League's Substances of Abuse, and Maryland Group Faculty Practice. Mr. Benford received a BA and BS in Social Work and Psychology at the University of Maryland, Baltimore County. He received his graduate degree in Social Work in 1984 from the University of Maryland, Baltimore. Mr. Benford has extensive experience working with federal offenders and defendants, professional athletes, and individuals with substance use disorders. Mr. Benford has been a trainer for the University of Maryland Baltimore's psychotherapy certificate program and Double Abuse Trainings focusing on the intersection of child maltreatment and substance use. Mr. Benford has clinical interests in disparities in criminal justice sentencing and healthcare, as well as working with high school, college, and professional athletes.

Laurel Berman, Ph.D., is the National Brownfields Coordinator with ATSDR Division of Community Health Investigations. Dr. Berman coordinates the ATSDR Land Reuse Health Program, which integrates public health and redevelopment from the early planning stages. She brings her skills to the Initiative from a long career as an environmental scientist and a community engagement specialist. Dr. Berman has led the Initiative in creating tools and resources to construct healthier communities through revitalization practices. These include an Environmental Health and Land Reuse curriculum and a community assessment tool (Action Model) that has led to the development of a unique data set of public health indicators associated with contaminated sites and redevelopment. Recently, Dr. Berman edited and co-authored the book, *Land Reuse and Redevelopment: Creating Healthy Communities* (ATSDR, 2020, in press). In addition, she has developed a North American expert consultancy group that provides free technical assistance to brownfields communities. Dr. Berman holds a Ph.D. and MS in Environmental and Occupational Health Sciences from the University of Illinois at Chicago School of Public Health, with a focus on industrial hygiene and toxicology. She is adjunct assistant professor in this program and currently teaches in the undergraduate program in public health. Dr. Berman is also adjunct faculty for DePaul University's (Chicago) Master of Public Health Program.

Rachel Berthiaume, MPH, is the Deputy Director of Distance Education for the Robert Wood Johnson Foundation's Clinical Scholars, a comprehensive leadership development program for healthcare providers from diverse fields. The providers work in interdisciplinary teams in cross-sector collaboration to tackle complex health problems in their communities. She administers the program's distance-based learning curriculum through an online learning platform, newsletters, webinars, web-based "book clubs," reflective online writing activities, and skill-building modules. Her career in public health began with Peace Corps service (Madagascar 2004–2006), and then continued with HIV/AIDS/STI prevention and treatment programs at health clinics in sub-Saharan Africa. She received her Master of Public Health in Health Behavior/Education from UNC-Chapel Hill's Gillings School of Global Public Health in 2012. Rachel previously managed health projects in Philadelphia, PA, and Michigan, examining intersections between communities and public agencies to improve maternal and child health service delivery, particularly in addressing equity and inclusion issues. Rachel can be reached at rberthia@email.unc.edu.

Slyving Bourdeau, LCSW, is a clinical social worker and received his BA in Social Work from Kentucky State University in 2005, his Master of Social Work from University of Central Florida in 2009, and is currently pursuing a Master of Business Administration. He was born and raised in Florida and is the youngest of four children. Mr. Bourdeau is a member of American College of Healthcare Executives. He entered the workforce in 2005 as a juvenile case manager providing appropriate services and/or interventions for children and adolescents displaying severe social, emotional, and/or behavioral disorders. Slyving Bourdeau's clinical experience is varied and includes time spent working on a medical and jail psychiatric unit with young adults, working in a grant funded substance prevention/treatment center, and operating a private healthcare consulting practice.

Kathleen (Katie) Brandert, MPH, CHES, worked for nearly a decade on a host of wicked maternal and child health issues, such as infant mortality, undoing racism, unintended pregnancy, health inequities, and more. There she realized her love for developing leaders who could take on the world's most pressing challenges. Since 2012, Katie has directed the Great Plains Leadership Institute (a year-long leadership training program) and served as Manager of Workforce Development and Leadership Programs in the College of Public Health, University of Nebraska Medical Center (UNMC). In that capacity, she is a team coach and faculty member in the Clinical Scholars Program (funded by the Robert Wood Johnson Foundation, led by the University of North Carolina, Chapel-Hill). Katie is also an adjunct faculty member at Nebraska Methodist College, and an instructor in Health Promotion at UNMC. Katie makes an impact with her skills in leadership development, coaching, and facilitation. She is certified in a number of personal assessments and tools, including 360 assessments, focused on personality and behavior, change, conflict, organizational culture, and intercultural development. Her areas of focus include training on leadership identity, building teams, public speaking, and the journey towards equity, diversity, and inclusion. She regularly provides executive coaching to leaders and facilitates (virtual and in-person) planning processes and strategy meetings for organizations across Nebraska and the country. Katie is a sought-after facilitator for difficult conversations, culture work, and organizational strategy. Katie lives in Omaha, Nebraska, where she loves to laugh, eat savory foods from Omaha's many chef-owned restaurants, grow tomatoes in her garden, crochet (but only in the winter), and raise her sons. She is currently completing her dissertation research in Leadership Studies at the University of Nebraska-Lincoln.

Natalie S. Burke, BS, is a nationally known speaker, "equity evangelist," strategist, master facilitator, and public health leader. Natalie provides executive leadership for CommonHealth ACTION whose mission is to develop people and organizations to produce health through equitable policies, programs, and practices. Since the mid-1990s, Natalie has held leadership positions focused on creating opportunities for health through community, institutional, systemic, and policy change. A graduate of the University of Maryland with a degree in Government and Politics, Natalie has been selected for numerous fellowships including the Emerging Leaders in Public Health Fellowship (hosted by the University of North Carolina's Schools of Business and Public Health) and New York University's Robert F. Wagner School of Public Service Lead the Way Fellowship for visionary and entrepreneurial leaders in the nonprofit sector. She also served as a W.K. Kellogg Foundation Fellow conducting federal health policy analysis at the National Health Policy Forum in Washington, DC. In 2012, she was selected to serve on the Council of Innovation Advisors for ConvergeUS, a national initiative focused on technology-based social innovation. Since 2015, Natalie has served as co-director of the Culture of Health Leaders National Program Center, funded by the Robert Wood Johnson Foundation; she directs the Kaiser Permanente Institute for Equitable Leadership in Baltimore; she is a member of the Institute for Healthcare Improvement's Equity Advisory Group; and she is a member of the NationSwell Council. Committed to the health and well-being of all people, Natalie views health as the product of complex interactions amongst systems and factors such as education, employment, environmental conditions, access to technology, housing, transportation, and healthcare. Throughout her career, she has sought to understand the root causes of ill-health including the delicate balance amongst genetics, personal health behaviors, and the systems and institutions that provide the contexts within which we live our lives and make our decisions. That understanding guides her work with corporate, academic, elected, and community leaders whose decisions produce health. For the past decade through curriculum development, education, and publications, she has focused on the roles that systemic privilege and oppression play in the production of the public's health, particularly health inequities, including serving as the primary architect for CommonHealth ACTION's nationally recognized Equity, Diversity, and Inclusion Training Institute.

Hope Bussenius, DNP, APRN, FNP-BC, FAANP, FAR, maintained a 26-year practice as a family nurse practitioner with a multidisciplinary history of being a clinical nurse practitioner and teacher in Haiti for 25 years, co-founder of Health Connection Primary Care Clinic, lieutenant in the US Navy Reserves, research coordinator II for the AIDS Research Consortium of Atlanta, and a legal nurse consultant at King & Spalding, LLC. Currently, as an assistant clinical professor at the Nell Hodgson Woodruff School of Nursing at Emory University. She received her Bachelor of Science in Nursing from the Medical College of Georgia in 1990, Masters in Nursing from Emory University in 1993, and completed her Doctor of Nursing Practice at Georgia Health Sciences University in 2012, specializing and developing a technology model called the Transformative Technology Evaluation and Assessment Model (2TEAM). As a pioneer in smartphone development, in 2010 she developed an award-winning smartphone application connected to a repository, Pedia BP, that has more than 80,000 downloads in 30 countries. She is the founder of Take2Heart

Initiative, a non-profit organization for pediatric hypertension, and received the 2018 BAYADA Award for Technological Innovation in Health Care Education and Practice. In 2016, she was awarded the Robert Wood Johnson Foundation Clinical Scholars Award for the wicked project Oral Health in Communities and Neighborhoods (OHICAN) and with her team, developed a second smartphone application connected to a repository. The OH-I-CAN app has more than 30,000 downloads in all 50 states. The 2TEAM has been adopted in the curriculum at Emory University, Georgia, and in the Lillian Carter Center for Global Health and Social Responsibility. Recently, she received the E. Louise Grant Distinguished Alumni Award from Augusta University, and was appointed as the National Collegiate Athletic Association (NCAA) Faculty Athletic Representative (FAR) of Emory University and named as the Division III FAR Fellow.

Caroline Chandler, MPH, is a doctoral student in the Department of Maternal and Child Health, Gillings School of Global Public Health, University of North Carolina at Chapel Hill. She earned a Master's in Public Health from the Gillings School of Global Public Health, and she is currently a predoctoral fellow at the Carolina Consortium on Human Development and a community engagement fellow at the Carolina Center for Public Service. Ms. Chandler has experience evaluating national media campaigns and programs designed to promote prevention and wellbeing. Ms. Chandler's research focuses on social–emotional health and development in children and adolescents in contexts of adversity, with an emphasis on participatory research methods.

Gail Christopher, DN, ND, is an award-winning social change agent with expertise in the social determinants of health and well-being and in related public policies. She is known for her pioneering work to infuse holistic health and diversity concepts into public sector programs and policy discourse. Dr. Christopher recently retired from her role as Senior Advisor and Vice President at the W.K. Kellogg Foundation (WKKF), where she was the driving force behind the America Healing initiative and the Truth, Racial Healing and Transformation effort. Dr. Christopher also served as Kellogg's Vice President for Program Strategy and worked on place-based programming in New Orleans and New Mexico. In 2015 she received the Terrance Keenan Award from Grantmakers in Health. She chairs the Board of the Trust for America's Health. In 2019, she became a Senior Scholar with George Mason University's Center for the Advancement of Well-Being. Dr. Christopher also became Executive Director of the National Collaborative for Health Equity in November 2019. She is the visionary for and architect of the WKKF led Truth Racial Healing and Transformation (TRHT) effort for America. TRHT is an adaptation of the globally recognized Truth and Reconciliation Commission (TRC) model. TRHT evolved from the decade long WKKF America Healing, racial equity and racial healing initiative, designed and led by Dr. Christopher. Over the last ten years she has had responsibility for several other areas of foundation programming. These include, food, health and well-being, leadership, public policy, community engagement, and place-based funding in New Orleans and New Mexico. In August 2017, Dr. Christopher left her leadership position with WKKF to launch the Maryland-based Ntianu Center for Healing and Nature and to devote more time to writing and speaking on issues of health, racial healing, and human capacity for caring. She is currently Chair of the Board of the Trust for America's Health. Dr. Christopher is a nationally recognized leader in health policy, with particular expertise and experience in integrative health and medicine, social determinants of health, health inequities, and public policy issues of concern to our nation's future. Her distinguished career and contributions to public service were honored in 1996 when she was elected as a fellow of the National Academy of Public Administration. In 2007 she received the Leadership Award from the Health Brain Trust of the Congressional Black Caucus for her work in reducing racial and ethnic health disparities; in 2009 she was named a Society for Public Health Education (SOPHE) Honorary Fellow, which is the highest recognition given to a non-SOPHE member who has made significant contributions to health education and to public health; in 2011 she was awarded the "Change Agent Award" by the Schott Foundation for Public Education; in 2012 she was the recipient of the Association of Maternal & Child Health Programs (AMCHP) John C. MacQueen Lecture Award for her innovation and leadership in the field of maternal and child health. Most recently in 2015 she was the recipient of the Terrance Keenan award for Grantmakers in Health. She is chair of the board of the Trust for America's Health. Gail has more than 30 years of experience in designing and managing national initiatives and nonprofit organizations. She brings extensive knowledge and experience in creating a comprehensive approach to well-being and is nationally recognized for her pioneering work to infuse holistic health and diversity concepts into public sector programs and policy discourse. A prolific writer and presenter, Dr. Christopher is the author or co-author of three books, a monthly column in the *Federal Times*, and more than 350 articles, presentations, and publications. Her national print and broadcast media credits are numerous, and include *The Washington Post*, *Los Angeles Times*, *Dallas, Times*, *National Journal*, *Essence*, *Good Morning America*, *The Oprah Winfrey Show*, *National Public Radio*, and documentaries on PBS and CBS. Prior to joining the foundation, Gail was vice president of the Joint Center for Political and Economic Studies' Office of Health, Women and Families in Washington, DC. There, she led the Joint Center Health Policy Institute, a multi-year initiative created to engage underserved, racial, and ethnic minorities in health policy discussions. Previously, she was guest scholar in the governance studies department at The Brookings Institution in Washington, DC and executive director of the Institute for Government Innovation at Harvard's John F. Kennedy School of Government in Cambridge, Massachusetts. She has additional experience at the National Academy of Public Administration, Howard University School of Divinity, Americans All National Education Program, and Family Resource Coalition of America. She has also launched, led, and managed three public commissions. Under her sponsorship, the landmark Dellums Commission research into conditions faced by young men of color-produced policy recommendations to reduce racial and ethnic health disparities. Gail holds a Doctor of Naprapathy from the Chicago National College of Naprapathy, Illinois, and completed advanced study in the interdisciplinary PhD program in holistic health and clinical nutrition at the Union for Experimenting Colleges and Universities at Union Graduate School of Cincinnati, Ohio.

Dean Coffey, PsyD, is Clinical Associate Professor of Pediatrics (Clinician Educator) in the Division of General Pediatrics, Children's Hospital Los Angeles (CHLA) and Keck School of Medicine of USC. As the Child and Family Program Area Lead in the outpatient Mental Health Center at CHLA, he manages a team of professionals providing mental health services to children ages 6 to 12 years and their families. Dr. Coffey has extensive experience implementing the Incredible Years Parent Program (IY) in both clinical and community-based settings. He is an Incredible Years Certified Agency Mentor and provides training and group supervision for parent group leaders in Southern California. Dr. Coffey is an alumnus of the Robert Wood Johnson Clinical Scholars Program (2016–2019) who continues to work in the Filipino communities throughout California to reduce the disparate high rates of teen suicidal ideation and suicide attempts by using IY to enhance parent–child relationship.

Marian Currens, CRNP, serves the city of Baltimore as a Nurse Practitioner for more than 30 years. She began her career at Johns Hopkins Bayview Medical Center where she grew to appreciate the many challenges of treating substance use disorders. Marian expanded her work experience to include outpatient methadone maintenance, suboxone maintenance, and drug-free intensive outpatient treatment. For the past 22 years, she has been the nurse practitioner managing the medical care for the inpatient chemical dependency services at UMMC Midtown Campus, formerly Maryland General Hospital. She also holds the position of Associate Medical Director for the Center for Addiction Medicine (CAM). Under her management, CAM has grown to include multiple levels of care while maintaining Joint Commission Certification. Marian is also an active board member (or chair) on several local associations including the Maryland Association for the Treatment of Opioid Dependence (MATOD), the Maryland Association of Chemical Dependency Nurses (MACDN), and the Maryland Addiction Directors Counsel (MADC). When Marian can find time, she enjoys kayaking and the great outdoors.

Gaurav Dave, MD, DrPH, MPH, is Associate Professor of Medicine and Associate Director of the Center for Health Equity Research at the University of North Carolina at Chapel Hill (UNC). He has more than 15 years of clinical, public health research, and evaluation experience. Dr. Dave's research focuses on reducing health disparities associated with cardiovascular diseases, specifically hypertension prevention, control, and management. He oversees implementation of the NIH-funded Heart Matters study, which aims to enhance uptake of cardioprotective behaviors and improve hypertension outcomes in Edgecombe and Nash counties in North Carolina. Dr. Dave is also an expert in the field of evaluation research, specializing in evaluating multi-level, complex initiatives and programs. He is Director of Evaluation for the NIH-funded North Carolina Translational and Clinical Sciences Institute and RWJF-funded Clinical Scholars National Leadership Institute at UNC. He also chairs the evaluation for HRSA's Southeast Regional Genetics Network at Emory University aimed to improve health equity and outcomes for individuals with genetic conditions. Dr. Dave has a medical degree from University of Pune, India, and worked as an emergency room physician in Mumbai. He also has master and doctorate degrees in Public Health, specializing in stakeholder engagement, participatory research, and evaluation.

Jed David, MS, OTR/L, SWC, is an occupational therapist at Children's Hospital Los Angeles and a Robert Wood Johnson Clinical Scholars Fellow. Jed completed his Public Policy, Management and Planning degree at the University of Southern California and his Occupational Therapy education at Columbia University. He received his national board specialty certification in the field of feeding, eating, and swallowing and serves multiple specialty care clinics at CHLA. Jed was born in Cebu, Philippines and grew up in the Historic Filipinotown and Silverlake area of Los Angeles. Jed is an active member of Kayamanan Ng Lahi Philippine Folk Arts and serves as their Associate Director of Programming. Jed aims to be a steward of the Filipino community by building a culture of mental health through an interdisciplinary and a culturally relevant approach such as the application of the Filipino core value of kapwa in clinical care and community health. He will continue to pursue his doctoral studies focused on the health and well-being of the Filipino community at Columbia University, and hopes he can inspire transformation among the next generation of Filipino-Americans to make a meaningful impact in health equity. He is the only son of four children and is proud of his Filipino roots and his family.

Asha Davis, MD, was born and raised in Houston, TX. She is the second daughter of four girls. From an early age, she knew she had an interest in medicine. This was strengthened during her undergraduate studies at Xavier University, New Orleans, Louisiana. Dr. Davis then attended Medical School at the University of Texas Medical Branch (UTMB), Galveston, Texas. Throughout her studies and medical training, she was ultimately led to a career in psychiatry. Her psychiatry residency was through Wake Forest Baptist Medical Center, Winston Salem, North Carolina. Through Wake Forest, she also completed a fellowship in Child and Adolescent Psychiatry. She is currently a board-certified adult as well as child and adolescent psychiatrist. Her current home base is in Miami, Florida. Dr. Davis's time is divided between working part time in an outpatient psychiatric clinic and through providing outpatient services via telepsychiatry. She self identifies as a doctor by day and a fashionista by night. When not engaged in clinical or fashion-related activity, she also enjoys traveling and spending quality time with friends and family.

Mark DeRuiter, MBA, PhD, is currently Director of the Clinical Doctorate in SLP program, Department of Communication Science and Disorders, University of Pittsburgh. While he was a clinical scholar he served as Associate Department Head for Clinical Education in the Department of Speech, Language and Hearing Sciences, University of Arizona. He holds a Certificate of Clinical Competence in Audiology and Speech-Language Pathology from the American Speech-Language-Hearing Association.

Nnemdi Elias, MD, MPH, was a Robert Wood Johnson Foundation Clinical Scholar at the time of this writing. Previously, she was at United Medical Center, the only hospital in southeast Washington, DC, as Senior Medical Director and founder of the office of Community Initiatives at United Medical Center and Medical Director of their HIV/AIDS clinic. Prior to that, she had served as Medical Director of the Comprehensive Clinical Center at UPO, a clinic for opioid dependency; Chief Medical Officer of the DC Department of Health/HAHSTA; and a senior staff member at the European and Developing Countries Clinical Trials Partnership in the Netherlands, an organization created by the European Commission. Under the President's Emergency Plan for AIDS Relief (PEPFAR) as Chief of the HIV/AIDS Care and Treatment section of the Centers for Disease Control and Prevention (CDC) Global AIDS Program in Tanzania, Dr. Elias oversaw the implementation of United States Government (USG) supported HIV care and treatment services. Before that she was at PEPFAR headquarters, within the Office of the Global AIDS Coordinator in the Department of State as a technical advisor. Dr. Elias was an assistant professor within the University of California, San Francisco (UCSF) Department of Medicine, Division of HIV/AIDS at SFGH. She obtained her medical degree from Yale University, completed residency in Internal Medicine/Primary Care at UCSF, and obtained a Master in Public Health from the University of California, Berkeley. She is involved in several programs in her local community.

Lia Garman, MPH, is a research assistant in the Maternal and Child Health Department at the UNC Gillings School of Global Public Health, where she recently completed her MPH. At UNC Lia supports the Clinical Scholars program as well as the Family Planning National Training Center, developing technical assistance materials for Title X grantee organizations. Lia previously worked at the Bixby Center for Global Reproductive Health at the University of California, San Francisco, where she supported training and research initiatives to expand access to contraception services. She graduated from UNC with a BA in Anthropology in 2012.

Melissa Green, MPH, is Deputy Director for Communication and Recruitment for the Clinical Scholars Program funded by the Robert Wood Johnson Foundation and is affiliated with the UNC Center for Health Equity Research (CHER). Melissa's experience includes 15 years managing research intervention studies in community settings using principles of community-based participatory research with and for African American and Latino populations. Her research interests include health disparities across the cancer continuum, peer support interventions, disease prevention, and factors that influence participation in health research. She received her Master of Public Health from the School of Public Health, University of North Carolina at Chapel Hill.

Seth Himelhoch, MD, MPH, received his medical degree at the University of Michigan School of Medicine (1994) and completed his residency training in general psychiatry at the University of California, San Francisco (1998). He completed a fellowship in health services research through the Robert Wood Johnson Clinical Scholars Program at Johns Hopkins School of Medicine (2003), where he concurrently received a master's degree in Public Health from the Bloomberg School of Public Health (2003). Dr. Himelhoch additionally completed a fellowship in Implementation and Dissemination Science through the Implementation Research Institute (2012). He is currently a Robert Wood Johnson Clinical Scholar (Cohort 2: 2017–2020).

Dr. Himelhoch's research focuses on developing and studying the efficacy of innovative strategies aimed at improving the health and welfare among people with co-occurring psychiatric and substance use disorders. He has a longstanding interest in evaluating behavioral interventions for people living with HIV/AIDS who have co-occurring substance use and psychiatric disorders. His current work seeks to evaluate the most promising behavioral and pharmacologic treatments aimed at achieving maximal efficacy for smoking cessation among people living with HIV/AIDS who smoke.

Dr. Himelhoch currently serves as professor and chair of the Department of Psychiatry at the University of Kentucky, College of Medicine. In that capacity, he is responsible for managing and overseeing inpatient and outpatient clinical, educational, and research-related services associated with the Department of Psychiatry and ensuring efficient management of clinical initiatives, educational training, and research portfolio.

Joyce R. Javier MD, MPH, MS, FAAP, is Associate Professor of Clinical Pediatrics at Children's Hospital Los Angeles, Keck School of Medicine, University of Southern California, and an attending physician at AltaMed General Pediatrics. She completed pediatrics residency training and a general academic pediatrics fellowship at Stanford University, California. She is a general pediatrician and physician scientist whose research over the past 18 years has focused on addressing health disparities among minority immigrant populations. Her most recent studies focus on recruitment of Filipino families in randomized controlled trials and using community-partnered participatory research to decrease mental health stigma and preventing adolescent depression and suicide among Filipino youth by partnering with parents and community stakeholders to implement and evaluate evidence-based parenting interventions. Her work has been funded by the National Institutes of Health NCATS KL2 and NICHD K23 awards, American Academy of Pediatrics (AAP), the SC CTSI, and the Robert Wood Johnson Foundation Clinical Scholars Program. She currently serves as an Executive Committee Member on the AAP Council on Community Pediatrics, co-chair of the Society for Pediatric Research Advocacy Committee, and a member of Pediatric Policy Council. In 2018, she received the AAP Local Hero Award and was named one of the 100 Most Influential Filipina Women in the World by the Filipina Women's Network. More information regarding research and advocacy can be found at filipinofamilyhealth.com

Jeffrey Karp, DMD, MS, is a board-certified pediatric dentist and residency program director at the University of Minnesota School of Dentistry. Jeff is an oral health advocate at the local, state, and national levels for individuals with special healthcare needs. As a dental academician, Dr. Karp teaches pediatric dentistry residents and dental students to provide a dental home for infants, children, and adolescents with complex medical conditions, physical, neurodevelopmental, and intellectual disabilities, and cleft and craniofacial differences.

Kent Key, MPH, PhD, is a Health Disparities Researcher specializing in Community Engaged Research in the Division of Public Health in the College of Human Medicine, Michigan State University and Executive Deputy Director of the Community Based Organization Partners (CBOP). Dr. Key is also founder of CBOP's Community Ethics Review Board in Flint, Michigan. He is the National Administrator of the Community Based Public Health Caucus of the American Public Health Association and a Robert Wood Johnson Foundation Fellow for the Culture of Health Leaders Program. Dr. Key also works to create pathways to careers in Public Health, Medicine and Research for urban youth.
Dr. Key has an interest in urban minority populations and uses qualitative methods to evaluate the perceptions and lived experience with a goal towards the development of community-driven solutions for health and equity.
His motto is "You have not lived until you have done something good for someone who cannot repay you!"

Alfred Larbi, MPH, is the grants officer at the Cambridge Clinical Trials Unit (CCTU) and interim research lead of the Patient Led Research Hub within the CCTU. He provides financial and methodological advice to researchers developing clinical research proposals, focused on a broad spectrum of treatment areas. He also supports the strategic operations and administrative functions of the unit.

Horacio Lopez, MD, is a board-certified community pediatrician who has served Historic Filipinotown in Los Angeles, California, for more than 25 years. Dr. Lopez served as the chairman of the Pediatric Department of Hollywood Presbyterian Medical Center for three terms. He was a fellow of the Robert Wood Johnson Clinical Scholars Program (Cohort 1: 2016–2019) and addressed mental health disparities of Filipino immigrants in Los Angeles. Dr. Lopez recognizes the importance of social–emotional health in children and incorporates the concepts of Incredible Years Parenting Program in his practice. He believes that Filipino immigrants can strengthen family relationships through recognizing the strengths of the Filipino culture while assimilating to the American way of life.

Charles Moore, MD, FAACE, received a Bachelor of Science from Union College and a medical degree from Harvard Medical School, Boston, Massachusetts. He subsequently completed residency training in Otolaryngology–Head and Neck Surgery and fellowship training in Craniomaxillofacial–Cranial Base, Facial Plastic and Reconstructive Surgery at the University of Michigan. Dr. Moore is a professor at Emory University, Atlanta, Georgia, and the Chief of Service in the Department of Otolaryngology–Head and Neck Surgery at Grady Health System. Dr. Moore has a longstanding and profound commitment to the training and development of learners from all backgrounds. His research focus has been in the investigation of factors involved in healthcare disparity with a particular focus on head and neck cancer incidence in medically underserved communities. He is the president and founder of Health Education, Assessment and Leadership (HEAL), Inc. This organization began in 2004 as a traveling educational resource out of the back of his personal vehicle. Through this organization, he strives to educate the community on health issues, assess its needs, and in the process build leaders from within the community to address those issues. This traveling resource has grown into the Healing Community Center (HCC), one of Atlanta's newest Federally Qualified Healthcare Centers. This center is a free and affordable medical facility with four separate locations that provide general adult medical care, pediatric medical care, specialty medical care, dental services as well as mental health services for the uninsured and disadvantaged. The HCC is focused on those who fall in the gap between public-funded healthcare and the privately insured. A primary emphasis is on preventative health, nutrition, and wellness. This center incorporates all of the major Atlanta academic institutions and community organizations in an integrated fashion to provide service-learning experiences while also providing the necessary care to those in need. Dr. Moore is the recipient of the American Medical Association Foundation Pride in Profession, Excellence in Medicine Award, the 2011 Gold Foundation Award for Humanism in Medicine, and the 2015 Jerome C. Goldstein, MD Public Service Award, awarded from National Academy of Otolaryngology. He is also the recipient of the Healthcare Georgia Foundation Award and the Zenith Award for Community Activism from the City of Atlanta and the Rollins School of Public Health, Goizueta Business School Martin Luther King Community Service Award Recipient for his work in impoverished communities. Dr. Moore is a Robert Wood Johnson Foundation Clinical Scholar and he received the Thomas Jefferson Award from Emory University for his distinguished leadership and service to the Emory and Atlanta community. He also recently received the National Medical Fellowship Excellence in Medical Education Award.

Cheryl Noble, MSW, MSPH, earned her BA in International Studies from Bethel University, St. Paul, Minnesota in 2003 and her MSW and MSPH from the University of North Carolina at Chapel Hill in 2011. Her areas of expertise include the development and implementation of research study protocols and instruments, collection and analysis of qualitative data, and program development and management. Ms. Noble has more than 8 years of experience in program development and management and 13 years' experience in the social services and health and human services arenas.

David Reznik, DDS, is a graduate of Emory College and Emory University's School of Dentistry, Atlanta, Georgia, and is Director of the Oral Health Center of Grady's Infectious Disease Program, a clinic he founded more than 28 years ago. He also serves as Chief of the Dental Medicine Service for the Grady Health System. Dr. Reznik is president and founder of the HIV Dental Alliance (HIVdent), a not-for-profit organization of concerned healthcare providers committed to assuring access to high quality oral healthcare services for people with HIV disease throughout the United States. Dr. Reznik has lectured and published extensively on HIV and oral health, infection control issues, and more recently antibiotic stewardship. He has also provided technical assistance to oral health programs throughout the United States for the Health Resources and Services Administration (HRSA) HIV/AIDS Bureau (HAB) grantees and serves as a clinical site visitor for HAB grantees. He has served as an outside consultant for malpractice cases for the HRSA Bureau of Primary Care. Dr. Reznik is a Robert Wood Johnson Foundation Clinical Scholar (Cohort: 1 2016–2019) alumni working with a multidisciplinary team to increase access to oral healthcare for adults and children throughout Georgia.

Peter Scal, MD, MPH, is a pediatrician and health services researcher. For the past 25 years he has partnered with youth and families, clinicians, researchers, advocates, and policy makers to improve health and healthcare for children and youth with special healthcare needs. The program described in this chapter highlights what we can accomplish when we partner with motivated communities. Thanks to all of you.

Avril (Apple) Sepulveda, OTD, OTR/L, BCP, is a board-certified pediatric occupational therapist with 20 years' experience in the field. She received her undergraduate degree in Occupational Therapy (OT) in the Philippines and master's degree in OT as San Jose State University as well as a doctorate in OT at University of Southern California. She is a fellow of the Robert Wood Johnson Clinical Scholars Program (Cohort 1: 2016–2019). She is also the Board Chair of 2020 Mom, a national non-profit organization dedicated to close the gaps in maternal mental healthcare. Apple's areas of expertise include occupational therapy interventions for infant development and feeding, pediatric feeding and swallowing in medically complex children, sensory processing and integration, lactation support, dysphagia, and maternal–infant mental health. Apple recognizes the value of mental health in fostering families through advocacy and program development and is involved working on decreasing mental health stigma in immigrant Filipino communities.

Anjali Taneja, MD, MPH, FASAM, is a family physician and DJ/musician who is passionate about reimagining healthcare and healing in the United States. She is Executive Director of Casa de Salud (@casadesaludnm), a culturally humble, anti-racist model of integrative healthcare that aims to transform the biomedical model into one of solidarity with community and collective care. Casa integrates accessible and dignified primary care, queer/transgender care, harm reduction, addictions treatment, acupuncture, reiki, massage, and healing circles for uninsured, immigrant, and other marginalized communities in Albuquerque, New Mexico. The clinic runs a rigorous health apprenticeship that trains primarily young women of color interested in healthcare and healing; many go on to become healthcare leaders. Anjali is board certified in family medicine and addiction medicine and is a fellow of the American Society of Addiction Medicine. Anjali holds an appointment as Community Faculty in the Department of Family and Community Medicine, University of New Mexico, and as Associate Medical Staff in the Emergency Room at Crownpoint Healthcare Facility, in the Navajo Nation. She previously served as a medical director for Iora Health, leading the clinical and operations work of an innovative clinic serving Culinary Workers Union members with severe, chronic illnesses, in Las Vegas, Nevada. She also previously served as the medical director for the Bernalillo County Metropolitan Detention Center's Jail Narcotics Treatment Program in Albuquerque, New Mexico, providing methadone treatment for inmates with opioid addictions. Her advocacy around preserving the program when a jail warden attempted to unilaterally shut it down led to her being escorted out of the jail as well as a community advocacy response that resulted in reinstatement and strengthening of the treatment program. Anjali completed her family medicine residency and fellowship at Harbor-UCLA Medical Center, Los Angeles, California; graduated from Rutgers New Jersey Medical School, Newark, New Jersey; and received her master's degree in Public Health from Columbia Mailman School of Public Health, New York City. While in medical school, she spent a year as the Jack Rutledge Fellow for Universal Health Care, at the American Medical Student Association. And upon graduation from medical school she was a founding board member of the National Physicians Alliance (NPA), an organization committed to healthcare access, professional integrity in the field of medicine, and health justice. She served a five-year term on the NPA board. She founded CureThis (2007–2013), an online community space bringing healthcare leaders, community members, and patients together for discussion around new models of care. She was a lead member of the Peoples Movement Assembly for Health, Healing Justice, and Liberation at the 2010 United States Social Forum, and oversaw the medic response team of volunteers at this event attended by more than 18,000 people. For the last decade she has worked with others who she is in deep study with to build an interactive timeline of the history of the medical industrial complex in the United States, and to develop tools and a digital strategy hub online, to gather and inspire healthcare workers who are intervening on the medical industrial complex. Anjali is a 2016–2019 Robert Wood Johnson Foundation Clinical Scholar; a Next City Vanguard 40 under 40 Urban Leader; and a member of the Creating Health Collaborative, an international collaborative of health innovators invited to share their ideas and visions of health beyond healthcare. She has served as Vice Chair of Bernalillo County's Addiction Treatment Advisory Board. She was recently selected as one of Go Magazine's 100 Women we Love 2020, and was recently appointed to the New Mexico Governor's Council on Racial Justice. Anjali sees her work as bridge work among healers, healthcare providers, and activists working to inspire new paradigms of care and safety. She also sees music as a creative outlet and a healing modality, and was a DJ at clubs around the country for 20 years. For several years, Anjali was a resident DJ at New York City's popular monthly MUTINY party featuring south Asian-inspired electronic, experimental, drum'n'bass, hip hop, and world music. Anjali lives in Albuquerque, New Mexico, and can be found on social media at @losanjalis.

MAJ Tonita Smith, MSN, is an author, entrepreneur, motivational speaker, mentor, and registered nurse. She is proudly serving on active duty as a public health nurse in the United States Army for the past 19 years. She recently returned to the United States after serving a hardship tour for 12 months in South Korea. Her role was Chief of Public Health Nursing. Tonita's most recent accomplishment is being the founder of a non-profit organization, St. Louis Prayer Project, Inc., whose mission is to educate, mentor, and teach coping skills, conflict resolution, and life skills to underserved youth 10–18 years of age. She is recognized as a Robert Wood Johnson Foundation Clinical Scholar Alumni where she volunteers her time in her community mentoring youth through an anti-violence awareness and prevention program. While in South Korea, Tonita developed and implemented a mentorship program and curriculum for youth. She has since been able to collaborate with local organizations in St. Louis, Missouri, to duplicate this program. Tonita is also known for her powerful, transparent book *The Power of Shut-up Grace*. She is transparent in sharing her journey about her once razor blade sharp tongue and her lack of control over her words. She admits she was once a foolish woman now delivered and transformed to a wise woman who walks in purpose. She is living proof that once you begin to operate in your passion you will meet your purpose and from there the sky is the limit. Tonita looks forward to retirement so that she can continue to pursue her passion of serving the youth in the community on a full-time basis as she continues to walk in her God-given purpose.

Amanda Stanec, Ph.D., was born and raised in Nova Scotia, Canada, and moved to the United States to teach and coach in Virginia. During this time she attended Virginia Commonwealth University where she attained a Master of Science with an emphasis in Physical Education and Sport Psychology. Completely devoted to her field, she enrolled in a PhD program in Kinesiology within the Curry School of Education, University of Virginia, where she was recognized as the outstanding doctoral student in her graduating year. Further achievements include the publication of more than 25 as well as co-authoring several book chapters related to physical education, sport, and health topics. In 2011, Amanda founded Move Live Learn, a company that conducts research, develops programs and curricula, and provides professional development for educators and coaches across the globe. Recent clients include the International Olympic Committee, the Association of the Summer Olympic International Federations, the Jackie Joyner-Kersee Foundation, United World Wrestling, NFL Play 60, Boys & Girls Clubs of America, and Wrestling Canada.

Derrick Stephens, LCSW, MBA, has been an advocate for vulnerable children and individuals living with a mental illness for the past 20 years, Mr. Stephens is dedicated to making sure that access to education, physical and mental wellness, and innovative technology such as virtual reality for foster youth and alumni are universal. Mr. Stephens is a licensed clinical social worker and obtained a Master of Social Work and a Master of Business Administration from the University of Central Florida. He is a recent graduate of the Robert Wood Johnson Clinical Scholar Fellowship where he worked to improve quality of life outcomes for foster youth and families. His passion comes from his own personal journey of spending his childhood in the foster care system due to a drug and alcohol addicted mother who also was diagnosed with schizophrenia and a father who committed suicide. Mr. Stephens is the founder of Underdog Dream, a 501c not-for-profit working to provide foster youth with the opportunity to imagine the possibilities, see a future filled with purpose and live with intention. He also serves as research faculty with Florida State University College of Medicine and is the president and CEO of Phoenix Healthcare Consultants.

William Wagner, LCSW, Ph.D., is a clinical social worker, psychotherapist, and medical anthropologist with extensive experience in public health advocacy, clinical service provision, and research. For more than 25 years he has worked as a clinician and researcher with immigrants and refugees experiencing serious mental illness and co-occurring substance abuse issues with a focus on the connections between broader public health and individual health concerns. His research in anthropology focuses on trauma, memory, identity, and mental health. He is the founder and executive director of Centro Sávila, a non-governmental, non-profit outpatient behavioral health and social service program in Albuquerque, New Mexico. He is a graduate of the University of Chicago and the University of New Mexico. Dr. Wagner is a Fulbright-Hays Scholar, a Robert Wood Johnson Foundation Clinical Scholar Alum, and the 2016 New Mexico Social Worker of the Year and the New Mexico Voices for Children 2019 Spirit of Hope recipient.

Kevin Washington (Mwata Kairi), Ph.D., is a licensed African-Centered psychologist in Florida and Washington, DC. He has taught/lectured at several colleges nationally and internationally. NewsOne has sought his expertise out with Roland Martin as well as *Essence*, *Black Entertainment Television* (*BET*) *News*, *Vocal Point*, and many other national and international organizations. He is a past president of the Association of Black Psychologists and is currently an associate professor and head of Sociology and Psychology at Grambling State University is the National Director of Black Marriage Day. As a Fulbright-Hays scholar Kevin researched the impact of socializing institutions on the healing or restructuring of post-apartheid South Africa (Azania). It was in South Africa where he researched Ubuntu and how it can inform mental health service delivery to people of African ancestry and others. Not only does he work on healing the psycho-spiritual wounds that are present within people as a result of Cultural and Historical Trauma, he continues developing healing paradigms for persons of African ancestry who have been impacted by Persistent Enslavement Systemic Trauma (PEST). This work is critical to his advancing of Ubuntu psychology/psychotherapy. He is the founder of Ubuntu Psychotherapy and Black Coaching. As the founder of Ubuntu Psychotherapy (Psychology) he advances a culturally sensitive modality for mental health counseling and psychotherapy for Black men and boys as well as Black/African families. He advances culturally relevant trauma-informed care and interventions to be utilized by psychotherapists that are culturally inclusive and particularized concomitantly. Through his research and writing he seeks to assist people to live life with power, purpose, and passion.

Eric Weintraub, MD, is Associate Professor of Psychiatry at the University of Maryland, School of Medicine where he serves as Director of the Division of Alcohol Abuse. He has extensive clinical experience in treating individuals with opioid use disorders (OUDs). Dr. Weintraub has been a national leader in developing innovative approaches to expand access to mediation-based treatments in underserved rural areas by utilizing the application of a variety of telemedicine approaches.

Carolyn Wolf-Gould, MD, attended Hamilton College, Clinton, New York, and Yale University School of Medicine, New Haven, Connecticut. She has been a family physician in Oneonta, New York, since 1994, and practicing transgender medicine as part of general primary care since 2007. She is the founder of the Gender Wellness Center at Susquehanna Family Practice, a center that has been growing rapidly to meet the needs of patients in upstate New York. She and her team of providers are the recipients of a Robert Wood Johnson Foundation Clinical Scholars Grant from 2016–2019 to create a rural-based Center of Excellence in Transgender Health for upstate New York. She is a member of the World Professional Association for Transgender Health (WPATH) and is the collaborating physician for Choices Counseling and Consulting. Dr. Wolf-Gould is committed to training healthcare professionals on how to include transgender health services as a part of primary care.

Contents

Preface

The Clinical Scholars National Leadership Institute, more commonly known as Clinical Scholars, was funded in 2015 with the mission to equip healthcare providers from every discipline with leadership tools centered on equity to transform their careers and the health of their communities. Our team set about to bring together the tools and the faculty needed to launch a top-tier experience that would integrate cutting-edge leadership development theory with sophisticated and nuanced tools to advance health equity in organizations and communities. On a very short schedule we began our recruitment and enrolled our first cohort of program fellows, making up nine teams from across the United States. As of the publication of this book, we have enrolled 161 fellows working on 44 different teams representing 26 states and territories. These individuals come from 15 different health professions and have experienced more than 65 career advancements, have been awarded more than 40 new grants to further support the sustainability and scalability of their work, and 47 of them have won awards for their work! Hundreds of publications have stemmed from their efforts to disseminate their findings. Data about their success and impact is a moving target as they continue to push forward and achieve amazing goals. Every week we hear news of how they are using their equity-centered leadership skills to advance health and health equity. As the co-project directors of Clinical Scholars, we can only say what a privilege and a pleasure it has been to have the opportunity of working with each and every fellow of the Clinical Scholars National Leadership Institute. The world is in dire need of changes to advance health equity. We have faith that we know just the healthcare professionals who can achieve that goal!

Towards the end of Cohort 1's three years of training, we came upon the idea of creating a collaborative book project to share both the outcomes of their projects and what we have all learned as we created this new experience of Clinical Scholars. Characteristically, these impressive leaders were game for the challenge and volunteered their time for the writing of their contributed chapters. Every single team's project is represented in this work.

This book project has been a joyous and labor-intensive journey—but not one that we as editors have traveled alone. Indeed, this project could never have come into being without an abundance of people who carried heavy loads and contributed to and supported the work along the way. Of course, we thank our fellows who put so much effort into both their projects and the chapters collected herein. Our grateful thanks go to Ms. Edith Amponsah, who committed nearly two years to this project as she finished her Master of Public Health degree and then beyond, prior to starting medical school. Edith served as the project manager, providing both research assistance and much appreciated editing help. Her work included not only formatting the final chapters but, in some cases,, making substantive contributions as well. Truly, this book would not exist without her deft hand and collaborative spirit! We also want to thank Ms. Lia Garman, who joined our project at the start of her Master of Public Health degree. Lia's ability to find just the right citations was appreciated by many of the authors as were her advice and substantive contributions. We had much appreciated editing assistance from Dr. Carol Lorenz and Dr. Gabriel Sealey-Morris. In particular, Dr. Lorenz helped to put the final polish on several of the chapters in this collection. Thank you all for your work in helping to bring this book to fruition. And thanks go to Suzanne Singer, who contributed to copyediting and formatting as the book came together.

We are forever indebted to the Robert Wood Johnson Foundation for its unique and bold vision to build a culture of health that centers on advancing health equity. The generous support from the Foundation has allowed for the in-depth training of literally hundreds of healthcare professionals, health equity activists, health equity researchers, and scholars to develop sophisticated and nuanced skills, to collaborate creatively with communities, and to produce meaningful, measurable, and replicable outcomes that demonstrate real change. We are grateful that they were enthusiastic of Clinical Scholars leading and supporting this project. In particular, we want to thank Dr. Kay Felix, Managing Director, Leadership for Better Health, for her unwavering commitment to this project and work, as well as our Project Officer, Sallie George. The directors (past and present) of the family of Culture of Health Programs have provided much needed encouragement as this project came into being, listing it as a top priority of the Core Strategy Team, for how the outcomes of our collective work might be disseminated broadly to encourage and inspire others. And so, with much warmth, we extend our thanks to Natalie Burke, Gail Christopher, and Brian Smedley of Culture of Health Leaders; Michael Oakes and Andriana Abariotes of Interdisciplinary Research Leaders; and Keshia Pollack Porter, Harolyn Belcher, and Thomas LaViest of Health Policy Research Scholars. We also would like to extend a grateful hand to Dr. David Krol and Ms. Melissa Nahm, who served as our initial Project Officers at RWJF and helped Clinical Scholars get off to such a strong start. Your wisdom and insight are woven throughout the program.

Support and encouragement for undertaking such a complex project is certainly important. There was no parallel for the outright enthusiasm for this book to that expressed by Cohort 1 of Clinical Scholars, the majority of whom elected to participate in this project. Without their absolute zeal and unwavering commitment, this work would never have come into being. This work includes chapters from participants in both the Clinical Scholars and the Culture of Health Leaders programs. Composing and contributing a chapter for this work was optional, and for most contributors was completed after they had graduated from their respective programs—and thus after the support from the programs had concluded. Written on their own time, these chapters represent labors of love, demonstrations of commitment and belief in sharing their findings with the larger community. They represent their hope that others will find inspiration herein to drive their own efforts to advance health equity in their own communities. It was an honor to work with you during the program. We look forward to many years of inspiration to come.

Claudia S.P. Fernandez, DrPH, MS, RD, LDN
Department of Maternal and Child Health,
Gillings School of Global Public Health,
The University of North Carolina at Chapel Hill,
North Carolina, United States

Giselle Corbie-Smith, MD
Center for Health Equity Research,
Department of Social Medicine,
School of Medicine,
The University of North Carolina at Chapel Hill,
North Carolina, United States

Introductory Chapter: A New Approach to Developing Leadership for Cross-Sector, Community-Based Change

Claudia S.P. Fernandez and Giselle Corbie-Smith

1. Introduction

Our world is changing...and changing rapidly. Change calls for new approaches and a new kind of leadership to help society face the deeply entrenched problems that continue to plague it and diminish the health of its populace. Traditional approaches have failed to move the needle on some of the most Wicked Problems [1, 2], particularly for marginalized groups, including problems such as maternal mortality, obesity, diabetes, and other scourges facing humanity. In the face of major scientific advances in medicine and healthcare over the last century, morbidity and mortality rates in the United States (US) are far behind those of its economic peers [3]. When compared with ten other high-income countries (e.g., United Kingdom), life expectancy rates in the US were the lowest while infant mortality and obesity rates were the highest, despite the US spending twice as much on healthcare [4]. In 2017, health care expenditures in the US reached $3.5 trillion, growing by 3.9 percent and accounting for $10,739 per person [3–5], higher than any other nation. Despite this fact, the US continues to lag behind on several major indicators of health including investment in preventive care and social services. The CDC's 2020 Healthy People Goal was to reduce the maternal mortality rate to 11.4 maternal deaths per 100,000 live births [6]. However, by 2018 that rate was not in sight, with a reported US maternal mortality rate at 17.4 deaths per 100,000 live births/year [7]. While this number is no exemplar for a high income country, the wide-ranging health inequities indicate an even sadder tale: as late as 2018 white s had a maternal mortality rate of 14.7/100,000 and Hispanic women a rate of 11.8/100,000, while black women faced a rate more than three times higher at 37.1/100,000 [7]. In 2015-2016 obesity rates hit 39.8%, making the US the world leader in this unhealthy statistic [8]. Again, these obesity rates evince wide disparities by race and ethnicity, with the lowest rate for non-Hispanic Asians (12.7%), as compared with non-Hispanic White (37.9%), Non-Hispanic Black (46.8%), and Hispanic populations (47%) [8].

Racial and ethnic minority populations in the US are disproportionately impacted by chronic conditions and related complications that impose major social and economic burdens of disability, morbidity, and mortality on individuals, families, communities, and the healthcare system [9–15]. These disparities are further perpetuated in rural versus urban areas [16–18], among sexual and gender minorities [19–21], and in those with disabilities [22]. The coronavirus pandemic of 2020 illustrates clearly how the brunt of morbidity and mortality are borne on the shoulders of marginalized communities [23] facing significant challenges in the social contributors to health [24]. Why does the US continue to lag far behind other economically developed peer nations despite its economic and political power? [3, 25] Why are whole segments of the US population consistently burdened by poor health? What can be done to ensure all people in the US have a fair chance of living a healthy life? Solutions to these vexing questions lie in shifting to a culture of health as opposed to the fragmented, often judgmental approach to health currently embraced by the US. Promoting a culture of health requires not only an understanding of health itself, but an appreciation of how social determinants of health contribute to the complexities and variations in health across geographic, economic, ethnic, and social sectors. Challenges inherent in moving toward a culture of health have no defined rules of play or clear end points; rather they are ever-evolving, ever-lasting challenges and thus require an "infinite mindset" on the part of leaders [26]. Such grand challenges have no single winners, but all can lose if the Wicked Problems identified earlier remain insufficiently addressed. An essential element in the shift to a culture of health in the US is leadership that eschews the "winner-take-all" values common in today's tribalized and polarized world. Developing leaders with the unique abilities required to live with an infinite mindset requires a new approach to cultivating leadership itself. Emerging leaders need not only to build tools and skills, but also explore and challenge their own and their organizations' values, perspectives, and attitudes. They need resilience to "thrive in an ever-changing world" [26]. Furthermore, they must develop as individuals while simultaneously developing collaborative teams that can be leveraged to work with larger groups to focus on the ever-changing needs of society.

2. A call for a new approach to leadership

In appreciation for the complexity that underlies pervasive health inequities, the Robert Wood Johnson Foundation (RWJF) committed to developing leaders across sectors, professions, and disciplines in and outside of health care to collaboratively address fundamental causes undergirding health inequities in the US. In 2014, RWJF unveiled their new vision for creating a Culture of Health in which "every person has an equal opportunity to live the healthiest life they can—regardless of where they may live, how much they earn, or the color of their skin" [27]. The Foundation called for "different sectors to come together in innovative ways to solve interconnected problems". Their Action Framework (**Figure 1**) helps describe their vision for impact.

The Action Framework embraces four interconnected Action Areas: Making Health a Shared Value; Fostering Cross-Sector Collaboration to Improve Well-being; Creating Healthier, More Equitable Communities; and Strengthening Integration of Health Services and Systems. In 2015 the RWJF funded four leadership development programs focused on health equity, diversity, and inclusion. The Foundation collectively named these programs Leadership for Better Health: Change Leadership Programs. Specifically, the four development programs are:

- Clinical Scholars, also known as the Clinical Scholars National Leadership Institute (https://clinical-scholars.org/ and at www.ClinicalScholarsNLI.org)

- The Culture of Health Leaders (https://cultureofhealth-leaders.org/)

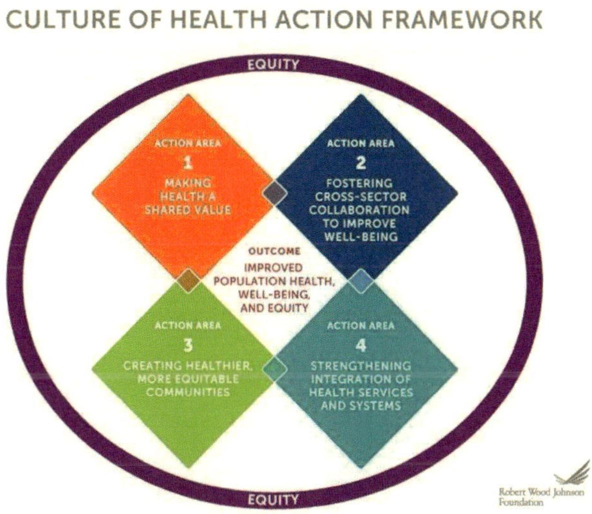

Figure 1.
Culture of health action framework.

- The Interdisciplinary Research Leaders (https://interdisciplinaryresearch-leaders.org/)
- Health Policy Research Scholars (https://healthpolicyresearch-scholars.org/)

All programs are centered on health equity and strive to foster innovative cross-sector collaboration, but each program is unique in that it delivers leadership development tailored to the target group. Participants enrolled in each program matriculate through a 3-year experience consisting of both onsite and distance-based engagement. Whether enrolled as individuals or as teams, each participant unit focuses their work in community settings with an aim to address root causes of health inequities that negatively impact the culture of health.

This book presents work from two of the mid-career development programs: *Clinical Scholars* and *Culture of Health Leaders*. You will be introduced to the two programs and their respective participants. Both programs strive to support development of a new type of leadership in which collaborative and systemic approaches bring teams of leaders together with others in the community to work toward common goals.

The first section of the book presents four chapters explaining the structure of the programs to give the reader an understanding of the participant experience. Chapters 1 through 3 detail the *Clinical Scholars* approach to leadership development, explaining the pedagogical structure (Chapter 1), how leadership and the concepts of equity, diversity, and inclusion are interwoven through workforce development efforts (Chapter 2), and the approaches implemented to evaluate outcomes of the *Clinical Scholars* program (Chapter 3). Chapter 4 introduces the reader to the *Culture of Health Leaders* program, explaining the structure and goals for developing community-based leaders who are enrolled.

These chapters are intended to enlighten those engaged in workforce development efforts and illustrate that real change comes from the combination of learning and doing. There are important ways workforce development programs engage mid-career participants as learners, building their skills and helping them expand their perspective and talents. This development enables them to focus their efforts on the kind of community engagement that creates meaningful change in collaboration with the communities being served. We hope these chapters illustrate how inspiration and resilience are as crucial as skills building in workforce development. As the Directors of the *Clinical Scholars* program, we have learned that fostering resilience in inspired and passionate leaders is crucial for them to continue their work despite obstacles and difficulties that continually arise--some on a personal level and others on a societal level. We hope our readers gain ideas and inspiration from this book for their own efforts in developing the leaders of today as well as tomorrow.

Chapters following the program overviews have been contributed by program participants, and in some cases their community partners. Program participants come from different places, circumstances, experiences, and perspectives. Some are academics and some are practitioners, some are community activists, some are at non-profits—and many cross several categories. What they all share is a desire to help make positive change in health equity at the local level by working with communities themselves. The reader will notice clear differences in the chapters compared with many typical project reports or research articles. Each chapter describes the health-equity related project that served as a focus of participant learning and engagement while enrolled in one of the three-year RWJF-funded development programs.

Clinical Scholars Fellows identified a Wicked Problem in their respective communities and developed and implemented community-based approaches to address the problems in a sustainable manner, hence the name Wicked Problem Impact Project. Their chapters describe the approaches, community partnering, and outcomes achieved through their leadership. Additionally, authors were asked to share resources through a Tool Kit, allowing interested readers who find inspiration from these projects to obtain useful information or strategies to assist them in making a similar difference in their own communities. Since *Clinical Scholars* and *Culture of Health Leaders* are both leadership development programs that made significant investments in the knowledge, skills, perspectives, and commitment of the participants, the authors were asked to share some reflections on leader learning through their engagement with their programs and the communities they served. Some authors shared insights as teams and others as individuals, all in the spirit of inspiring others to become engaged in the Wicked Problems facing their own communities. The front page of each chapter identifies the RWJF program in which the chapter authors participated.

As you read through this book, you'll learn how individuals and teams addressed some of the most pressing health equity issues facing communities in the United States. Participants from both programs tackled entrenched Wicked Problems. Projects ranged from taking on the creation of health care structures for transgender and other gender-nonconforming individuals in the midst of healthcare deserts (Chapter 5), and addressing disparities that challenge children with special health care needs or other marginalized communities in getting needed dental care (Chapters 6 and 7), to interventions focused on life skills for youth, parenting, youth-mentoring, and violence prevention (Chapters 8, 9, 10 and 11). These leaders in the quest for health equity detail their work in projects ranging from developing peer-based community mentoring and health-education programs for marginalized adult communities (Chapter 12), to structuring community based efforts to combat the opiate addiction crisis in rural communities (Chapters 13 and 14), and community reclamation of environmentally blighted areas (Chapter 15).

Topics and communities engaged are diverse. The chapters present not only the approach and findings of the projects, but also advice and Tool Kits to help others who face similar health equity issues get a proverbial leg-up on addressing the crises in their own communities. Indeed, a goal of this book is that readers will identify similar challenging issues (Wicked Problems) in their spheres and be inspired to engage their own talents in addressing them.

Further, we hope sharing the structure and design of the RWJF leadership development programs will provide workforce development experts with useful ideas to incorporate in their programs, and help their participants become innovative and effective champions for health and health equity.

The most important outcome for all these programs—and the measure of whether they are worth the considerable investment of the Robert Wood Johnson Foundation—is the ultimate impact of each project on its community and the participant's continuing influences on health equity through the course of their careers. We know lasting change is evolution not revolution. While more distal outcomes may take several years to culminate in population health changes, the observable changes reported in the chapters in this volume are impressive—and penned at the conclusion of participants' three-year development experience. Yet we know these projects will endure beyond this experience just as these newly-minted culture of health champions will continue collaborating to address health disparities and help make an America in which every person has the opportunity to live a healthy life.

We hope these chapters inspire, instruct, and guide you as you work to address the complex problems in the culture of health in your own communities. While efforts of each project will have ripple effects for years to come, one of the greatest outcomes would be to extend the impact of the Leadership for Better Health programs into a movement by which all of us are engaged in healing our communities nationwide.

Author details

Claudia S.P. Fernandez[1]* and Giselle Corbie-Smith[2]

1 Gillings School of Global Public Health, University of North Carolina at Chapel Hill, North Carolina, United States

2 School of Medicine, University of North Carolina at Chapel Hill, North Carolina, United States

*Address all correspondence to: claudia_Fernandez@unc.edu

References

[1] Rittel HWJ, Webber MM. Dilemmas in a General Theory of Planning. Policy Sciences. 1973;4(2):155-169. DOI: 10.1007/bf01405730.

[2] Churchman CW. Wicked Problems. Management Science 1967;14(4): B141-B146 DOI:10.1287/mnsc.14.4.B141.

[3] Kassebaum NJ, Barber RM, Bhutta ZA, Dandona L, Gething PW, Hay SI, Kinfu Y, Larson HJ, Liang X, Lim SS, Lopez AD. Global, regional, and national levels of maternal mortality, 1990-2015: A systematic analysis for the Global Burden of Disease Study 2015. The Lancet. 2016;388(10053):1775-812. DOI: 10.1016/S0140-6736(16)31470-2.

[4] Papanicolas I, Woskie LR, Jha AK. Health care spending in the United States and other high-income countries. Jama. 2018;319(10):1024-39. DOI:10.1001/jama.2018.1150.

[5] Centers for Medicare and Medicaid Services. National Health Expenditure Data: Historical [Internet]. 2019. Available from: https://www.cms.gov/research-statistics-data-and-systems/statistics-trends-and-reports/nationalhealthexpenddata/nationalhealthaccountshistorical.html. [Accessed 2020-05-28].

[6] HealthyPeople.gov. 2020 Topics & Objectives: Maternal, Infant, and Child Health [Internet]. Available from: https://www.healthypeople.gov/2020/topics-objectives/topic/maternal-infant-and-child-health/objectives. [Accessed 2020-06-14].

[7] Hoyert DL, Miniño AM. Maternal mortality in the United States: Changes in coding, publication, and data release, 2018. National Vital Statistics Reports. 2020;69(2):1-16.

[8] Hales CM, Carroll MD, Fryar CD, Ogden CL. Prevalence of obesity among adults and youth: United States, 2015-2016. NCHS Data Brief. 2017;288:1-8.

[9] Institute of Medicine. Unequal treatment: confronting racial and ethnic disparities in health care. Washington, DC: The National Academies Press; 2003. 780 p. DOI:10.17226/10260.

[10] Lu MC, Kotelchuck M, Hogan V, Jones L, Wright K, Halfon N. Closing the black-white gap in birth outcomes: A life-course approach. Ethnicity & Disease. 2010;20(1 Suppl 2):S2-76.

[11] Avery RB, Rendall MS. Lifetime inheritances of three generations of whites and blacks. Am J Sociol. 2002;107(5):1300-1346. DOI: 10.1086/344840.

[12] Warren-Findlow J. Weathering: Stress and heart disease in african american women living in Chicago. Qualitative Health Research. 2006;16(2):221-237. DOI: 10.1177/1049732305278651.

[13] Geronimus AT. The weathering hypothesis and the health of african-american women and infants: Evidence and speculations. Ethnicity & Disease. 1992;2(3):207-221.

[14] Thorpe RJ, Fesahazion RG, Parker L, et al. Accelerated health declines among African Americans in the USA. Journal of Urban Health: Bulletin of the New York Academy of Medicine. 2016;93(5):808-819. DOI: 10.1007/s11524-016-0075-4.

[15] Dickman SL, Himmelstein DU, Woolhandler S. Inequality and the health-care system in the USA. Lancet. 2017;389(10077):1431-1441. DOI: 10.1016/S0140-6736(17)30398-7.

[16] Halverson JA, Barnett E, Casper M. Geographic disparities in heart disease and stroke mortality among black and

white populations in the Appalachian region. Ethnicity & Disease. 2002;12(4):S3-91.

[17] Mainous AG 3rd, King DE, Garr DR, Pearson WS. Race, rural residence, and control of diabetes and hypertension. Annals of Family Medicine. 2004;2(6):563-568. DOI: 10.1370/afm.119

[18] Egede LE, Gebregziabher M, Hunt KJ, Axon RN, Echols C, Gilbert GE, Mauldin PD. Regional, geographic, and racial/ethnic variation in glycemic control in a national sample of veterans with diabetes. Diabetes Care. 2011;34(4):938-943. DOI: 10.2337/dc10-1504.

[19] Perszyk DR, Lei RF, Bodenhausen GV, Richeson JA, Waxman SR. Bias at the intersection of race and gender: Evidence from preschool-aged children. Development Science. 2019:e12788. DOI: 10.1111/desc.12788.

[20] Laiti M, Pakarinen A, Parisod H, Salanterä S, Sariola S. Encountering sexual and gender minority youth in healthcare: An integrative review. Primary Health Care Research & Development. 2019;20:e30. DOI: 10.1017/S146342361900001X.

[21] Valdiserri RO, Holtgrave DR, Poteat TC, Beyrer C. Unraveling health disparities among sexual and gender minorities: A commentary on the persistent impact of stigma. Journal of Homosexuality. 2019;66(5):571-589. DOI: 10.1080/00918369.2017.1422944.

[22] Krahn GL, Walker DK, Correa-De-Araujo R. Persons with disabilities as an unrecognized health disparity population. American Journal of Public Health. 2015;105(S2):S198-S206. DOI: 10.2105/AJPH.2014.302182.

[23] Weiner S. The new coronavirus affects us all. But some groups may suffer more [Internet]. 2020. Available from: https://www.aamc.org/news-insights/new-coronavirus-affects-us-all-some-groups-may-suffer-more. [Accessed 2020-05-25].

[24] Penman-Aguilar A, Talih M, Huang D, Moonesinghe R, Bouye K, Beckles G. Measurement of health disparities, health inequities, and social determinants of health to support the advancement of health equity. Journal of Public Health Management and Practice. 2016;22(Suppl 1):S33. DOI: 10.1097/PHH.0000000000000373.

[25] Martin N, Montagne R. U.S. has the worst rate of maternal deaths in the developed world [Internet]. Available from: https://www.npr.org/2017/05/12/528098789/u-s-has-the-worst-rate-of-maternal-deaths-in-the-developed-world. [Accessed 2020-05-25].

[26] Sinek S. The Infinite Game. Penguin. 2019. 272 p. 151.

[27] Plough AL. Measuring What Matters: Introducing a New Action Framework in Culture of Health [Internet]. 2015. Available from: https://www.rwjf.org/en/blog/2015/11/measuring_what_matte.html. [Accessed 2019-06-11].

Chapter 1

Clinical Scholars: Effective Approaches to Leadership Development

Claudia S.P. Fernandez, Giselle Corbie-Smith, Melissa Green, Kathleen Brandert, Cheryl Noble and Gaurav Dave

Abstract

The Clinical Scholars (CS) National Leadership Institute (CSNLI) equips interprofessional teams of health care professionals through equity-centered leadership training, preparing them to be change leaders working to advance health equity in communities across the US and its territories. At the time of this writing, four cohorts consisting of 131 Fellows from 14 different disciplines, participating in 36 different teams of two to five members are working on "Wicked Problem Impact Projects", an implementation science-based approach to action learning projects. This chapter reports on the design of the 3-year CS experience, the onsite and distance-based training support, and the subsequent learning responses of 98 participants, 30 of whom had completed the 3-year training (Cohort 1), 34 of whom had completed 2-years of the training (Cohort 2), and 34 who had completed 1-year of the training (Cohort 3). The training program is guided by 25 competencies that weave leadership and equity throughout, which are divided into four families: Personal, Interpersonal, Organizational, and Community & Systems. Learning outcomes indicated that Fellows are highly satisfied, with all participants rating their experience at 6.10-6.77 on a 7-point scale across all sessions, all years. Retrospective pre-and post-tests assessed learning gains on the competencies, indicating statistically significant changes from baseline to midpoint in participant knowledge, attitude, use, and self-efficacy in each of the 25 competencies and large and significant gains by competency family. The Clinical Scholars Program presents an in-depth, longitudinal, state-of-the-art approach to promoting the cultivation and development of a large and sophisticated set of skills that intentionally integrate leadership competencies with a focus on health equity. Taken together, these outcomes show how a logical and structured process, using widely available tools, can contribute to both learning and implementation of skills that lead to real world impacts in communities. Given the results reported at the close of their Clinical Scholars experience, the data suggest that investing in robust, intensive leadership development of interprofessional teams is a smart decision for impacting the culture of health in communities nationwide.

Keywords: leadership development, competencies, curriculum, workforce development, culture of health, leadership, return on investment

1. Introduction

A broad range of health-related professions have called for or implemented leadership training as an essential component of workforce development, increasingly recognizing it as a core skill. Such fields of practice include post-graduate training in medicine, nursing, and other professions [1–12], academia and academic administration [8, 10, 13], and public health [5, 14–25]. Even at the pre-professional level [26, 27], and notably at the advanced degree training in health professions [5, 9, 28–32], leadership development has enjoyed decades of experimentation and implementation.

Studies of the impact of leadership training illuminate the topics of common focus, the learning of participants [3, 11–16], and some studies address the outcomes participants achieve as they employ the skills honed in their development programs [3, 13, 14, 16, 28, 29]. Health and healthcare has embraced the call for leadership development [8–10, 17, 30, 33, 34], with an emphasis typically on training physicians and nurses. Some programs have emphasized the importance of interdisciplinary training [9, 14, 28, 29]. Others have called for leadership training to occur over time and in practice-focused settings for maximum and lasting impact [13, 35–37].

Built upon insights gained from a long history of leadership programs at the University of North Carolina's School of Public Health [1, 3, 4, 13–15, 29, 38–44] and elsewhere [11, 16, 22, 34, 36], the Clinical Scholars National Leadership Institute (CSNLI, online at www.ClinicalScholarsNLI.org) also referred to broadly as Clinical Scholars (CS) and as the Clinical Scholars Program, aims to significantly expand the skills in leadership, health equity, public health, and the breadth of enrolled interdisciplinary Fellows. Of the three mid-career leadership development initiatives funded in 2015 under the Robert Wood Johnson Foundation's (RWJF) Culture of Health family of programs, the Clinical Scholars National Leadership Institute focuses on mid- to senior-level health professionals who are tackling complex, or "wicked", problems [45–47] that are impacting US communities. The University of North Carolina at Chapel Hill (UNC) serves as the National Program Center (NPC) for the Clinical Scholars Program.

The Clinical Scholars Program prepares health professionals to be change leaders. As trusted members of their communities, Fellows learn to partner with stakeholder groups to address the fundamental issues and root causes that underlie poor health among populations or communities in the United States. To do so, they require sophisticated and nuanced skills in a variety of areas that encompass and integrate leadership and domains of equity, diversity and inclusion (EDI). This chapter describes the pedagogical construction of the CS Program, addressing the overarching program goals, the skill-development approaches implemented, and a brief examination of the subsequent skill outcomes documented. Subsequent chapters in this section address the development and integration of competencies related to EDI (Chapter 2); the evaluation approach to Clinical Scholars (Chapter 3), which provides a deeper examination of program outcomes; and a series of chapters that present the outcomes of the Wicked Problem Impact Projects (WPIP) of the Clinical Scholars teams from the initial cohorts enrolled in the program (Chapters 5-9, 11-14).

2. The Clinical Scholars National Leadership Institute

Clinical Scholars is a 3-year leadership development program which accepts up to 35 Fellows in each cohort. Potential participants apply in teams of between two to five members. All applicant teams propose a WPIP [46], which identifies an intractable, multifaceted issue around health equity made more complex by the very real contributions of politics, policy, behavior, environment and other complicating social and economic factors. This WPIP serves as a focus point for Fellow development and as the applied-implementation science project for the team's work throughout the program.

Selection of teams is based on competitive applications and follows a multi-stage process (**Figure 1**). Multi-pronged recruitment efforts reach health professionals through the health professional organizations in which they are networked, the health profession educational communities in which they were trained, and the public and private healthcare systems in which they are employed, through list-servs, in-person convenings, public webinars, and word of mouth. Applications are accepted annually from January to March via the RWJF website. Completed applications are reviewed by a National Advisory Committee (NAC), RWJF project officers and staff, and the Co-Directors and staff of the CS Program. In the semi-finalist stage teams participate in video-based live interviews with selection committee representatives. The NAC recommends the final slate of candidate teams to the NPC, which are officially accepted by the RWJF. Typically, about 10% of completed applicants are selected and named as Fellows of Clinical Scholars and enrolled into a cohort. New cohorts launch each fall.

Once enrolled, Fellows engage in both onsite and distance-based learning. Teams accepted into the Clinical Scholars Program receive a funding award of $35,000 per team member for each of the three years they matriculate through the CS program. This funding is intended to support their time for learning and development and to support costs associated with the implementation of their WPIPs.

This chapter includes data from the first three cohorts of Clinical Scholars, representing a total of 98 individual Fellows (Cohort 1: 30 Fellows, Cohort 2: 34 Fellows; Cohort 3: 34 Fellows) from 25 states and US territories. The demographics of enrolled Fellows in the first four cohorts is presented in **Figure 2**, representing the enrolled participants at the time of this writing.

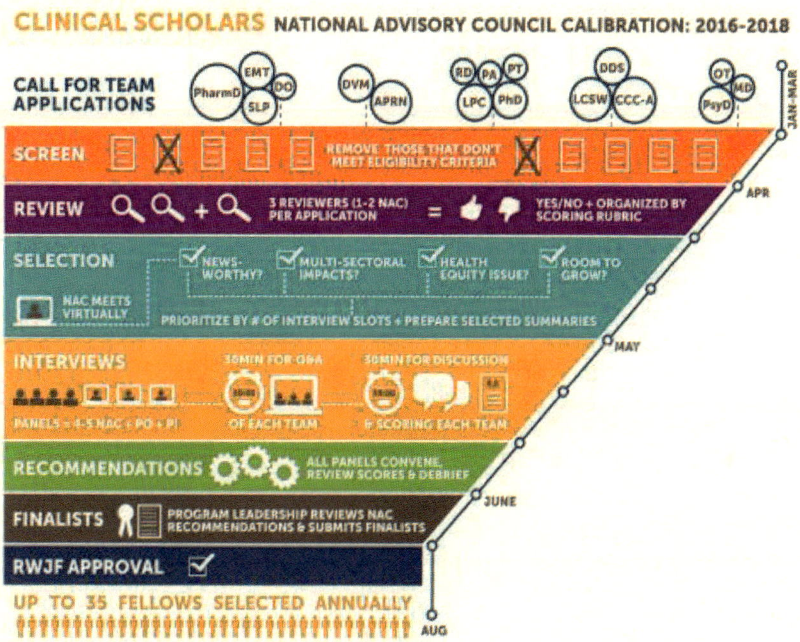

Figure 1.
The clinical scholars selection process.

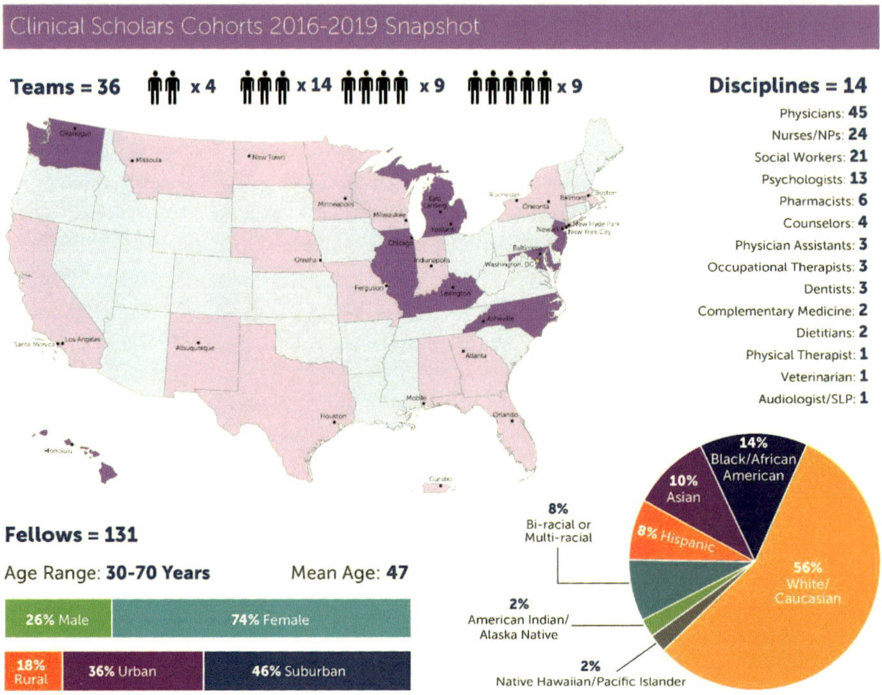

Figure 2.
Demographics of Enrolled CS Program Fellows, Cohorts 1-4.

2.1 Goals of the clinical scholars program

Clinical Scholars has been strategically created to enable a diverse cohort of mid-to-senior career healthcare professionals to broaden their perspective and skills to become leaders and change agents over the remainder of their careers. Eight overarching goals guide the program's curricula across both the integrated leadership and health equity cores of the program (**Table 1**).

2.2 Core competencies of the Clinical Scholars National Leadership Institute

To gain the nuanced and sophisticated skills needed to move their WPIPs forward, 25 leadership competencies stand at the core of the Clinical Scholars training experience and stem from these overarching goals (**Figure 3**). These competencies were developed after reviewing core competencies successfully implemented in similar leadership programs [1, 3, 4, 13–15] and expanded to integrate domains of health EDI [2, 47, 48]. The Clinical Scholars program groups these competencies into four meta-categories of Leadership Skills: *Personal, Interpersonal, Organizational*, and *Community and Systems* (see **Figure 3**). Sessions provided throughout the program are cross-walked against these competencies to ensure that these critical areas are addressed multiple times throughout the training, each time with an added nuance, facet or deepening of the content to reinforce skill development.

Clinical Scholars represents a highly robust program that couples "hard skills" drawn from health services research, public and population health, engaged scholarship, health equity research, and cultural sociology with methods developing individual and team "boundary-spanning leadership skills" shown to significantly impact participant development [1, 3, 4, 13–15, 36], interdisciplinary effectiveness [28, 29] and project-related real-world outcomes, as described in subsequent chapters of this work.

By the End of Training the Clinical Scholars Participants Will:
Understand leadership styles and how to be increasingly effective in leading and managing others while working collaboratively and inter-professionally.
Advocate for positive change within teams, organizations, community, or in policy.
Promote creative thinking, innovation, and thought diversity.
Understand how to appraise, synthesize, and use best evidence to guide practice and policy recommendations.
Communicate effectively with both technical and non-technical stakeholders in multiple formats.
Negotiate to create win/win outcomes for all stakeholders.
Engage in project-focused learning with a strong lens on healthy equity and implementation science.
Positively impact complex issues that create "Wicked Problems" around achieving a culture of health and health equity across the country, demonstrating effectiveness in project outcomes.

Table 1.
Overarching goals of the clinical scholars program.

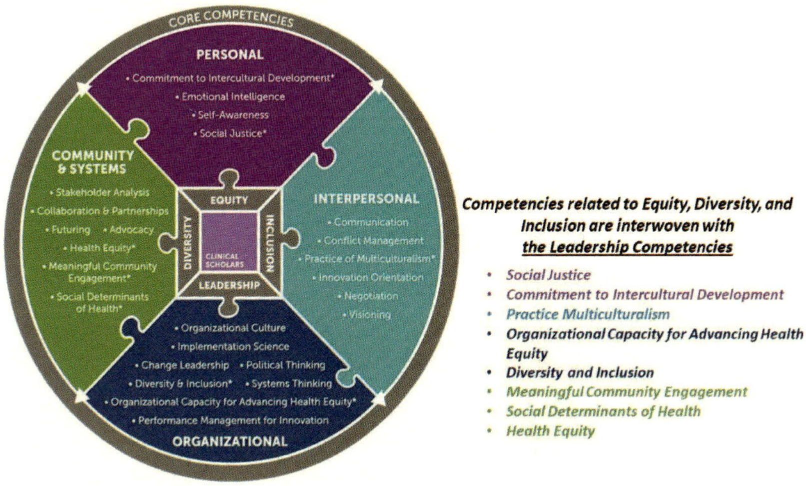
CORE COMPETENCIES
PERSONAL
• Commitment to Intercultural Development*
• Emotional Intelligence
• Self-Awareness
• Social Justice*
COMMUNITY & SYSTEMS
• Stakeholder Analysis
• Collaboration & Partnerships
• Futuring • Advocacy
• Health Equity*
• Meaningful Community Engagement*
• Social Determinants of Health*
INTERPERSONAL
• Communication
• Conflict Management
• Practice of Multiculturalism*
• Innovation Orientation
• Negotiation
• Visioning
EQUITY
DIVERSITY
INCLUSION
LEADERSHIP
CLINICAL SCHOLARS
• Organizational Culture
• Implementation Science
• Change Leadership • Political Thinking
• Diversity & Inclusion* • Systems Thinking
• Organizational Capacity for Advancing Health Equity*
• Performance Management for Innovation
ORGANIZATIONAL
Competencies related to Equity, Diversity, and Inclusion are interwoven with the Leadership Competencies
• Social Justice
• Commitment to Intercultural Development
• Practice Multiculturalism
• Organizational Capacity for Advancing Health Equity
• Diversity and Inclusion
• Meaningful Community Engagement
• Social Determinants of Health
• Health Equity

Figure 3.
The 25 Core competencies of the clinical scholars program.

2.3 Pedagogical design of the Clinical Scholars National Leadership Institute

The Clinical Scholars program delivers professional training and development through two main components of the program: onsite face-to-face intensive development programs (retreats) and a robust distance-based "Continuous Learning Program" (CLS), occasionally similarly described in the literature as a Personalized Learning Cloud (PLC) [35]. Fellows progress through the 7 onsite curricula (**Figure 4**), which progressively teach the leadership and health equity skills targeted in the program. Retreats are labeled to follow the visible color spectrum (Red, Orange, Yellow, Green, Blue, Indigo, Violet) in order to clearly differentiate between them, as the curricular content is unique to each intensive onsite training and builds across the entire experience. Core themes thread throughout all the onsite retreats and lead to overall outcomes at the individual participant level, the team level and at the WPIP level. These onsite intensive retreats meet in fall and spring throughout the 3-year experience (approximately 14 days of in-person training/year). Each retreat is typically about five days in length. The

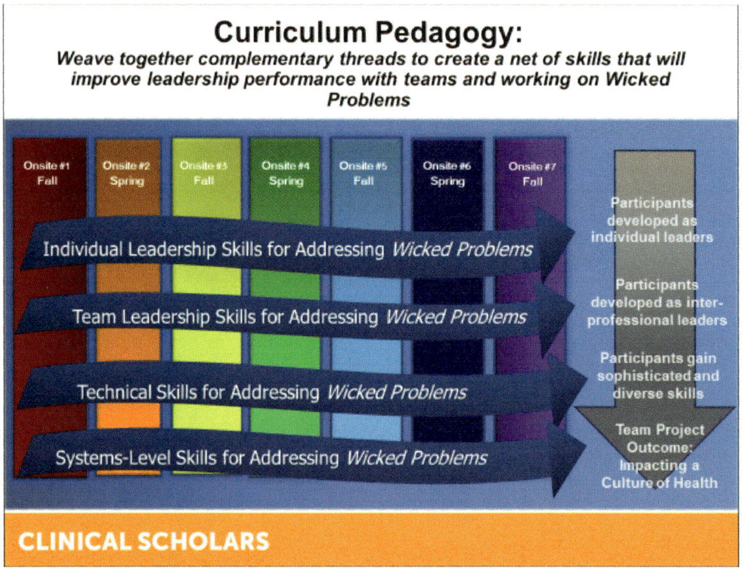

Figure 4.
Clinical scholars onsite curriculum structure and timeline for cohorts.

full curriculum provides approximately 210 contact hours of continuing education per participant over the three-year experience. Each year CS provides nearly 7000 contact hours of face-to-face training and approximately 10,000 hours of self-paced, distance-based education to the participating healthcare professionals.

2.4 Onsite retreats

Onsite retreats are grounded in current leadership and health equity science and utilize a variety of psychological and leadership assessments, including a 360-degree multi-rater feedback survey, which is administered in the "Orange" retreat program [1, 2, 4, 13, 15, 18, 29, 39–44, 47–49]. In all, the Clinical Scholars Program includes 12 different leadership and psychological assessment tools, each of which provides different insights into leadership behavior and effectiveness. All tools are debriefed initially at the onsite retreats and participants can continue to seek insight from the assessment in working with the personal executive coach assigned to them for the duration of the three-year program. The Clinical Scholars team includes seven team members and partners who are certified in many of the assessments used and experienced in delivering the simulations. **Figure 5** depicts the assessments currently included in the curriculum.

Based on principles of adult learning theory, the Clinical Scholars Program also emphasizes experiential learning, in addition to the WPIP-focused learning. A variety of simulation exercises, group based experiential learning through role-play, scenarios or situations that demonstrate behaviors or skills, are built into the program and utilized at most retreats. These sessions typically either teach skills with immediate application or participants engage in simulation-based learning with intermittent debriefs. More than ten simulations are embedded throughout the onsite portion of the program (**Figure 5**). While the didactic sessions impact participant knowledge and the experiential practice sessions develop skills, the simulation activities help change attitudes, values, and perspectives.

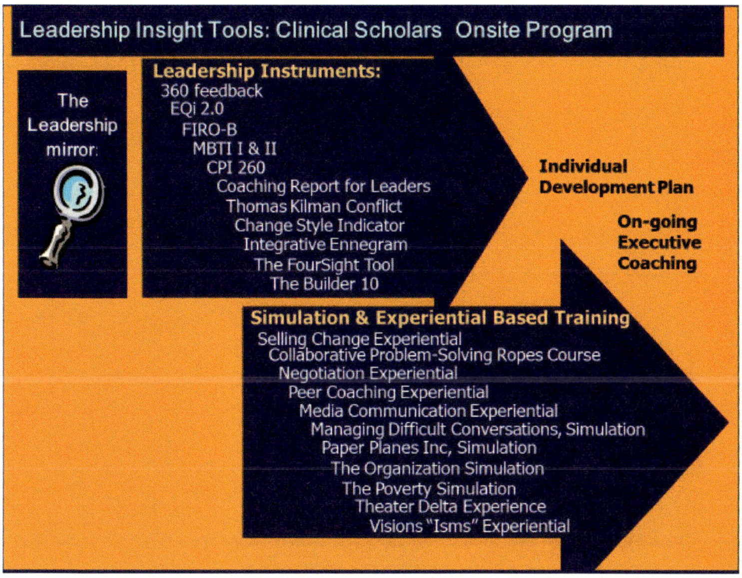

Figure 5.
Leadership assessment, experiential training and simulations used in the clinical scholars National Leadership Institute.

2.5 The distance-based continuous learning system

Between the intensive retreat programs, Fellows return to their home communities and engage in the multi-platform, distance-based CLS, which includes web, phone, print, and video/audio-based participation strategies that work at the levels of individual, team, small group and entire cohort learning. **Figure 6** depicts the Continuous Learning System's "Learning Wheel" with its 14 experiential components.

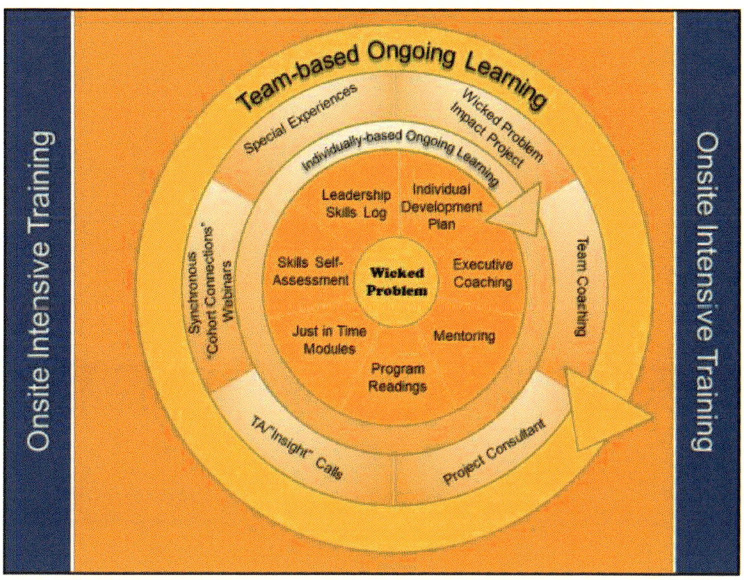

Figure 6.
The continuous learning system wheel of the clinical scholars program.

This system is highly customizable to both individual and team learning needs as a wide variety of experiences are offered, with Fellows required to complete a minimum subset of learning events of their own choosing within each component that align with their learning goals and team needs (**Table 2**). The outside layer of the wheel illustrates the team-based learning strategies while the inside layer of the wheel presents the individual learning strategies, all of which ultimately contribute

Components of the Continuous Learning System			
	Component	**Description**	**Minimum Completion Requirement**
Individual Based CLS Work	Leadership Skills Self-Assessment	Self-rating on the 25 program competencies	25, completed at program start, midpoint, and end
	Leadership Skills Log	Behavioral examples of implementing the program competencies	18 behavioral descriptions of competency statements (6/year)
	Individual Development Plan	Stated goals for self-development with action plans and outcome statements	1 set
	Executive Coaching	1:1 phone-based sessions, between 4 and 8 per year	4 per year
	Mentoring	Fellow identified, initiated and managed mentoring relationship	1 mentor required
	Program Readings/ Book Club	~3 books/onsite session usually with 2 selected for follow-on phone-based book club (3 Fellows/book assigned to lead book club)	1 required for selected Fellows
	Just-in-Time Modules	Commercially available online leadership library with half-hour modules directly related to core leadership and health equity lessons taught in program (FastTrack, Inc., Chapel Hill, NC)	18 modules required (6/year)
Team Based CLS Work	Project Consultant	Budget available to support team-identified consultant(s) to foster WPIP progress	Optional
	Technical Assistance Call	Hour-long phone calls of selective interest to cohort, 5 offered per year	10 per year (split between TA calls and Webinars)
	Program Webinars	Hour-long webinars of general interest to cohort, 5 offered per year	
	Team Executive Coaching	Bi-monthly coaching support calls, with support available at the onsite intensives	5 per year
	Special Onsite Experiences	Optional 2-day onsite trainings in special topics such as structural racism, communications, health policy and advocacy, etc.	Optional
	Wicked Problem Impact Projects	Team identified problem-based learning projects in partnership with community, focused on a "wicked problem" in that community	1 required per team

Table 2.
Clinical scholars CLS component descriptions.

to the team's Wicked Problem Impact Project. Each component of the CLS Learning Wheel is briefly defined in **Table 2**. Throughout the 3-year experience, Executive Coaches deepen skills development at the individual level, while Team Coaches support team development and progress on the WPIPs and the deliverables. All coaches provide feedback to the UNC-based Clinical Scholars team of emerging participant needs to inform the content of technical assistance and webinar topics.

While founded on evidence-based strategies for developing the competencies listed in **Figure 3**, Clinical Scholars also uses rapid-cycle innovation to tailor and modify the learning opportunities to be responsive to the Fellows' needs, interests and changing conditions in economic, political, social and health systems over the course of the program. For example, Peer Coaching was initially conceived as a team-to-team activity that would take place within cohorts, however through experimentation, the program will institute it as an individual-learning based cross-cohort activity.

Participation is tracked in the varying CLS components. Minimum levels of participation in the Clinical Scholars program require approximately 2-3 hours per week on the part of each individual participant. Program Fellows spend additional time on their team projects. The $35,000 learning grant awarded per team member to each team is intended to support both individual and team learning as well as the project focused work required by their WPIPs. Internal evaluation data indicate that during the first three years of the Clinical Scholars program being implemented, each Fellow spent between 509 and 600 hours per year engaged in the Clinical Scholars Program. Data indicate that 80-85% (411-510 hours) of this time was spent on Team WPIPs, the activities of which are integrated with their workplace duties because of the structure of the grant support from the RWJF. Ten to 14% (62-71 hours) were spent in onsite session convening. Fellows report 10-12 hours of coaching and/or mentoring per year and an additional 17-21 hours of individual learning, per individual. Time spent in individual learning is highest in the first year of the program and time spent in the team based WPIP is highest in the final year of the program.

3. Key learning events

3.1 WPIP and team progress

As a learning competency, communication and the ability to effectively present materials to both technical and non-technical stakeholders in multiple formats is strongly valued in the Clinical Scholars Program. Thus, program Fellows present the evolving outcomes of their WPIPs, as early as their very first retreat ("Red"). At each retreat, teams provide a brief update to their cohort and the NPC representatives of their progress to date. In the Green retreat, this presentation becomes more formalized with each team presenting a poster session, which all current cohorts of Clinical Scholars attend, as well as a variety of invited guests, including Robert Wood Johnson Foundation (RWJF) representatives.

3.2 Presentation of participant-generated outcomes

In their third year of the program, teams present their outcomes and WPIP impacts at a separate meeting, convened by the RWJF which brings together four different branches of the Leadership for Better Health programs (Health Policy Research Scholars, Interdisciplinary Research Scholars, Culture of Health Leaders, and Clinical Scholars). During the Clinical Scholars "Blue" and "Indigo" retreats the Fellows learn how to use social and digital media to present the outcomes of their learning, incorporating B-roll in video-based presentations that they can then use to disseminate their WPIP programs and activities. In the "Violet" retreat each team presents the next generation idea that has grown from the team WPIP in a short "Big Idea Talk", based on the TED talk format. These presentations are digitally captured and made available on the web. Each team also creates a Tool Kit that describes their WPIP and provides tools and advice for those in other communities who are facing similar health equity challenges. These tool kits are also available at the Clinical Scholars website (www.ClinicalScholarsNLI.org/community). In addition, all Clinical Scholars teams in Cohort 1 and select teams from Cohort 2 were invited to contribute a chapter to this volume.

4. Pedagogical impact: findings of participant satisfaction and learning outcomes

The difficulty of evaluating leadership development programs is a common challenge in the field [49–53]. Chapter 3 in this volume addresses a) the complex issues

Participant Feedback Scores and Comments

Retreat	Overall Onsite Session Satisfaction Score (out of 7.0 possible	Number of participant session ratings	Cohorts included in rating	Example participant quote (session title, session rating)
Red	6.5	631	1, 2, 3	"It is empowering to be a part of this network of professionals doing important work to create a culture of health." (Team Wicked Problem Impact Project Presentations, Score: 6.71)
Orange	6.43	131	1, 2, 3	"Practical, applicable, engaging, skills-based." Communicating in High Stakes Situations, Score: 7.0)
Yellow	6.10	353	1, 2	"Thank you so much for allowing us the time and the space to talk and listen to one another." (Year 2 Planning Score: 6.75)
Green	6.37	93	1, 2	"Visual and interactive scenarios. Made me more aware of my biases and assumptions." (Experiential Teaching Health Disparities and Racism, Score: 6.77)
Blue	6.75	285	1	This session has given me a lot of great knowledge on language, framework, and tools to incorporate into culturally responsive programs. (Moving Beyond Recruitment: Utilizing a Culturally Responsive Approach to All Levels of Evaluation Design and Execution, 6.63)
Indigo	6.37	52	1	This is so powerful for clinicians who are accustomed to presenting via data and clinical knowledge. (Presenting Your Best You, 6.89)
Violet	6.77	38	1	-It really has been the best professional development experience of my life, and I feel like it will be. Any others will pale in comparison to this. Thank you!

Participants are asked to rate their experience at the Onsite Retreat on a 7-point Likert-type scale (1 = Very Poor, 7 = Outstanding);

Table 3.
Overall participant satisfaction with onsite retreat sessions.

in program evaluation, b) the approach used in evaluating the CS Program, and c) a deeper look at program impacts. The below examination of the broad measures observed-to-date help link the pedagogical structure with findings and contribute to elucidating the impact programs such as CS have on participant experience and skill development.

4.1 Program-related measures: participant satisfaction and fellow learning

The Clinical Scholars program tracks a variety of program-related outcomes. Data presented are for Cohorts 1-3, with Cohort 1 (n = 30) completing three years of the program, Cohort 2 (n = 34) completing two years of the program and Cohort 3 (n = 34) completing just one year of the program.

4.2 Participant satisfaction

At each retreat, participants complete evaluations at the end of each program session. Additionally, Fellows rate their overall experience for each retreat. Ratings are made on an anchored 7-point scale. Across all retreats, Program Fellows rate the experience highly, with overall session ratings ranging between 6.10-6.77 on a 7-point scale (**Table 3**), covering each of the retreats in the curriculum. The distance-based CLS portion of the program does not formally evaluate each specific component in order to reduce respondent burden.

5. Fellow learning

Assessments of learning gains by competency are made utilizing a retrospective pre- and post-test method [54–56], examining participant knowledge, attitude, use, and self-efficacy in each of the target competencies. Participants complete a survey at start, midpoint and end of the program. This approach is described more fully in Chapter 3. At publication, findings in the competency assessment are promising, in that Fellows are reporting significant growth in all 25 target competencies. **Figure 7**

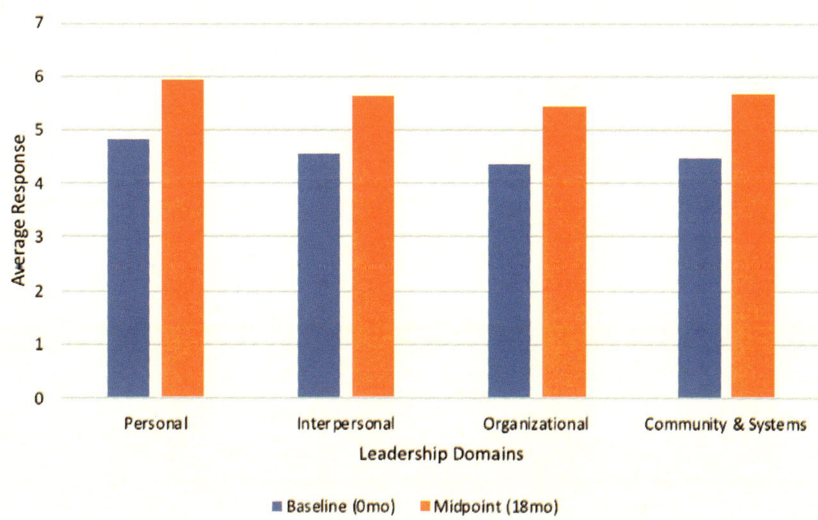

Figure 7.
*Competency changes from baseline to midpoint in cohorts 1 and 2 of the clinical scholars program by competency family. *See Chapter 3 for a detailed explanation of the Clinical Scholars Competency Assessment. **Based on a 7-point Likert-type scale. ***Data is presented as a composite of four dimensions of growth (knowledge, attitude, use, and self-efficacy) and grouped into competency domains.*

depicts the change in competency scores in each competency family for Cohorts 1 and 2 from baseline to 6 months into the program. Data are collected utilizing a retrospective pre/post approach (see Chapter 3 for more detail).

In addition to these competency-gain measurements, the evaluation approach also measures session knowledge, captures behavioral implementation of the competencies, engages in concept mapping with Fellow cohorts, and assess community engagement and network development. Chapter 3 provides an in-depth description of the evaluation efforts of the CS Program.

6. Discussion

The Clinical Scholars Program presents an in-depth, longitudinal, state-of-the-art approach to promoting the cultivation and development of a large and sophisticated set of skills that intentionally integrate leadership competencies with a focus on health equity. While the integration of leadership and equity competencies is an innovation, the pedagogical approaches and components of Clinical Scholars are similar to other prominent UNC-based national or global leadership programs, including the Maternal and Child Health Public Health Leadership Program (MCHPHLI.org), the Food Systems Leadership Institute (FSLI.org), and the ACOG-Robert C. Cefalo Leadership Institute (ACOGLeadershipInstitute.org). Each of these programs has previously published on similar learning impacts in audiences also focused on serving the greater good, and collectively these programs illustrate how significant gains in learning can be achieved in relatively short onsite development experiences, particularly when those experiences are supported by pedagogically-connected distance-based activities. Taken together, these outcomes show how a logical and structured process, using widely available tools, can contribute to both learning and implementation of skills that lead to real world impacts in communities (please refer to the chapters 5-9, 11-14 in this volume).

Approaching leadership development in the Clinical Scholars method is the product of partnership, and not solely reliant on the resources of two large academic institutions (the University of North Carolina at Chapel Hill and the University of Nebraska). This ability to achieve the high level of leadership training was accomplished through partnering with both nimble and agile businesses [57–60] as well as community-based organizations [61] and professional organizations [62], all highlighted as important considerations by the Macy Foundation [63]. In this way, the program itself role models the expectations given to the program Fellows: partnering across sectors to create successful outcomes. In 2017, Grimm, et al. [64] distinguished between *leader* development and *leadership* development, with the former focused on individual improvement and the latter focused on how teams, organizations, and communities share in the impact of the efforts. While the data shown in this chapter present only a limited view of the Clinical Scholars as leaders who are gaining knowledge and abilities as individuals, the program is, in reality, a strong blend of both *leader* and *leadership* development. As detailed in Chapter 2, leadership and the concepts of equity, diversity and inclusion cannot be separated from one another in the experience. Nor can the teams and their projects be separated from the community. The Clinical Scholars Program invests deeply both in leader and leadership development. Indeed, the latter can hardly be attained in the absence of the former. Evaluating outcomes on so many levels goes far beyond the scope of the pedagogical data presented here. However, in Chapter 3, the evaluation approach which robustly assesses many components of leadership development and the involvement of communities and systems is documented. The chapters in this work which are written by the Clinical Scholars themselves (Chapters 5-9, 11-14) clearly illustrate the many involvements, outcomes, and impacts of their work in the communities they serve and further help to elucidate how the CS Program promotes leadership development.

Creating a robust pedagogical underpinning that supports and drives achieving complex project outcomes by participants is crucial in meeting the visions and goals of organizations leading the call for impacting health equity in the United States. In 2014, The Robert Wood Johnson Foundation unveiled their new vision for creating a Culture of Health in which "every person has an equal opportunity to live the healthiest life they can—regardless of where they may live, how much they earn, or the color of their skin" [65]. Rather than try to achieve change by engaging in "doing more of the same", the RWJF held that a "new vision for a healthy population will require different sectors to come together in innovative ways to solve interconnected problems". To that end, the Foundation introduced their Action Framework (see *Leading Community-Based Changes in the Culture of Health in the US: Experiences in Developing the Team and Impacting the Community*). The Framework translates the broad range of sectors and people involved in building a Culture of Health into four interconnected Action Areas: Making Health a Shared Value, Fostering Cross-Sector Collaboration to improve well-being, Creating healthier, more equitable communities; and Strengthening integration of health services and systems. Clinical Scholars answers this call by developing a cadre of interprofessional leaders with a multitude of skills in integrated teams of health professionals working on complex, community-based wicked problems in the culture of health. Outcome data illustrate that participants enjoy the intensive learning experience, they significantly improve their skills on twenty-five competencies related to the RWJF framework, and they implement those skills in real-world settings to create notable impacts in communities (Chapters 5-9, 11-14). These data, taken along with the reports of most significant change stories and qualitative comments of the program Fellows (data presented elsewhere), lend to the conclusion that the pedagogical design of the Clinical Scholars Program has greatly facilitated the ability of these health professionals to contribute to furthering the vision of the RWJF in their own communities.

While those at the Gillings School of Global Public Health at the University of North Carolina at Chapel Hill have been engaged in this type of workforce development for literally decades, others have also sought to improve health by "better aligning health professions education with societal needs", thus echoing the call from the Robert Wood Johnson Foundation [1, 3, 4, 15, 18, 28, 29, 40–44, 47]. For example, in 2018, the Josiah Macy Jr. Foundation [63] highlighted the following priority areas: interprofessional education and teamwork; education for the care of underserved populations; new models of clinical education along with a focus on career development; rigorous research and expanded scholarship to improve health professions learning environments; and organizational commit to diversity, equity and inclusivity. While more specific than the Culture of Health Framework, this alignment is an example of trends in leadership development in health professions [47, 48, 64]. This trend recognizes the need for pedagogical approaches that prepare leaders for the quickly changing and complex system of care in which they practice. These leaders need to be equipped to work effectively in teams and to lead change within and outside of healthcare systems to ensure just opportunities for a healthy life for all people. The Clinical Scholars program answers this call for new curriculum content through the integration of leadership and health equity training, an emphasis on boundary spanning leadership skills, and project-focused work in partnership with communities to address health inequities.

We believe that it is no accident that more health care and philanthropic organizations are calling for innovative and robust ways for developing leaders that share a serious commitment to creating a culture of health. Yet meeting the need for this type of leader brings its own challenges. The sheer number of communities in distress and facing serious health inequity can seem overwhelming. While the CS Program represents a demonstrated impactful training program, it cannot possibly meet the needs of the tens of thousands of potential candidates who would benefit from this type of development. It is the belief of these authors, given our combined decades of experience in the field, that serious leadership development requires a serious investment in the individual and the team--both leader and leadership development. Equivalent experiences, skills development and self-insight does not result from reading a book, attending webinars or an afternoon lecture—it comes from intensive training focused on the needs of the learner(s) at the time of learning and applied to real world problems. These types of experiences are intensive and infrastructure heavy, and thus are impossible to deliver on a massive scale. A significant limitation of leader development efforts, in general, is that by their very nature they are focused on the individual. Adding interpersonal relationships and leadership development, such as by working in teams adds another layer of complexity. Intentionally integrating complex content, like addressing health equity, further complicates the process, making the intervention even less appropriate to mass application. Clinical Scholars advances a further step down the path of complexity in that each of the enrolled teams partners with the local communities they serve to address community-identified problems, making these truly community-based participatory projects and truly examples of leadership development. While it would be an ideal outcome to take the insights learned from developing participants in the Clinical Scholars Program and apply them on a broad scale, an inherent limitation to this approach is that this development is most effective when done in cohort-sized groups in which a networked community is formed. Our experience suggests that the idea size of this community is between 25 and 35 members.

The most important outcome for Clinical Scholars—and the measure of whether the program is worth the considerable investment of the Robert Wood Johnson Foundation—is the ultimate impacts of both the Fellow Teams' WPIPs and their continued influences through the course of their careers. While these outcomes may take several years to culminate in measurable changes, the observable changes reported in their chapters in this volume are impressive—and penned at the conclusion of their 3 year Fellowship-based Wicked Problem Impact Project, but not at the conclusion of how those projects endure beyond this Fellowship experience. Given the results reported at the close of their Clinical Scholars experience, the data suggest that investing in robust, intensive leadership development of interprofessional teams is a smart decision for impacting the culture of health in communities nationwide.

Author details

Claudia S.P. Fernandez[1*], Giselle Corbie-Smith[2], Melissa Green[2], Kathleen Brandert[3], Cheryl Noble[4] and Gaurav Dave[2]

1 Gillings School of Global Public Health, University of North Carolina at Chapel Hill, North Carolina, United States

2 School of Medicine, University of North Carolina at Chapel Hill, North Carolina, United States

3 College of Public Health, University of Nebraska Medical Center, Nebraska, United States

4 Independent Evaluation Consultant, California, United States

*Address all correspondence to: claudia_fernandez@unc.edu

References

[1] Fernandez CSP, Steffen D. Leadership for public health. In: Shi L, Johnson, JS, editors. Novick and Morrow's Public health administration: Principles for Population Based Management. 3rd ed. Sudbury, MA: Jones and Bartlett Publishers; 2013. p. 241-265.

[2] Fernandez CSP, Steffen D, Upshaw, V. Leadership for public health. In: Shi L, Johnson, JS, editors. Novick and Morrow's Public health administration: Principles for Population Based Management. 4th ed. Sudbury, MA: Jones and Bartlett Publishers; *in press 2020.*

[3] Fernandez CSP, Noble CC, Jensen ET, Chapin J. Improving leadership skills in physicians: a six-month retrospective study. J Leadership Studies 2016;9(4): 6-19. DOI:10.1002/jls.21420.

[4] Fernandez CSP, Peterson HB, Holmstrőm SW, Connolly AM. Developing emotional intelligence for health care leaders. In: Di Fabio A, ed. Emotional Intelligence—New Perspectives and Applications. New York, NY: InTech; 2012:239-260.

[5] Baer MT, Harris AB, Stanton RW, Haughton B. The future of MCH nutrition services: A commentary on the importance of supporting leadership training to strengthen the nutrition workforce. Maternal and Child Health Journal. 2015;19(2);229-235.

[6] Freshman B., Rubino L. Emotional intelligence: A core competency for health care administrators. The Health Care Manager. 2002;20(4):1.

[7] Schwartz RW, Pogge C. Physician leadership: Essential skills in a changing environment. The American Journal of Surgery. 2000;180(3):187-192. DOI: 10.1016/S0002-9610(00)00481-5.

[8] Graham EA, Wallace CA, Stapleton FB. Developing women leaders in medicine at the grass roots level: evolution from skills training to institutional change. Journal of Pediatrics. 2007;151:1-2.

[9] Mallon WT, Grigsby RK. AAMC. Leading: Top Skills, Attributes, and Behaviors Critical for Success. 2nd ed. American Association of Medical Colleges: Washington, DC. 2016.

[10] Morahan PS, Gleason KA, Richman RC, Dannels S, McDade SA. Advancing women faculty to senior leadership in U.S. academic health centers: Fifteen years of history in the making. Journal of Women and Gender in Higher Education. 2010;3(1):137-162.

[11] Awad SS, Hayley B, Fagan SP, Berger DH, Brunicardi FC. The impact of a novel resident leadership training curriculum. The American Journal of Surgery. 2004;188(5),481-484. DOI: 10.1016/j.amjsurg.2004.07.024

[12] Cummings GG, MacGregor T, Davey M, Lee H, Wong CA, Lo E, Stafford E. Leadership styles and outcome patterns for the nursing workforce and work environment: A systematic review. International Journal of Nursing Studies. 2010;47(3):363-385. DOI: 10.1016/j.ijnurstu.2009.08.006

[13] Fernandez CSP, Noble CC, Jensen ET, Martin L, Stewart M. A retrospective study of academic leadership skill development, retention and use: The experience of the Food Systems Leadership Institute. J Leadership Education 2016b;15(2 Research):150-171. DOI: 1012806/V15/I2/R4.

[14] Fernandez C, Noble CC, Jensen E, Steffen D. Moving the Needle: A Retrospective Pre- and Post-analysis of Improving Perceived Abilities Across 20 Leadership Skills, Maternal and Child Health Journal. 2014;19(2):343-352.

[15] Fernandez CSP, Noble C, Jensen E. An examination of the self-directed online leadership learning choices of public health professionals: the MCH PHLI experience. Journal of Public Health Management and Practice. 2017. DOI: 10.1097/PHH.0000000000000463

[16] Saleh SS, Williams D, Balougan M. Evaluating the effectiveness of public health leadership training: The NEPHLI experience. American Journal of Public Health. 2004;94(7):1245-1249. DOI: 10.2105/AJPH.94.7.1245

[17] Health Resources and Services Administration. Maternal and Child Health Leadership Competencies Version 4.0. [Internet]. 2019. Available from: https://mchb.hrsa.gov/training/documents/MCH_Leadership_Competencies_v4.pdf [Accessed 2019-12-16].

[18] Fernandez C, Kavanagh L, Walker DK. Letter from the Editors, Introduction to the Special Issue on Leadership Development for the MCH Workforce. Maternal and Child Health Journal. 2015;19(2):227-28. DOI: 10.1007/s10995-014-1660-3.

[19] Grason H, Kavanagh L, Dooley S, Partelow J, Sharkey A, Bradley KJ, Handler A. Findings from an assessment of state Title V workforce development needs. Maternal and Child Health Journal. 2012;16(1):7-20. DOI: 10.1007/s10995-010-0701-9.

[20] Streeter N. Workforce Crisis in MCH Leadership. Maternal and Child Health Journal. 2015;19:240-243. DOI:10.1007/s10995-014-1621.

[21] Reynolds MC, Birzer M, St. John J, Wells N, Anderson B, Walker DK. Family Leaders and Workforce Leadership Development. Maternal and Child Health Journal. 2015;19(2):252-256. DOI: 10.1007/s10995-014-1617-6.

[22] Treviño E, Mains D, Gonzalez A and Reimer D. Comparison of Public Health Leadership Institutes in the United States: A Descriptive Study. Leadership in Public Health. 2004;6(4): 37-50.

[23] Institute of Medicine. The Future of Public Health. Washington: National Academy Press; 1988. 240 p. DOI: 10.17226/1091

[24] Gebbie K, Rosenstock L, Hernandez LM, editors. Who will keep the public healthy? Educating public health professionals for the 21st century. Washington, DC: National Academy Press; 2002. 320 p. DOI:10.17226/10542.

[25] Roper WL. Strengthening the public health system. Public Health Reports. 1992;107(6):609-15.

[26] Belcher HME, Stone JD, McFadden JA, Hemmingson TA, Kreutzer C, Harris LG, Wheeler BY, Van Osdel J, Avila M, Yorker B, Hoffman BR, Turner-Musa JO. Evaluating Maternal and Child Health and Leadership Competencies in Emerging MCH Leaders: The MCHC/RISE-UP Experience. Maternal and Child Health Journal. 2015; 19:2560-2567.

[27] Lachance JA, Oxendine JS. Redefining Leadership Education in Graduate Public Health Programs: Prioritization, Focus, and Guiding Principles. American Journal of Public Health. 2015;105(Suppl 1):S60-64.

[28] Rosenberg A, Zuver D, Kermon S, Fernandez C, Margolis L. Reflections on the contributions of self-advocates to an interdisciplinary leadership development program for graduate students in health affairs, Disability and Health Journal. 2018;11(2):293-297. DOI:10.1016/j.dhjo.2017.09.002.

[29] Dodds J, Vann W, Lee J, Rosenberg A, Rounds K, Roth M, Wells, M, Evans E, Margolis, LH. The UNC-CH MCH Leadership Training Consortium: Building the Capacity to Develop Interdisciplinary MCH Leaders.

Maternal and Child Health Journal. 2009;14(4):642-648 DOI: 10.1007/s10995-009-0483-0

[30] Association of Schools and Programs of Public Health. MPH Core Competency Model. [Internet]. 2020. Available from: https://www.aspph.org/teach-research/models/mph-competency-model/. [Accessed: 2019-05-28].

[31] Council on Education for Public Health. Accreditation Criteria: Schools of Public Health and Public Health Programs. [Internet]. 2016. Available from: https://storage.googleapis.com/media.ceph.org/wp_assets/2016.Criteria.pdf. [Accessed: 2019-05-24].

[32] Public Health Foundation. Core Competencies on Public Health Professionals. Council on Linkages Between Academia and Public Health Practice. [Internet]. 2014. Available from: http://www.phf.org/resourcestools/Documents/Core_Competencies_for_Public_Health_Professionals_2014June.pdf. [Accessed: 2019-05-24].

[33] Association of American Medical Colleges. AAMC Leadership programs [Internet]. 2019. Available from: https://www.aamc.org/members/leadership. [Accessed: 2019-06-11].

[34] Geerts JM, Goodall AH, Agius S. Evidence-based leadership development for physicians: A systematic literature review. Social Science & Medicine. 2020;246:112709. DOI:10.1016/j.socscimed.2019.112709.

[35] Moldoveanu, M; Narayandas, D. The Future of Leadership Development. 2019. Available from : https://hbr.org/2019/03/educating-the-next-generation-of-leaders. [Accessed 2019-06-01].

[36] Lacerenza C, Reyes DL, Marlow SL, Joseph DL, Salas E. Leadership training design, delivery, and implementation: A meta-analysis. Journal of Applied Psychology. 2017;102(12):1686 –1718. DOI: 10.1037/apl0000241.

[37] McAlearney AS. Executive leadership development in U.S. health systems. Journal of Healthcare Management. 2010;55(3):206-222.

[38] Umble K, Steffen D, Porter J, Miller D, Hummer-McLaughlin K, Lowman A, Zelt S. The national public health leadership institute: Evaluation of a team-based approach to developing collaborative public health leaders. American Journal of Public Health. 2005;95(4):641-644. DOI:10.2105/AJPH.2004.047993.

[39] Margolis LH, Rosenberg A, Umble K, Chewning L. Effects of interdisciplinary training on MCH professionals, organizations and systems. Maternal and Child Health Journal. 2013;17(5):949-958. DOI: 10.1007/s10995-012-1078-8.

[40] Umble KE, Baker EL, Woltring C. An evaluation of the national public health leadership institute - 1991-2006: part 1. Developing individual leaders. Journal of Public Health Management and Practice. 2011a;17(3):202-213. DOI: 10.1097/PHH.0b013e3181f1e3dc.

[41] Umble K, Baker EL, Diehl SJ, Haws S, Steffen D, Frederick S, Woltring C. An evaluation of the national public health leadership institute--1991-2006: part II. Strengthening public health leadership networks, systems, and infrastructure. Journal of Public Health Management and Practice. 2011b;17(3):214-224. DOI: 10.1097/PHH.0b013e31820759d0.

[42] Umble KE, Orton S, Rosen B, Ottoson J. Evaluating the impact of the management academy for public health: Developing entrepreneurial managers and organizations. Journal of Public Health Management and Practice. 2006;12(5):436-45. DOI: 10.1097/00124784-200609000-00006.

[43] Orton S, Umble K, Zelt S, Porter J, Johnson J. Management academy for public health: Creating entrepreneurial

managers. American Journal of Public Health. 2007;97(4):601-5. DOI: 10.2105/AJPH.2005.082263.

[44] UNC Gillings School of Global Public Health. North Carolina Institute for Public Health: Leadership Programs [Internet]. Available from: https://sph.unc.edu/nciph/leadership-programs/ [Accessed 2019-06-11].

[45] Churchman CW. Wicked Problems. Management Science 1967;14(4): B141-B146 DOI:10.1287/mnsc.14.4.B141.

[46] Rittle HWJ, Webber MM. Dilemmas in a General Theory of Planning. Policy Sciences. 1973;4(2):155-169. DOI: 10.1007/bf01405730.

[47] Upshaw V, Rice D, Cipriani K, Fernandez CSP. Equity, Diversity and Inclusion in Public Health Practice. In: Shi L, Johnson, JS, editors. Novick and Morrow's Public health administration: Principles for Population Based Management. 4th ed. Sudbury, MA: Jones and Bartlett Publishers; *in press 2020.*

[48] Brandert K, Corbie-Smith G, Berthiuame R, Green M, Fernandez CSP. Clinical Scholars: Making Equity, Diversity and Inclusion Learning an Integral Part of Leadership Development. In: Fernandez CSP, Corbie-Smith G, editors. Leading Community Based Changes in the Culture of Health in the US: Experiences in Developing the Team and Impacting the Community. InTech Publishers; 2021.

[49] Dave G, Noble C, Chandler C, Corbie-Smith G, Fernandez CSP. Clinical Scholars: Using Program Evaluation to Inform Leadership Development. In: Fernandez CSP, Corbie-Smith G, editors. Leading Community Based Changes in the Culture of Health in the US: Experiences in Developing the Team and Impacting the Community. InTech Publishers; 2021.

[50] Dvir T, Eden D, Avolio BJ, Shamir B. Impact of transformational leadership on follower development and performance: A field experiment. The Academy of Management Journal. 2002;45(4):735-744. DOI: 10.2307/3069307.

[51] Frese M, Beimel S, Schoenborn S. Action training for charismatic leadership: Two evaluations of studies of a commercial training module on inspirational communication of a vision. Personnel Psychology. 2006;56(3):671-698. DOI:10.1111/j.1744-6570.2003.tb00754.x

[52] Malling B, Mortensen L, Bonderup T, Scherpbier A, Ringsted C. Combining a leadership course and multi-source feedback has no effect on leadership skills of leaders in postgraduate medical education. An intervention study with a control group. BMC Medical Education. 2009;9(1):1-7. DOI:10.1186/1472-6920-9-72.

[53] Packard T, Jones L. An outcomes evaluation of a leadership development initiative. Journal of Management Development. 2015;34(2):153-168. DOI:10.1108/JMD-05-2013-0063.

[54] Pratt CC, Mcguigan WM, Katzev AR. Measuring program outcomes: Using retrospective pretest methodology. American Journal of Evaluation. 2000;21(3):341-349. DOI:10.1177/109821400002100305.

[55] Hill LG, Betz DL. Revisiting the retrospective pretest. American Journal of Evaluation. 2005;26(4):501-517. DOI:10.1177/1098214005281356

[56] Howard GS, Ralph KM, Gulanick NA, Maxwell SE, Nance DW, Gerber SK. Internal invalidity in pretest-posttest self-report evaluations and a re-evaluation of retrospective pretests. Applied Psychological Measurement. 1979;3(1):1-23. DOI:10.1177/014662167900300101

[57] FastTrack Leadership Development Inc. Online leadership module library

[Internet]. Available from: www.WeTrainLeaders.com. [Accessed 2019-12-22].

[58] InsideOut Enneagram. Available from: http://www.insideoutenneagram.com/home.html. [Accessed 2020-01-02].

[59] Mitchen Leadership and Organization Development. Available from: www.mitchen.net. [Accessed 2020-02-23].

[60] Compass Consultation. Available from: www.CompassConsultation.com. [Accessed 2020-02-23].

[61] Community Campus Partnerships for Health. Available from: https://www.ccphealth.org/. [Accessed 2020-01-02].

[62] Academy Health. Available from: https://www.academyhealth.org/. [Accessed 2020-01-02].

[63] Macy Foundation. Improving environments for learning in the health professions: Recommendations from the Macy Foundation conference. In: Conference Recommendations; 15-18 April 2018; Atlanta, GA; 2018.

[64] Grimm B, Tibbits M, Maloney S, Johansson P, Siahpush M. Suggestions for strengthening the public health leadership development model. Journal of Pedagogy in Health Promotion. DOI: 10.1177/2373379917721721.

[65] Plough AL. Measuring What Matters: Introducing a New Action Framework in Culture of Health [Internet]. 2015. Available from: https://www.rwjf.org/en/blog/2015/11/measuring_what_matte.html. [Accessed 2019-06-11].

Chapter 2

Clinical Scholars: Making Equity, Diversity and Inclusion Learning an Integral Part of Leadership Development

Kathleen Brandert, Giselle Corbie-Smith, Rachel Berthiaume, Melissa Green and Claudia S.P. Fernandez

Abstract

The plethora of persistent and pervasive health inequities in the United States is a Wicked Problem which threatens the health and wellbeing of all people. To dismantle them is no easy task, and requires a health care workforce practiced in leadership skill sets embracing a deep focus on areas of equity, diversity and inclusion (EDI). This chapter describes how the core competencies and curriculum of the Clinical Scholars Program have been designed to offer this set of skills. To start, the program's foundational set of 25 competencies cover four domains (Personal, Interpersonal, Organizational, and Community & Systems) and include both more traditional leadership competencies as well as contemporary competencies focused on equity, diversity, and inclusion. The curriculum takes the set of 25 leadership and EDI competencies and breaks them down into learning sessions where participants listen, practice, and apply the ideas, behaviors, and mindsets. The leadership core and the EDI core of the curriculum exist both in tandem and in unison to provide the full Clinical Scholars experience. At times, sessions focus on one core or the other, and at times, both leadership and EDI are present in the learning of a session. Example learning sessions for each core and the weaving of the cores together are provided. Four challenges to creating an equity-centered leadership program are identified: 1. The personalized nature of the journey of self-development; 2. Shifting Mindsets and Skill Sets; 3. Piloting an evidence-based curriculum on EDI; and 4. Maintaining engagement with participants over time and across distance. A set of top recommendations for weaving EDI and Leadership learning are also offered. The chapter details the importance of meaningfully focusing on EDI when tackling modern, wicked problems.

Keywords: equity, diversity, leadership development, competencies, curriculum, workforce development, culture of health, leadership

1. Introduction

In their 1973 article, Rittel and Webber introduced the idea of 'wicked problems' [1]. They described wicked problems as being ill-defined, without clear explanation for their existence or clear solution for their eradication. They differentiate these problems from more "benign" problems by explaining that wicked problems are malignant, socially complex, and impacted by multiple systems. Benign problems—though they may be difficult—can be clearly solved with tools we have at the ready. Wicked problems are those we have no identified solutions for, that have no ready-made fix, instead they require a new combination of tools and skills to successfully tackle them [1]. Poverty, climate change, food security, and the balance between technological advance and personal privacy are all examples of wicked problems.

Decades later, in 1998, Ronald Heifetz introduced the concept of "Adaptive Leadership", which, over subsequent decades, grew into a predominant framework for applying leadership to intractable problems [2–4]. This framework identifies "technical problems" as being separate from "adaptive problems", in which the solutions are unclear and require learning and mobilization of stakeholders to address. In the adaptive leadership model, all parties must grow, adapt, and change as they learn new information and apply that learning to the challenge. Thus Adaptive Leadership does not rely on historical or pre-defined strategies to address these complex challenges, but rather recognizes that the strategies need to be developed through mutual understanding, collaboration, and often invention. Adaptive leadership strategies are useful in addressing wicked problems faced by society.

A wicked problem faced by our health and healthcare workforce—threatening the health and wellbeing of all people—is the plethora of persistent and pervasive health inequities in the United States. These inequities begin at birth—starting with which babies are more likely to be carried to term and celebrate their first birthday [5–8] —and continue compounding through a person's life. For example, we know there are differences in which patients receive treatment for health problems and what treatment options they receive [9–14], and the literature indicates that a person's zip code is an important predictor of the length and the quality of their life [15–17]. These inequities are rooted in historic policies, continued through current-day operation of our social systems and institutions, and perpetuated by the myth that responsibility for an individual's health outcomes lies solely within that individual's sphere of control. While these inequities are not solely created within the health care system, the health and health care workforce has particular responsibility and opportunity to address them.

Like other wicked problems, there is no easy fix, no magic bean, and no one-size-fits-all solution for the policies, practices, and biases that cause and perpetuate health inequities. To dismantle them requires a health care workforce practiced in leadership skill sets embracing a deep focus on areas of equity, diversity and inclusion (EDI).

The Clinical Scholars National Leadership Institute (CSNLI, online at ClinicalScholarsNLI.org), known more broadly as Clinical Scholars (CS) or the Clinical Scholars Program, is a leadership development experience for clinician leaders that weaves the concepts of leadership, equity, diversity and inclusion together in a three year, robust curriculum. The mission of the program is to "*develop adaptive leaders from all health disciplines to extend their influence and impact through transformative leadership training centered in equity, diversity, and inclusion*." At the heart, the Clinical Scholars Program teaches adaptive leadership strategies to health care professionals so they may have positive influence on the wicked problem of persistent health inequities in their communities and across the span of their careers.

While Chapter 1 of this book describes the overall pedagogy of the Clinical Scholars Program, this chapter describes how the program's core competencies and curriculum have been designed to develop a health care workforce with the skills needed to take on these wicked problems. It details the creation of this content and its intentional formats, challenges that emerged in the process, and the importance of meaningfully focusing on EDI when tackling modern, wicked problems.

2. A call for something more

In 2009, the Center for Creative Leadership (CCL) announced a shift in their leadership development focus towards the idea of "Boundary Spanning Leadership", characterizing it as *"the capability to create direction, alignment, and commitment across boundaries in service of a higher vision or goal."* [18]. CCL found five categories of boundaries in their research that leaders need to be able to span to address today's evolving challenges: vertical, horizontal, stakeholder, demographic, and geographic. Similarly, in 2013, leadership development experts at the University of North Carolina's Gillings School of Global Public Health wrote about the role of public health and health care providers serving as "boundary spanning leaders" [19] and published the outcomes of programs focused on training leaders in these skill sets [20–23]. More recently, the de Beaumont Foundation, along with partners in the public health field, released the report, *Building Skills for a More Strategic Health Workforce: A Call to Action* [24]. In the report, they identify eight domains of "Strategic Skills" the health workforce needs to invest in to address the complex problems currently in front of us: systems thinking; change management; persuasive communication; data analytics; problem solving; diversity and inclusion; resource management; and, policy engagement. Collectively, these bodies of work are suggesting a critical shift— the need to move beyond trying to address *wicked* problems with solutions intended to solve benign ones. To make this shift, we need leaders who have the skill set and the mindset to develop new solutions that better match these wicked problems.

So what would leadership development designed for such leaders actually look like? In Clinical Scholars, our charge is to create and support networks of visionary leaders who can break down silos, tackle the root causes of health inequities, and lead in a rapidly evolving landscape. We have created a program that supports our participants, referred to as "Fellows", to change the culture of health in their communities by building bridges between public health, health care and other systems that have enormous influence on an individual's well-being and their opportunity to be healthy—education, neighborhoods, transportation, income, faith, and others. We have developed a curriculum to help these leaders transform culture at every level, putting health and equity at the core. Clinical Scholars does this by challenging traditional ideas of leaders and conventional teachings in leadership development programs to include concepts of EDI as integral to the concept of leadership itself.

For Clinical Scholars, equity, diversity and inclusion are more than buzz words spoken at a boardroom table. They are concepts ingrained into the fibers of our program. We define *Equity* as the fair provision and distribution of resources and power so all people may realize their full potential. To reach equity means we have eliminated privilege and advantage of historically included groups, and the oppression, disparities, and disadvantages of historically excluded groups (adapted from CommonHealth ACTION, VISIONS) [25, 26]. We see *diversity* as the representation and mix of identities, differences, and similarities, both collectively and as individuals. These differences may include race, ethnicity, gender identity, disability, sexual orientation, socio-economic status, personal historical experiences, philosophical approaches and paradigms, among others (adapted from CommonHealth ACTION, Ford Foundation, VISIONS) [25–27]. *Inclusion* is the conceptual state by which all voices, perspectives, and people can contribute, be heard, and their talents utilized. It is not merely a seat at the table; it is full participation, engagement, and belonging (adapted from CommonHealth ACTION, VISIONS) [25, 26].

What makes the Clinical Scholars Program unique is that while other leader and leadership development programs might give a nod to EDI through discreet session content, CS weaves EDI concepts into the entire curriculum, focusing on how to lead the diverse communities in which our clinician leaders live, grow, work, play and pray. In other well-known executive leadership experiences, EDI curriculum is absent, optional, or lacks the robust integration needed for a more complete response to modern social complexities [28–30]. In CS, we recognize that a one-time conversation on cultural differences will not produce the change needed to address health care inequities; we set out to do better by our clinician leaders by preparing them with an integrated skill set to lead change in our current system of care. EDI is not just one of the competency focus areas, but is a foundational principle addressed alongside and equal to traditional leader development competencies. Clinicians in the CS Program receive equal emphasis on emotional intelligence and intercultural sensitivity, on managing difficult conversations and on addressing racism in communities, and on feedback using traditional leadership assessment tools and considering the power and equity dynamics at play in organizations. Our desired outcomes include graduates with the skill set and the mindset to approach their practice and their work within their community in more equitable ways and to challenge the paradigms they see that lead to inequity and health disparities. The program gives clinicians the knowledge and opportunity to recognize the systemic and institutional barriers and "-isms" which play a significant role in health outcomes, and to create innovative and community-oriented solutions for change.

3. Core competencies

In order to impart the nuanced and sophisticated skills needed to create a culture of health in communities, 25 leadership competencies stand at the core of the Clinical Scholars Program and stem from the overarching goals described in Chapter 1 of this book. The program groups these competencies into four domains: *Personal, Interpersonal, Organizational*, and *Community & Systems* (see **Figure 1**). Additionally, the competencies marry traditional leadership skill sets with contemporary skill sets in the areas of equity, diversity and inclusion.

To develop our complete list of 25 competencies the CS leadership team and partners from Community-Campus Partnerships for Health looked to institutions of higher learning and clinical practice to identify the most important behaviors and skills clinician leaders need to best address the wicked problems plaguing their

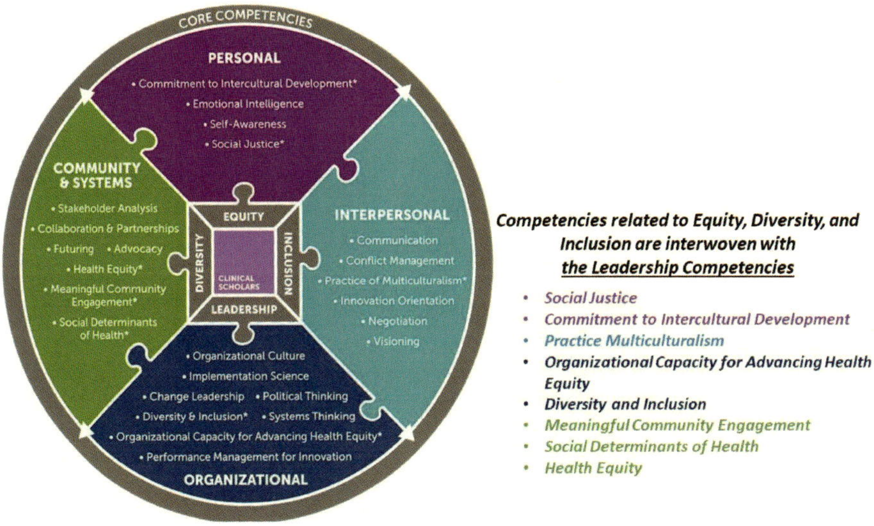

Figure 1.
The 25 Core competencies of the clinical scholars program.

communities. Those findings were combined with existing competency sets from other long-standing and successful leadership institutes, including the Maternal and Child Health Public Health Leadership Institute [20] the ACOG-Robert C. Cefalo Leadership Institute [22, 31], the Food Systems Leadership Institute [21], and the UNC Leadership for Neurodevelopmental Disabilities (LEND) program [32, 33]. Other competencies were culled from the literature on equity, diversity and inclusion, as well as from the work of national partners and organizations working on EDI in communities. The CS leadership team and partners reviewed and revised the existing core leadership competencies, added competencies specific to EDI core principles, and provided guiding definitions for each. (See Clinical Scholars Competencies and Definitions, Appendix A).

4. Curriculum

Over the course of the three-year program (See the pedagogical framework discussed in Chapter 1), participants are challenged to learn, try on, and then step fully into new and enhanced behaviors and mindsets that help them grow from being individual contributors into being leaders of teams, communities, and systems. To do this, the Clinical Scholars curriculum takes the set of 25 leadership and EDI competencies and breaks them down into learning sessions where participants listen, practice, and apply the ideas, behaviors, and mindsets. Session formats vary depending on the declared learning objectives. Formats utilized in the program include didactic lectures, small and large group discussions, case study debriefs, practice scenarios, and simulation experiences, among others.

A leadership core and an EDI core of the curriculum exist both in tandem and in unison to provide the full Clinical Scholars experience. At times, sessions focus on one core or the other, and at times, both leadership and EDI are present in the learning of a session. Here, we highlight the origins of each core curriculum alongside an example of that curriculum in action. One example is from our leadership core, one example illustrates our EDI core, and the third example shows how the cores come together to provide a deeply rich learning experience.

4.1 The leadership Core

Overall, the Clinical Scholars leadership core couples "hard skills" drawn from health services research, public and population health, engaged scholarship, health equity research, and cultural sociology with methods that develop individual and team "boundary-spanning leadership skills" shown to significantly impact participant development. Many of the sessions in the leadership core were adopted and adapted from other successful national leadership programs that illustrated significant participant learning [20–22, 31], encouraged interdisciplinary effectiveness, [32, 33] and showed real-world outcomes connected to projects undertaken as a part of the training [20, 21].

Leadership Core Example: *The Discovery Leadership Profile™.*

CS Competencies Covered:

- Change Leadership/Change Management
- Communication
- Emotional Intelligence
- Self-Awareness

The CS offers a total of up to 12 assessments to Fellows over the course of the three-year program (see Chapter 1). Many of these assessments address leadership core competencies. A prime example of the leadership curriculum and one of the most robust assessments in the program is a 360 assessment called the Discovery Leadership Profile (produced by Multi-Health Systems Inc.), which Fellows complete six months into the program. Long-standing components of leadership development programs, 360 assessments are multi-rater tools that gather feedback on key leadership areas. These assessments help identify strengths and developmental needs. Similar to other 360 tools, the Discovery Leadership Profile reflects standardized and validated questions around leadership. The assessment experience offers participants a full wrap-around experience of increasing awareness of one's self, and is paired with executive coaching in its debrief to foster improvement and personal advancement. To start the process, Fellows identify approximately 12–20 people that are above, across, and below them in the hierarchy of their organizations—along with community partners outside their organization as appropriate—who frequently see their leadership style in action. In a 80-minute session at the Orange Retreat (the second in the series of seven intensive in-person training programs, see Chapter 1), faculty explain the 360 tool, offer guidance on how to understand and interpret results, and provide reflection time for Fellows to digest what the results are telling them. Later in the retreat, following time to reflect and consider the meaning of the data, Fellows meet with an executive coach certified in the assessment to debrief and discuss their personal results. Coaches are charged with helping the participants move towards actionable behavioral changes that reflect their results.

4.2 The EDI Core

We believe that leadership development involves not only enhancing skill sets, but transforming mindsets as well. Too often, leadership programs fail to make lasting change in program participants. This happens when programs focus on changing behaviors that show up on the surface, but neglect to address the underlying mindset that explains the behavioral choices being made [34]. Addressing mindsets requires a new conversation about the root cause of current behavior. It requires uncovering and questioning the subconscious thought patterns and implicit bias each training participant comes into the program with. It requires offering a new lens from which to view the world. We see this challenge as being evident in equity, diversity and inclusion work.

The intention was set from the beginning: Clinical Scholars curriculum would incorporate knowledge, skills, attitudes, behaviors, and mindsets focused on EDI equally with those concentrated on more traditional leadership areas. While the leadership core of CS is based on decades of research focused on leadership and leadership development, the same historic body of knowledge in academic/scholarly literature is not available for EDI training and development, especially as a leadership skill. In our search of the literature and online curricula, we could not find a clear curriculum either with the integration of EDI and leadership content equally, or with a main focus on EDI with leadership as a subset of the content. You can find leadership development programs that provide isolated EDI content, but no publicly available curriculum weights EDI equally with leadership, or smoothly integrates the two together throughout the program.

A critical success factor in developing the program's combined content was an EDI curriculum retreat held early on in the program's tenure (July 2017). Participants of the retreat included the Clinical Scholars program development team, along with partners--Community-Campus Partnerships for Health,

Behavioral Impact Aims
• Engage in a personal EDI journey (e.g. see and address self-limiting behaviors)
• Recognize and interrupt 'isms' (e.g. understand historical context of privilege and oppression)
• Incorporate EDI into their Wicked Problem Impact Projects (e.g. intentionally integrate community perspectives)
• Use strategic skills for group and organization level change (e.g. conflict and negotiation skills in cross-cultural groups)
• Catalyze health equity change with communities (e.g. apply principles of authentic partnership)
• Influence public policy (e.g. understand nuts and bolts of public policy advocacy)

Table 1.
EDI behavioral impact aims of the clinical scholars National Leadership Institute.

VISIONS, Inc.--well versed in EDI training content and methodologies. Through a facilitated process, the group discussed their vision for what the EDI curriculum could look like, identified potential components for the curriculum and sources for those components, and created the beginnings of a library of high-quality, skill development-focused content. Two significant products of the retreat were: 1) a deep understanding of the desired behaviors, language, and techniques the program wanted participants to exhibit by the end (Behavioral Impact Aims), and 2) the first version of an evolving EDI Curriculum Map.

It was essential to understand at a deep level exactly what we hoped would be enduring take-aways around EDI when the Fellows graduated from the program. To that end, a facilitated discussion at the retreat began with critically examining the initial EDI competency set identified, and ended by achieving consensus around the following question: "*Given these competencies and our visions, at the end of year 3, what do we want Clinical Scholars to know, understand and do?*" The collective responses of the group fell into six categories (labeled Behavioral Impact Aims) and clarified the behaviors and developments we want to see in the Fellows upon their completion of the program (see **Table 1**).

The formation of an EDI curriculum map followed. By looking at the identified Behavioral Impact Aims and the EDI core competencies, retreat participants were able to develop suitable learning objectives to meet intended goals of the program. The map outlined which learning would take place at what point in the three-year curriculum. Conversations revolved around which skills were more foundational and which skills would add valuable layers to already understood concepts. The map also indicated which learning needed a face-to-face experience and which could be done through distance-methods.

EDI Core Example: *The Community Action Poverty Simulation.*

CS Competencies Covered:

- Advocacy
- Change Leadership/Change Management
- Commitment to Intercultural Development
- Communication
- Emotional Intelligence
- Organizational Capacity for Advancing Health Equity

- Organizational Culture
- Political Thinking
- Social Determinants of Health
- Social Justice
- Systems Thinking

Clinical Scholars layers EDI concepts over the course of the three-year program. A prime example of the EDI curriculum and one of the most robust experiential components of the curriculum is called "The Poverty Simulation," produced by the Missouri Community Action Network. In the Yellow Retreat (3rd in the in-person training series), participants explore the experience of "personal agency" through role-play of individuals living under conditions common to the working poor in a 4-hour simulation experience. Participants must navigate complex and conflicting family dynamics, unsympathetic workplace demands, and emergent neighborhood crises, along with compounding barriers caused by inadequate public systems (transportation, schools, healthcare, etc.). The simulation consists of several short "weeks" of experience from which participants report both significant stress and perceived accuracy in the imitation of the lives of the working poor. An extensive debrief of the session helps to further the objective lessons about how the social determinants of health play a significant role in an individual's health and regularly overpower personal agency under these conditions. The learning objectives for this session revolve around increasing appreciation of the effects of poverty and its impact on health equity, helping participants explore misconceptions of the experience of poverty, and identifying how the experience of poverty can impact the communities engaged by the Fellows' Wicked Problem Impact Project (WPIP).

4.3 Weaving the two cores

Overall, the CS curriculum can be seen as a piece of woven fabric. Simply-constructed woven fabrics are produced by interlacing two sets of thread with one another; the repeating pattern of interlacing is called the weave. In the CS Program the Leadership Core and the EDI Core are the sets of threads. As the curriculum draws each piece in, interlacing the threads together by building on, nesting with, and linking to other components, the weave of the fabric is made. In weaving fabric, both sets of thread are important to creating textile that is useful, performs well, and is pleasing the eye; the same is seen in the Clinical Scholars Curriculum. The two curriculum cores of leadership and EDI are equally important to the viability, lasting behavioral impact, and ultimately, the success of the program. While some Clinical Scholars sessions may focus more heavily on either traditional leadership or contemporary EDI competencies and skill sets, other sessions weave these threads together into complex and multifaceted learnings.

Weaving Example: *Applying an Equity Lens.*

CS Competencies Covered:

- Advocacy
- Change Leadership/Change Management
- Commitment to Intercultural Development

- Communication
- Organizational Capacity for Advancing Health Equity
- Organizational Culture
- Political Thinking
- Social Justice
- Systems Thinking

Health care systems and organizations can take a leadership role in ensuring that everyone has the opportunity to be healthy [35]. In particular, health care organizations have the ability to not only address health disparities directly at the point of care but also to influence the social and economic determinants that result in health disparities. The Institute for Healthcare Improvement (IHI) has developed a framework for health care organizations to promote health equity in the communities they serve [35]. There are five key components of the framework: 1) Make health equity a strategic priority; 2) Develop structure and processes to support health equity work; 3) Deploy specific strategies to address the multiple determinants of health on which health care organizations can have a direct impact, such as health care services, socioeconomic status, physical environment, and healthy behaviors; 4) Decrease institutional racism within the organization; and, 5) Develop partnerships with community organizations to improve health and equity. At the Blue Retreat (5th in the in-person training series), faculty discuss the business and moral case for applying an equity lens to organizational policy in healthcare. In the two-hour session, Fellows are asked to think about the leadership skills they have acquired and how they might apply the IHI framework to their work or advocate for its application in their organizations. In small groups, Fellows brainstorm each component of the framework and use a gallery walk methodology to share out and discuss examples.

5. Challenges and lessons learned

The development of a new training program and curriculum comes with its challenges and lessons learned. There are four areas of our work in the Clinical Scholars curriculum that challenged the program staff to think in new ways about leadership development.

5.1 Challenge #1: the personalized nature of the journey of self-development

The CS team built the curriculum very thoughtfully and intentionally, from information collected from the literature, institutions of higher learning, organizations widely respected for their equity work, and team and partners' expertise and knowledge. We anticipate and are confident that this curriculum will spur improved and successful behaviors and approaches by Fellows within their clinic settings and community-based work. At the same time, we recognize the personal nature of one's growth-journey in EDI is brought about by one's own identities, background, and readiness to advance their EDI proficiency. While we select for participants and teams that center equity as an approach to their Wicked Problem Impact Project, we have found the continuum of values and beliefs, behaviors and practices is not narrow. We have seen the unevenness of how a session's learning can land for a cohort of Fellows. For some, content is new and can feel paralyzing, while for others the content might feel familiar, and even too rudimentary. Additionally, we have learned that Fellows can fall prey to assumptions about how their own beliefs are directly reflected in learning sessions, and how both challenging and enlightening it can be to gain insight into where one stands on the EDI growth-journey in a relative sense. The program is called to support all Fellows by helping those earlier in the growth-journey to feel brave enough to continue the work, and those who are further in the journey to show both grace to others and humility to see this journey has no end, as there is always more to understand, know and do.

The ways we support all Fellows are through intentional program structure and design. Building strong relationships between the participants from the start helps them to challenge one another and foster their individual and collective growth. Another tool we use is safe and open cohort-based discussions about EDI session content; these discussions often provide insights to previously uninvestigated assumptions and attitudes that allow everyone to move to a new place in their EDI learning journey. Most importantly, we work to react well to the variety of responses to content by providing sufficient supports for individuals no matter where they are on the growth-journey. The characteristics of the Fellows described earlier mirror the characteristics of the CS staff team; the EDI growth-journey is something all invested in this program are participating in. To better shore up the sensitivity with which we respond, the CS staff team is encouraged and has dedicated funding to further develop their own EDI skills and awareness through workshops, training, and conferences.

This challenge we are describing is further exacerbated as the program strives to include lessons from all 25 competencies within the in-person and distance-based sessions and activities. This leads to a packed schedule, which might not meet the learning styles of all participants. While clinicians are familiar with this type of intensity in professional trainings, the nature of EDI topics elicits more emotional response and calls on more mental and emotional energies than traditional leadership topics. As CS staff saw this play out in both the EDI and leadership in-person sessions, the curriculum and schedule were modified to have dedicated reflection and preparation times and tools to support the Fellows for the unique work needed for EDI area advancement. Providing more space and time to process content, and balancing the delivery of new content and the time allotted for digestion of that information, have been two essential approaches for effective EDI competency training. In addition, Fellows are provided with more than a dozen books addressing EDI and leadership topics over the three years and weekly "self-reflection prompts" are sent via email to all Fellows, providing structure and guidance for continuing this growth-journey in between the onsite retreat sessions.

We acknowledge that leadership growth is a personalized intellectual and emotional journey that needs immediate and ongoing attention. Related formally scheduled sessions focus on stress management and managing difficult conversations. The program team incorporates breaks for reflection and self care and pairs Fellows with peers in other cohorts for peer support. Executive and team coaches are present during onsite meetings to offer additional support. Fellows have access to an open space to practice yoga or Zumba and often assemble for group outdoor walks and runs. The structured and iterative nature of the program allows the CS team and Fellows to learn from Fellow's experiences and reflections. For example, an optional Structural Inequalities training offered by our partners, Community-Campus Partnerships for Health, included an expedited and condensed photovoice activity in which participants presented self-captured and selected photographic images representing inequality in their communities and shared the structural context of the photo. Fellows and other participants via consensus selected a photo reflecting injustice and engaged in guided discussion about the underlying factors using the SHOWED method [36] meant to engage groups in critical dialog about vital shared community issues. Hours after the training, one of the guest youth participants was detained from entering the event's hotel by security. Learning of this incident, participants discussed their roles and action steps as actors, allies, and accomplices in social justice, recognizing that the systems that they work and live in are not set up to readily support these EDI concepts.

5.2 Challenge #2: shifting mindsets and skill sets

Teaching negotiation tactics--a traditional leadership development topic--is about strategy and skill. Teaching how to meaningfully engage in authentic partnerships with communities--an EDI competency--is about strategy, skill, and *shifting mindsets*. The case for "why we need leadership" is ingrained in the American way. It is underneath so many of the lessons in our school systems, and is embedded in the language of organizations. The case for "why we need equity, diversity, and inclusion" has not permeated the language and minds of school, organizations, and communities in the same way. While many organizations in the last several years have begun to understand and make the business case for EDI, it is not a universally accepted core principle. The need to act in ways that are fair, just, and equitable to all people despite their differences is not ingrained in people, in the organizations they participate in, or in the systems in which they live. This adds to the burden and the importance of the EDI core. Participants will not take in or hone skills around EDI if they do not first have the shift in mindset needed to appreciate difference, celebrate it, and leverage it so they can see why those skills are important in the first place.

Furthermore, there is a push and pull of issues that need attention in healthcare. Racism is the most critical--it bookends the other oppressed identities in our nation's historic past--but it is not the only source of oppression. Sexism, ableism, classism, elitism, ageism, and others are also present in our systems and unfairly advantage some while disadvantaging others [26]. Each person is coming in with their own experience and identity, and in their own place in the journey. And, the journey is multi-dimensional in multiple ways. First, for the most part, Fellows come into the program understanding some areas of disadvantage, but not all. If a Fellow comes into the program with a very deep understanding of structural racism, but has not learned about disability issues, the work of the program is to assess where they are in the journey and what axis they are on in terms of thinking about oppression. The role of the program is to then create the space and elevate the need to broaden the lens each Fellow brings. Additionally, each Fellow themselves holds multiple identities, some of which might offer them privilege and others which disadvantage them. The intersectionality of identities presents further need to expand program learning to discuss the ways in which each "ism" works individually and is interconnected in the system. And finally, there will be times in their leadership work that a Fellow may not hold a particular identity that is being oppressed (e.g. Black, female), but because of that they have an obligation to advocate for others in those oppressed groups because of the advantaged position they hold. So we teach allyship as an important social lever we can pull to ensure the equity and diversity we are talking about.

Over and above that, the program meets these challenges by offering a variety of opportunities and examples over time and across competency sets to explore these issues in a safe and welcoming environment. We endeavor to put many illustrations of the complexities of inequality and difference in front of the Fellows, both as individuals, in their project teams, and across the entire group. Some examples of this follow. As mentioned, the program offers a Special Experience which focuses on structural racism and historical trauma. In our seven consecutive training intensives, sessions endeavor to weave the intersectionality of multiple issues throughout. The poverty simulation, described above, contrasts Fellow's daily experience with those living under both the conditions of poverty and the prejudice against it. In our Blue retreat (5th in the program series), a session specifically addresses the competition between diversity issues and how that can be destructive to anti-isms work and health equity coupled with skill building for being an ally. Additionally, sessions in the leadership core are based on the concept of "thought diversity" with several focused specifically on the differences in personality types that lead to differences in behaviors. The wide range of ways the program highlights differences (in personality, in social identity and culture, in experience) helps Fellows create organizational and team cultures that embrace differences more clearly, positively and openly.

Finally, we speak and model at every turn in the curriculum the grace we need in order to understand each other and support each other in the journey of reaching equity, diversity and inclusion in our lives, our workplaces, and our communities.

5.3 Challenge #3: piloting an evidence-based curriculum on EDI

It has been a challenge to find an evidence-based curriculum that embraces the breadth of leadership, equity, diversity and inclusion mandated by the charge of the RWJF funding. Piloting a newly designed, never vetted, 3-year EDI curriculum has held its share of challenges. While CS staff and partners brought a wealth of session topic examples and speaker ideas for the leadership core, the same level of tested topics and speakers was simply not available for the EDI core. Following the development of the Behavioral Impact Goals and Curriculum Map (see more information on both above), the team spent an incredible amount of time, energy and resources looking into already existing curriculum on EDI topics, and through the personal networks of staff and partners, for the bits and pieces that would fit within our EDI Leadership ideals. Sources for components of our curriculum that are widely available include trainings available from VISIONS, inc, a non-profit training and consulting agency specializing in diversity and inclusion (https://www.visions-inc.org/) and the *Transforming White Privilege* curriculum, a joint project of The Center for Assessment and Policy Development (CAPD), MP Associates, and World Trust Educational Services, funded by The W.K. Kellogg Foundation (https://www.racialequitytools.org/module/overview/transforming-white-privilege).

Furthermore, the topics of racism, sexism, classism, intersectionality, privilege and oppression can be quite charged. Any given session in our curriculum has a limited time frame, in an effort to meet the requirements of the program funders and the overall program goals. We cannot address everything that could be addressed, leaving some topics to be addressed in more superficial ways than would otherwise be needed to truly dig deeper into any given form of oppression/privilege dichotomy. A third struggle in piloting this curriculum has been around evaluating its effectiveness. Identifying the evaluation concepts overall to measure the desired competencies, and identifying measures of speaker success and content appropriateness has been challenging.

We have also experienced the challenge of making and implementing a curriculum with longevity in the face of an evolving societal awareness and response to new thinking around EDI concepts and terms. In order to avoid stagnation and teaching dated viewpoints, the Clinical Scholars team continually scans the larger landscape of key EDI discussions and research for important updates to the curriculum. The curriculum itself is designed with embedded flexibility for such updates, while maintaining proven methods and formats. Outside of the set curriculum, we offer other learning opportunities where unfolding information and new resources can be shared, such as weekly journal prompts and popular and scholarly articles and books.

5.4 Challenge #4: maintaining engagement with participants over time and across distance

The inclusive national nature of CS involves healthcare professionals distanced by geography (to date-25 states, Washington, DC, and Puerto Rico), discipline, and focus area, which creates challenges to engagement and building a sense of community. A hybrid in-person and distance-based leadership program can be challenging for all learners but especially so for providers who maintain full time employment and busy households. What unites these diverse Fellows is a common sense of purpose and commitment to make a positive impact on health well-being within their communities.

Research conducted of online learning demonstrates that learning effectiveness is optimized by learning formats in which learners interact with both instructors and classmates and actively participate in activities [37–39]. The CS program team strives for continuity, engagement, and responsiveness to leadership development in the context of real-life. While participants only convene in person three times a year (biannual CS intensives plus an RWJF-sponsored Annual Leadership Institute), contact is maintained with each Fellow cohort weekly with updates on program components and news about peers. News of Fellow accolades, promotions, professional and personal accomplishments are publicly acknowledged in the weekly updates to build comradery. Fellows are oriented to the online learning management system to communicate with staff, coaches, and each other, view the distance and in-person schedules, make travel arrangements, and access/submit program requirements.

Adaptations to the curriculum are responsive to Fellow real-life demands and feedback that some requests were duplicative and not harmonized. Fellow onboarding evolved into an integrated process coordinated between the CS Deputy Directors. The integration was needed to streamline contact with and requests from RWJF and their affiliates, communicate required and optional components of the program, prepare Fellows for their first in-person session and online session, introduce the online learning environment, and properly acknowledge and introduce Fellows on our website. Online monthly webinars were reduced from three a month to one every four to six weeks. Similarly, team coaches created a team coaching guide to anticipate the needs and potential experiences of teams throughout the three years of the program. Fellows received annual requirements framed as asynchronous learning to be completed annually, with suggestions to complete them on a regular basis over 2–3 hours per week. Fellows received individual quarterly progress reports of their completion of requirements.

External to program components, the Clinical Scholars team connects Fellows with mutual interests, approaches, challenges, and disciplines. Fellows organically make similar connections during onsite sessions and Fellows also facilitate connections within the Clinical Scholars program and across their networks serving as assigned or automatic peer mentors during and following the program.

5.5 Top recommendations for weaving EDI and leadership learning

- Support Fellows in developing detailed Group Agreements (See **Table 2**). These kinds of agreements can create the container that will hold the group's trust and fears, can be used to frame difficult conversations and learning across the program, and can be referred to when group norms are violated by staff, speakers, or participants.

- Ensure all persons connected to the program (leads, staff, speakers, coaches) also hold the important EDI values being fostered in this program.

Example Group Agreements		
• Be a humble learner • We have/are responsible for "stuff", conscious and unconscious (bias, "accessories", etc.) • Assume best intent & respect impact • Take risk to be vulnerable • Practice self focus (I believe, I feel) • It's OK to be YOU (be authentic) in this space, in your growing edge. (see other guidelines) • Allow growth for self and others • Listen with intensity usually reserved for speaking	• Move in/Move out of the interaction (neither dominate nor abdicate) • Be present in the room • Be gracious, not grumpy • Have one another's backs • Stay focused on 'big idea' • Allow quieter voices to be heard • Non-judgmental/curiosity • Welcome and seek out thought diversity • Practice patience... • Compassionate feedback • Extend grace to others	• Words matter • Practice "both/and" thinking • Try things on • Have fun! • Experience joy! • Keep confidences • **And,** ***confidentiality*** **means:** • Take away themes and A-HAs • No attribution to others • No sharing other's stories • No telling stories about others • Also, be vulnerable, but share comfortably

These agreements were created by the fellows themselves (developed by Cohort 4 in fall 2019) over the course of multiple, iterative discussions in the first onsite experience of the program, and are brought back to each experience moving forward.

Table 2.
CS cohort 4 group agreement.

- Create a protocol for staff to follow that offers a road map if, within a session or event, a Fellow is triggered, then staff move to offer any needed support to that participant.

- Create a protocol for staff to follow if a speaker's content or examples used within a session rub against the very EDI mindset you are working to achieve (e.g. use of microaggressions).

- Be prepared to stop other content-based programming to support the emotional and mental health needs of participants.

- The program will have missteps. Be humble enough to acknowledge, and agile enough to find a more effective path.

- Fellows will misstep. Create a trusted, safe, and brave space from the beginning to both hold missteps to account, and to extend the grace needed for continued self-focus and learning in the process.

6. Conclusions

Leadership development programs can be found in every industry and every field. A 2012 report showed that US companies spend $14 billion annually in this area [40]. These programs are often exclusive to traditional concepts of leaders focusing on conflict management, negotiation, and communication skill sets. The Robert Wood Johnson Foundation intentionally funded Clinical Scholars to expand the traditional model of leadership development to include equipping health care professionals with tools around equity, diversity and inclusion so that they could meaningfully impact the social determinants of health in their own communities. The Clinical Scholars National Leadership Institute team has found that the blending of leadership and EDI work is crucial to preparing leaders to face the health equity problems of today.

One participant wrote:

Not only have I grown as a leader, but also in terms of self-confidence and awareness that I can make change happen. I have found my voice, in advocating for change. I have found lasting friendships and partnerships, with individuals that have a shared sense of purpose. Through my individual growth, as well as growth within my team, we have made a change in the lives of those we serve, and within our communities. – Asha Davis, MD.

Appendix A: clinical scholars competencies and definitions

Personal Level Competencies
***Commitment to Intercultural Development**: continually increase one's awareness, content knowledge, cognitive sophistication, and empathetic understanding of the complex ways individuals interact within systems and institutions; develop and demonstrate an active, intentional, and ongoing engagement with diversity: in people, in the team, in populations, and in communities, with respect to ability, intellectual, social, cultural, geographical [41].
Emotional Intelligence: Ability to assess and understand the emotions of one's self, others and groups; the ability to relate to others beyond technical concerns; the ability to implement soft skills in interpersonal or organizational settings and manage stress [42, 43].
Self-Awareness: Assessing and understanding your personal leadership strengths and development areas (weaknesses); being aware of how personal preferences and leadership style differ from others; understanding what you still need to learn; the ability to "own" mistakes; use self-examination and reflection to create a life-long leadership learning plan [44].
***Social Justice:** Develop the knowledge, skills, and disposition needed to create environments that foster equitable participation and self-determination of all groups while seeking to address and acknowledge issues of oppression, privilege, and power [45].
Inter-Personal Level Competencies
Communication: Effectively communicate with individuals and groups representing diverse stakeholders both within and without the organization; speak in a clear and concise manner in both routine and high tension situations, with individuals, groups, and the press.
Conflict Management: Use dialog to solve critical problems; implement alternative dispute resolution strategies; successfully manage conflict between people or groups.
Innovation Orientation: Implement interpersonal strategies to promote the generation of new ideas, approaches, and processes; engage in innovation and entrepreneurship at a personal level in addressing wicked problems that impede achieving a culture of health.
Negotiation: Engage in productive dialog to resolve disputes between either people or organizations; represent/defend the interests of your organization/self when crafting agreements with other parties while creating new opportunities for partnerships and collaboration.
***Practice of Multi-Culturalism:** articulate and readily integrate into their work the concepts of identity, culture, equity, diversity and inclusion; examine and build respect and appreciation for individual differences (e.g., personality, learning styles, and life experiences) and group/social differences (e.g., race/ethnicity, class, gender, sexual orientation, country of origin, and ability as well as cultural, political, religious, or other affiliations) that can be engaged in the service of learning and working together [46].
Visioning: Create a compelling, engaging vision that embraces a holistic perspective of a chosen concept; integrate the vision with the mission of the larger organization; inspire others to work towards achieving that vision as well [47].

Organizational Level Competencies
***Organizational Capacity for Advancing Health Equity**: Understand and develop techniques, approaches and strategies to advocate for transformation of systemic power structures and policies such that shared power arrangements, increased community access and engagement, and equitable outcomes result [48].
Organizational Culture: Create an organizational culture that embraces varying skills and perspectives to capitalize on the contributions of various members; impact the organizational culture of groups such that members are engaged and mission-focused; create a work environment where group member satisfaction is high and people feel valued, engaged, and utilized to their full potential
***Diversity and Inclusion:** Foster cultures that support diversity and inclusion; employ language and behaviors that acknowledge that a community or institution's success is dependent on how well it values, engages and includes the rich diversity of its members or constituents [49, 50].
Implementation Science/Evidence-based practice: Identify and utilize factors and methods to examine the process of implementation to effectively operationalize proven interventions and produce positive outcomes [48].
Performance Management for Innovation: Develop measures of performance improvements; develop and/or implement performance standards which foster accountability and facilitate innovation; link performance measures and standards to a potential strategic plan/innovation plan for the organization; implement systems to promote innovation at the team or organizational level
Change Leadership/Change Management: Understand personal change style and personal preferences when navigating change; identify the need for organizational change; understand the cycle of organizational change; implement processes to bring necessary changes and achieve organizational sustainability [44].
Systems Thinking: Identify systems influences of wicked problems in planning solutions; implement systems theories to address organizational change and transformation; build organizational capacity to envision and select system-wide strategies to address acute problems.
Political Thinking: Developing and implementing political strategies both within the organization and externally.
Community & Systems Level Competencies
Advocacy: Influence groups, policy, public policy, and resource allocation decisions within political, economic and social systems and institutions; create persuasive dialog to support one's issue or goal.
Collaboration and Partnerships: Recognize and reconcile emotional and rational elements in collaboration-building and strategic planning; create opportunities for individual, team, and organizational success through the development of creative partnerships internal to and external to the organization; link partnership development with community impact, positive revenue streams and sustainability.
Futuring: Assess current trends for potential future developments in programs, concerns, political agendas, or concepts that are aimed at building a culture of health; contribute to creating the relevant systems of the future through technology, innovation, partnerships, and political influence.
***Health Equity**: Pursue the highest possible standard of health for all people, with special attention to the needs of those at greatest risk of poor health, based on social conditions; champion and advocate for interventions or policies that advance the opportunity for all to attain their highest level of health [48, 51].
***Meaningful Community Engagement:** Employ the four specific elements of authentic community engagement - 1) Guiding Principles of Partnership, 2) Quality Processes, 3) Meaningful Outcomes and 4) Transformative Experience(s) while working collaboratively with and through groups to address issues affecting the well-being of those people to build trust, enlist new resources and allies, create better communication, and improve overall health outcomes [48, 52].
***Social Determinants of Health:** Understand how the social determinants of health impact both individuals and communities; integrate intervention strategies and policies to address social determinants of health into approaches of the Wicked Problem Impact Project [53].
Stakeholder Analysis: Assess and analyze important players/factors that contribute to or impede individual, team, or organizational success; develop and implement strategies to align stakeholders to organizational mission and vision [54].

**Designate EDI focused competencies.*

Author details

Kathleen Brandert[1*], Giselle Corbie-Smith[2], Rachel Berthiaume[3], Melissa Green[2] and Claudia S.P. Fernandez[3]

1 Office of Public Health Practice, College of Public Health, University of Nebraska Medical Center, Nebraska, United States

2 School of Medicine, University of North Carolina at Chapel Hill, North Carolina, United States

3 Gillings School of Global Public Health, University of North Carolina at Chapel Hill, North Carolina, United States

*Address all correspondence to: kbrandert@unmc.edu

References

[1] Rittel HWJ, Webber MM. Dilemmas in a general theory of planning. Policy Sciences. 1973;4(2):155-169. DOI: 10.1007/bf01405730.

[2] Heifetz RA. Leadership without Easy Answers. Boston, MA: Harvard University Press; 1998. 348 p.

[3] Heifetz RA, Marty L. Leadership on the Line: Staying Alive through the Dangers of Leading. Boston, MA: Harvard Business School Press; 2002. 241 p.

[4] Heifetz RA, Linsky M, Grashow A. The Practice of Adaptive Leadership: Tools and Tactics for Changing your Organization and the World. Boston, MA: Harvard Business Press; 2009.

[5] Lu MC, Kotelchuck M, Hogan V, Jones L, Wright K, Halfon N. Closing the black-white gap in birth outcomes: A life-course approach. Ethnicity & Disease. 2010;20(1 Suppl 2):S2-76.

[6] Smith IZ, Bentley-Edwards KL, El-Amin S, Darity W. Fighting at Birth: Eradicating the Black-White Infant Mortality Gap. Oakland, CA: Duke University. 2018.

[7] Wallace M, Crear-Perry J, Richardson L, Tarver M, Theall K. Separate and unequal: Structural racism and infant mortality in the US. Health & Place. 2017;45:140-144.

[8] Willis E, McManus P, Magallanes N, Johnson S, Majnik A. Conquering racial disparities in perinatal outcomes. Clinics in Perinatology. 2014;41(4):847-875.

[9] Smedley BD, Stith AY, Nelson AR, editors. Unequal Treatment: Confronting Racial and Ethnic Disparities in Health Care. Washington, DC: National Academies Press; 2003. 780 p.

[10] Council on Ethical and Judicial Affairs. Black-white disparities in health care. JAMA. 1990;263(17):2344-2346. DOI:10.1001/jama.1990.0344017 0066038.

[11] Andrews RM, Elixhauser A. Use of major therapeutic procedures: Are Hispanics treated differently than non-Hispanic whites. Ethnicity & Disease. 2000;10(3):384-394.

[12] Balsa AI, McGuire TG. Statistical discrimination in health care. Journal of Health Economics. 2001;20(6):881-907. DOI:10.1016/s0167-6296(01)00101-1.

[13] Allison JJ, Kiefe CI, Centor RM, Box JB, Farmer RM. Racial differences in the medical treatment of elderly Medicare patients with acute myocardial infarction. Journal of General Internal Medicine. 1996;11(12):736-743. DOI:10.1007/BF02598987.

[14] Abreu JM. Conscious and nonconscious African American stereotypes: Impact on first impression and diagnostic ratings by therapists. Journal of Consulting and Clinical Psychology. 1999;67(3):387-393. DOI:10.1037//0022-006x.67.3.387

[15] Weeks WB, Kazis LE, Shen Y, Cong Z, Ren XS, Miller D, Lee A, Perlin JB. Differences in health-related quality of life in rural and urban veterans. American Journal of Public Health. 2004;94(10):1762-1767. DOI: 10.2105%2Fajph.94.10.1762

[16] Drewnowski A, Rehm CD, Solet D. Disparities in obesity rates: Analysis by ZIP code area. Social Science & Medicine. 2007;65(12):2458-2463. DOI: 10.1016/j.socscimed.2007.07.001.

[17] Wang F, McLafferty S, Escamilla V, Luo L. Late-stage breast cancer diagnosis and health care access in Illinois. The Professional Geographer. 2008;60(1):54-69. DOI: 10.1080/00330120701724087.

[18] Yip J, Ernst C, Campbell M. Boundary Spanning Leadership: Mission Critical Perspectives from the Executive Suite. Center for Creative Leadership Organizational Leadership White Paper. 2009. Available from: https://ssrn.com/abstract=1490462

[19] Fernandez CSP, Steffen D. Leadership for public health. In: Shi L, Johnson JA, editors. Novick and morrow's Public Health Administration: Principles for Population-Based Management. 3rd ed. Santa Barbara, CA: Jones and Bartlett Publishers; 2013. p. 241-265.

[20] Fernandez CSP, Noble CC, Jensen E, Steffen D. Moving the needle: A retrospective pre- and post-analysis of improving perceived abilities across 20 leadership skills, Maternal and Child Health Journal. 2015;19(2):343-352. DOI: 10.1007/s10995-014-1573-1.

[21] Fernandez CSP, Noble CC, Jensen ET, Martin L, Stewart M. A retrospective study of academic leadership skill development, retention and use: The experience of the Food Systems Leadership Institute. Journal of Leadership Education. 2016;15(2 Research):150-171. ERIC Number: EJ1131981.

[22] Fernandez CSP, Noble CC, Jensen ET, Chapin J. Improving leadership skills in physicians: A six-month retrospective study. Journal of Leadership Studies. 2016;9(4):6-19. DOI:10.1002/jls.21420.

[23] Fernandez CSP, Noble C, Jensen E. An examination of the self-directed online leadership learning choices of public health professionals: The MCH PHLI experience. Journal of Public Health Management Practice. 2017;23(5):454-460. DOI: 10.1097/PHH.0000000000000463.

[24] De Beaumont. Building Skills for a more Strategic Public Health Workforce: A Call to Action [Internet]. 2017. Available from: https://www.debeaumont.org/news/2017/building-skills-for-a-more-strategic-health-workforce-a-call-to-action/

[25] CommonHealth ACTION. Equity, Diversity, and Inclusion Training Institute – Living Glossary. 2015.

[26] Visions Inc. Is Reconciliation Possible? The Question Remains: Bridging the Troubled Waters – Lessons from Combatting Modern Racism in the US and South Africa [Internet]. 2017. Available from: https://www.visions-inc.org/uploads/1/1/7/0/117018765/is-reconciliation-possible-july-2017-3.pdf.

[27] Ford Foundation. Diversity, Equity, and Inclusion [Internet]. 2018. Available from: https://www.fordfoundation.org/about/people/diversity-equity-and-inclusion/

[28] eCornell. Stand Apart with a Leadership Certificate from Cornell University [Internet]. https://info.ecornell.com/leadership?creative=188485597906&keyword=executive%20leadership%20development%20program&matchtype=e&network=g&device=c&utm_campaign=ldrshp_US+-+EXM+-+Executive+Leadership&utm_source=google&utm_medium=cpc&utm_term=executive%20leadership%20development%20program&utm_content=g_188485597906_e&creative=188485597906&keyword=executive%20leadership%20development%20program&matchtype=e&network=g&device=c&url=https%3A%2F%2Finfo.ecornell.com%2Fleadership%3Fcreative%3D188485597906%26keyword%3Dexecutive%2520leadership%2520development%2520program%26matchtype%3De%26network%3Dg%26device%3Dc&target=&position=1t2&gclid=CjwKCAjwhbHlBRAMEiwAoDA3441dAvad42JPfo43JClcqKt_IcUOqdQftcpaJwrzsLcXJt_MZtolshoCKIoQAvD_BwE.

[29] Harvard Business School. Program for Leadership Development – Curriculum Guide [Internet]. Available from: https://www.exed.hbs.edu/Documents/leadership-development-curriculum.pdf

[30] Center for Creative Leadership. The Leadership Development Roadmap: A Guide for Developing Successful Leaders at All Levels [Internet]. 2016. Available from: https://www.ccl.org/wp-content/uploads/2016/09/leader-development-roadmap-center-for-creative-leadership.pdf

[31] Fernandez C, Noble C. Report to the American college of obstetricians and gynecologists (ACOG) on cohort 8 six-month follow up study of 10 core leadership skills. Unpublished manuscript. 2014.

[32] Dodds J, Vann W, Lee J, Rosenberg A, Rounds K, Roth M, Wells M, Evens E, Margolis LE. The UNC-CH MCH leadership training consortium: Building the capacity to develop interdisciplinary MCH leaders. Maternal and Child Health Journal. 2010;14:642-648. DOI: 10.1007/s10995-009-0483-0

[33] Rosenberg A, Zuver D, Kermon S, Fernandez C, Margolis L. Reflections on the contributions of self-advocates to an interdisciplinary leadership development program for graduate students in health affairs. Disability and Health Journal. 2018;11(2):293-297. DOI: 10.1016/j.dhjo.2017.09.002.

[34] Gurdjian P, Halbeisen T, Lane K. Why leadership-development programs fail. McKinsey Quarterly. 2014;1(1):121-126.

[35] Wyatt R, Laderman M, Botwinick L, Mate K, Whittington J. Achieving Health Equity: A Guide for Health Care Organizations. IHI White Paper. Cambridge, Massachusetts: Institute for Healthcare Improvement. 2016.

[36] Wang C, Burris MA. Photovoice: Concept, methodology, and use for participatory needs assessment. Health Education & Behavior. 1997;24(3), 369-387. DOI: 10.1177/10901981970 2400309

[37] Bento R, Schuster C. Participation: The online challenge. In: Aggarwal A, editors. Web-Based Education: Learning from Experience. Hershey, Pennsylvania: Idea Group Publishing; 2003. p. 156-164.

[38] Webster J, Hackley P. Teaching effectiveness in technology-mediated distance learning. Academy of Management Journal. 1997;40(6): 1282-1309.

[39] Hrastinski S. A theory of online learning as online participation. Computers & Education. 2009;52(1): 78-82.

[40] Loew L, O'Leonard K. Leadership development factbook 2012: Benchmarks and trends in US leadership development. Bersin by Deloitte. 2012.

[41] Association of American Colleges & Universities. Diversity, Equity, & Inclusive Excellence [Internet]. Available from: https://www.aacu.org/resources/diversity-equity-and-inclusive-excellence

[42] MHS Assessments. Emotional Quotient-Inventory 2.0 [Internet]. Available from: https://storefront.mhs.com/collections/eq-i-2-0.

[43] Fernandez CSP, Peterson HB, Holmstrom SW, Conolly A. Developing emotional intelligence for healthcare leaders: New perspectives and applications. Annamaria Di Fabio; Intech Publishers. 2012. DOI: 10.5772/31940. Available from: http://www.intechopen.com/books/emotional-intelligence-new-perspectives-and-applications/developing-emotional-intelligence-for-healthcare-leaders

[44] Center for Creative Leadership. Addressing the Leadership Gap in

Healthcare: What's Needed When It Comes to Leader Talent? [Internet]. 2016. Available from http://insights.ccl.org/wp-content/uploads/2015/04/addressingLeadershipGapHealthcare.pdf

[45] American College Personnel Association, National Association of Student Personnel Administrators. Professional Competency Areas for Student Affairs Educators [Internet]. 2015. Available from: http://www.naspa.org/images/uploads/main/ACPA_NASPA_Professional_Competencies_FINAL.pdf]

[46] Davies H, Sacks J. The dignity of difference: How to avoid the clash of Civilisations. Medicine Conflict and Survival. 2003;19(1):72-73.

[47] Last J, editor. A dictionary of public health. 1st ed. Oxford University Press; 2007.

[48] Centers for Disease Control and Prevention. A Practitioner's Guide for Advancing Health Equity: Community Strategies for Preventing Chronic Disease [Internet]. Available from: http://www.cdc.gov/nccdphp/dch/pdf/HealthEquityGuide.pdf.

[49] The Cultural Center. Advancing Diversity & Inclusive Excellence [Internet]. Available from: http://www.du.edu/cme/resources/inclusive-excellence.html;

[50] Rochester Institute of Technology. Framework for Inclusive Excellence [Internet]. Available from: https://www.rit.edu/diversity/inclusive-excellence-framework.

[51] Braveman P. What are health disparities and health equity? We need to be clear. Public Health Reports. 2014;129(Suppl 2):5-8. DOI: 10.1177/00333549141291S203.

[52] CCPH Board of Directors. Position Statement on Authentic Partnerships [Internet]. 2013. Available from: https://www.ccphealth.org/principles-of-partnership/.

[53] HealthyPeople.gov. Social Determinants of Health [Internet]. 2020. Available from: https://www.healthypeople.gov/2020/topics-objectives/topic/social-determinants-of-health]

[54] Schmeer K. Stakeholder Analysis Guidelines [Internet]. Available from: http://www.who.int/workforcealliance/knowledge/toolkit/33.pdf

Chapter 3

Clinical Scholars: Using Program Evaluation to Inform Leadership Development

Gaurav Dave, Cheryl Noble, Caroline Chandler, Giselle Corbie-Smith and Claudia S.P. Fernandez

Abstract

Leadership development programs are notoriously difficult to evaluate, and when evaluations are attempted, they often do not go beyond measuring low-level, short-term outcomes of the impacts experienced by participants. Many leadership development programs do not systematically assess changes that are catalyzed within the organizations, communities and systems in which participants lead. To address these challenges, evaluators of the Clinical Scholars National Leadership Institute (CNLI) have designed a comprehensive, mixed-methods evaluation approach to determine the effectiveness of the training and explore the impacts of participants in the spheres in which they lead. Guided by Michael Patton's Developmental Evaluation approach and framed by Kirkpatrick's Training Evaluation Model, the CSNLI evaluation collects data on multiple levels to provide a robust picture of the multiple outcomes of the program. The approach focuses on individual participant outcomes, by measuring competency changes over time and exploring how participants use the competencies gained through the training in their work. Social network analysis is utilized to measure the development and expansion of participants' networks and collaboration within the teams, cohorts, and across sectors and disciplines throughout their time in the CSNLI. The Most Significant Change methodology and semi-structured alumni interviews are used to measure impacts participants identify as occurring as a result of their participation. Finally, Concept Mapping is implemented to explore how Fellows make meaning of the foundational concepts and values of the CSNLI. The outcome and impact evaluation activities employed by the CSNLI, in combination with quality improvement-focused process evaluation, support innovation and excellence in the provision of a health equity-grounded leadership development program.

Keywords: leadership, process evaluation, outcome evaluation, impact evaluation, mixed method evaluation

1. Introduction

As discussed in depth in "Chapter 1: Clinical Scholars: Effective Approaches to Leadership Development," leadership training has been identified as an essential component in talent development in a wide range of sectors, including health care and public health. In the case of the Clinical Scholars National Leadership Institute (CSNLI), online at ClinicalScholarsNLI.org, more broadly known as Clinical

Scholars (CS) or the Clinical Scholars Program, leadership training is considered a catalyst to address social determinants of health and mitigate disparities (see Chapter 2). The Clinical Scholars Program is funded by the Robert Wood Johnson Foundation (RWJF), as a component of their investment to build a Culture of Health in the United States – by equipping clinical leaders with the necessary skills, commitment, and mindset to tackle some of the most complex health issues of our time, to ensure good health is available to all [1].

A common challenge facing leadership training programs is how to meaningfully measure program outcomes. It is widely accepted that leadership development programs are difficult to evaluate beyond process-type measures. There are a number of reasons why this is so – difficulty finding suitable control groups, lack of evaluation funding, attribution errors, biases introduced by self-report methods, and others [2–5]. In fact, a recent report found that only 24% of organizations utilize some form of impact measurement of their leadership programs, and that the most popular measurement tool is the satisfaction survey [6, 7]. However, there are ways to gather valuable outcome data for multi-level leadership development programs that can be used to provide a well-rounded picture of the longer term outcomes and possible impacts of the training efforts.

In the case of the Clinical Scholars Program, a comprehensive, multi-level evaluation plan is essential. Evaluation aims of a program of this scope include monitoring whether the program is being delivered effectively, determining whether the program's intended outcomes are being reached, determining cost-effectiveness of dollars spent on leadership training, and to ultimately (in the case of RWJF's Culture of Health initiative,) identifying whether good health is becoming more accessible to all people in the US [1].

As with any training program, when measuring leadership development programs that address complex leadership challenges such as health disparities, expanding quality health care services to marginalized populations, and building interdisciplinary teams to address social determinants of health, among others, evaluation plans must be robust and comprehensive, addressing three key types of evaluation:

1. *Process evaluation*, to inform program staff of participants' levels of satisfaction with the training and short-term learning;

2. *Outcome evaluation*, to measure the stickiness of the program and changes in learning and engagement over the course of the training program; and

3. *Impact evaluation*, as a marker of the translation of the program into population-level outcomes and changes that may occur after the training is complete.

This chapter uses the Clinical Scholars Program as a case study of how to design and implement an evaluation of a multi-level leadership development program. In this chapter, we will provide a brief description of the Clinical Scholars Program, describe theoretical underpinnings of our approach, outline the methods we have selected to measure goal achievement, and explore implications of our approach.

1.1 Program description

The Clinical Scholars Program is described in detail in Chapter 1. It is a three-year, multidimensional leadership development program created for mid-career clinicians who practice in a wide-variety of disciplines (e.g. medicine, social work, veterinary medicine, and nursing, among others) that address health across multiple levels across the social ecological model [8, 9]. Funded by the Robert Wood Johnson Foundation (RWJF), the Clinical Scholars Program is part of a broader Foundation-led initiative to build a Culture of Health in the United States to ensure that all people have access to good health [10]. Candidates apply for the program in interdisciplinary teams of 2-5 clinicians and selected teams implement a "Wicked Problem Impact Project" (WPIP) throughout the three-year program. Each team's WPIP is designed to provide an intervention to address a specific, complex health problem in their home community. Participants in the program are referred to as "Fellows".

The Clinical Scholars Program curriculum focuses on four main goals:

1. improving leadership skills
2. developing and strengthening interdisciplinary collaboration,
3. strengthening engagement and partnership with community stakeholders, and
4. expanding skills to make equity, diversity and inclusion (EDI) actionable in their leadership projects and activities

The curriculum addresses learning through multiple modalities, including biannual intensive onsite leadership retreats, robust distance learning activities, team and personal executive coaching, mentoring, and active utilization of leadership skills through the implementation of the Wicked Problem Impact Project. Through the Clinical Scholars Program, participants also develop a nationwide network of clinicians who are working to create a culture of health in communities across the United States.

As described in detail in Chapter 1, the pedagogical focus of the Clinical Scholars Program is to equip clinicians with boundary spanning leadership skills, which add to the discipline-specific skills obtained through formal clinical education programs. The Clinical Scholars Program has identified 25 evidence-based Leadership Competencies that guide curriculum development. The 25 competencies are organized into four practice domains: Personal, Interpersonal, Organizational, and Community and Systems (see **Figure 1**). Because the Clinical Scholars Program places high value on the development of Equity, Diversity, and Inclusion (EDI) as a foundational aspect of building a Culture of Health (Chapter 2), EDI competencies are interwoven throughout all four domains.

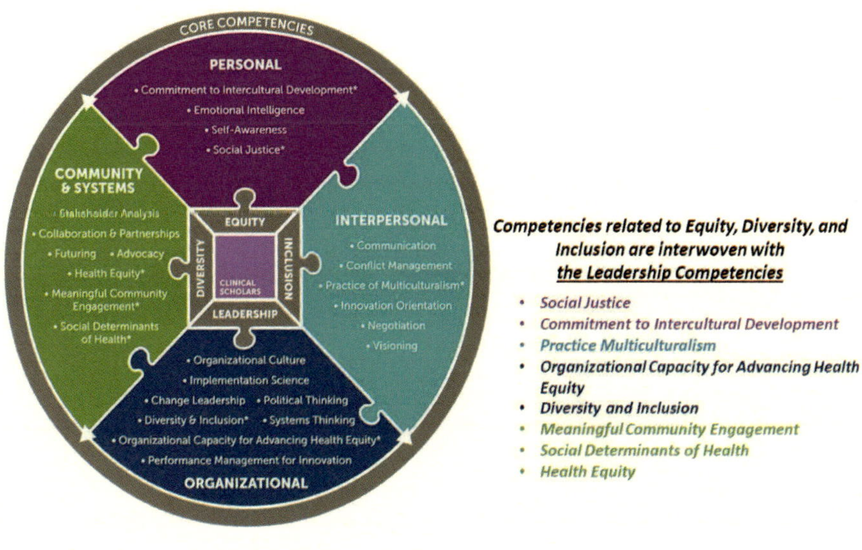
CORE COMPETENCIES
PERSONAL
• Commitment to Intercultural Development*
• Emotional Intelligence
• Self-Awareness
• Social Justice*
COMMUNITY & SYSTEMS
• Stakeholder Analysis
• Collaboration & Partnerships
• Futuring • Advocacy
• Health Equity*
• Meaningful Community Engagement*
• Social Determinants of Health*
INTERPERSONAL
• Communication
• Conflict Management
• Practice of Multiculturalism*
• Innovation Orientation
• Negotiation
• Visioning
ORGANIZATIONAL
• Organizational Culture
• Implementation Science
• Change Leadership • Political Thinking
• Diversity & Inclusion* • Systems Thinking
• Organizational Capacity for Advancing Health Equity*
• Performance Management for Innovation
EQUITY
DIVERSITY
INCLUSION
LEADERSHIP
CLINICAL SCHOLARS
Competencies related to Equity, Diversity, and Inclusion are interwoven with the Leadership Competencies
• Social Justice
• Commitment to Intercultural Development
• Practice Multiculturalism
• Organizational Capacity for Advancing Health Equity
• Diversity and Inclusion
• Meaningful Community Engagement
• Social Determinants of Health
• Health Equity

Figure 1.
The 25 Core competencies of the Clinical Scholars Program.

1.2 Evaluation theoretical approach

The Clinical Scholars Program recognizes that individual participants work in the context of their team environment, community environment, and training environment. These different contexts require us to define and measure multiple potential domains influenced by the Clinical Scholars Program that are based on the social ecological model [8, 9]. Throughout the Clinical Scholars Program curriculum, participants are provided with opportunities to build leadership capacity, apply knowledge, develop networks, and engage with communities with the goal of developing a new cadre of clinical leaders at the individual participant level, social/program level, and community/systems level to improve the culture of health in each participant's home community.

We employ Kirkpatrick's Four Level Training Evaluation model to evaluate the individual, social, and program-level impact of the Clinical Scholars Program [11, 12]. Kirkpatrick's model includes four domains. For the purposes of the Clinical Scholars Program evaluation, we have defined each level as follows:

- Level 1: Reaction – Clinical Scholars participants' rating of their experience of all program components in regard to satisfaction, relevance, and utility.
- Level 2: Learning – participants' self-report of gains in knowledge, self-efficacy, skills, and attitudes as a result of participation in the Clinical Scholars Program.
- Level 3: Behavior – tangible actions participants report taking as a result of the knowledge and skills obtained through participation in the Clinical Scholars Program and
- Level 4: Results – the impacts experienced by participants in their individual leadership, organizations, and communities.

Our evaluation design mirrors the theory and conceptual framework of the Clinical Scholars Program to measure program-attributable change in key areas – competencies, community engagement, networks and other complementary assessments.

Michael Patton's Developmental Evaluation provides the principles for how we approach the evaluation of the Clinical Scholars Program. This approach gives evaluators the role of a long-term partner with those who are delivering innovative initiatives, where evaluative questions are designed to "provide feedback and support developmental decision-making and course corrections along the emergent path [13]." Such partnerships between evaluators and program staff support real-time learning in complex and emergent situations, and are useful for programs such as Clinical Scholars with high levels of innovation, fast-paced decision making and areas of uncertainty. This style represents a more flexible and adaptive style of evaluation than a traditional evaluation. As such, the Clinical Scholars Program's evaluation plans regularly evolve to support emerging program outcomes.

Each of the theories briefly described above guide and provide a foundation for the methods employed to evaluate the multiple components of the Clinical Scholars Program. Our evaluation logic model Appendix A outlines the various short-, intermediate-, and long-term outcomes addressed through our approach.

1.3 Evaluation methods

Data collection is dispersed throughout the three-year Clinical Scholars curriculum, with particular consideration given to the spacing of data collection, in order

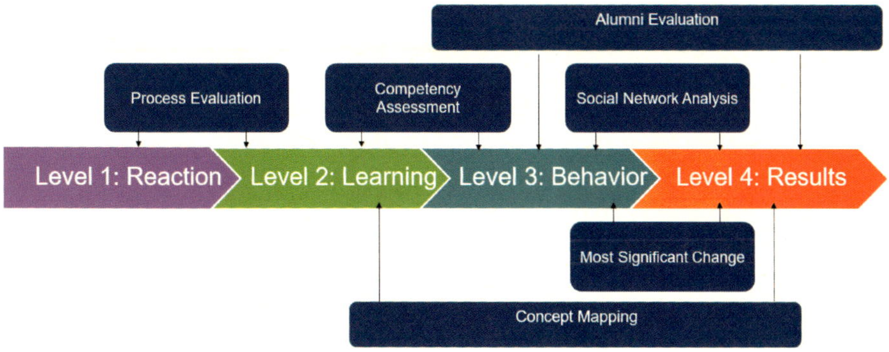

Figure 2.
The evaluation of the clinical scholars program using Kirkpatrick's training evaluation model.

to avoid overwhelming participants with evaluation asks. Our main evaluation activities include:

- Process Evaluation
- Competency Assessment
- Social Network Analysis (SNA)
- Community Stakeholder Assessment
- Concept Mapping
- Most Significant Change (MSC)
- Alumni Evaluation

In order to ensure we address all levels of training evaluation, we have mapped each of our evaluation activities onto the Kirkpatrick Four-Level Training Evaluation Model (**Figure 2**). A large portion of our evaluation efforts are directed at measuring changes in Levels 3 (Behavior) and 4 (Results), in order to provide a deeper understanding into how the Clinical Scholars Program is affecting participants' leadership growth and impact. The following sections describe each of our evaluation activities in detail.

2. Process evaluation

As with any training program, process evaluation is an essential piece in helping programs assess the success of an intervention. Process evaluation helps to enhance the likelihood of success by providing indications of what happened during the program, and if those activities were successful or not for various stakeholders. Process evaluation assists in informing program improvement, increasing participants satisfaction, and understanding the human capital involved in implementing the multiple components of a training program [14]. The two main process areas we focus on in the Clinical Scholars Program are onsite trainings and exit interviews.

2.1 Onsite trainings

Participants attend seven onsite retreats throughout the Clinical Scholars Program. During each retreat, participants are required to attend all learning sessions (Range 9-20 sessions per retreat) designed to teach and engage participants with leadership skills and equity topics (see Chapter 1 for a detailed description of the onsite curriculum). Immediately following each session, participants are asked to complete an 11-item survey that includes two open-ended questions for additional feedback about the session and feedback on the retreat overall. Items on overall session satisfaction, relevance, presenter delivery, presenter knowledge, usefulness of information, and knowledge and ability before and after each session are asked on 7-point Likert scales. We calculate means for all quantitative items and draw common themes from the open-ended feedback for each session. Summary reports for each session support rapid cycle learning by informing retreat debriefing sessions and discussions about aspects of sessions that can be improved for future cohorts.

Two of the items included on the session evaluation survey address learning: knowledge and ability. Knowledge and ability questions are developed using the session specific learning objectives provided by presenters. A retrospective pre/post design is utilized for the knowledge and ability questions. This approach is widely used in training programs, and the literature suggests this approach is often more reliable than the standard pretest, posttest approach and can help decrease response shift bias [15–22]. Knowledge and ability items are analyzed using a paired sample t-test to measure whether the difference between knowledge and ability before and after each session is statistically significant. Additional analyses are conducted to identify additional trends that surface over time, such as impact of topic relevance or speaker ability on changes in knowledge or ability.

2.2 Exit interviews

Exit interviews are utilized to provide an opportunity for participants to reflect on their experience in the Clinical Scholars Program. Six months after completion of the Clinical Scholars Program, interviews are scheduled with the most recently graduated participants. The exit interviews were designed using Moustakas' Phenomenological Research Approach [23, 24]. This approach was chosen for its ability to help the evaluation team understand the phenomenon of participants' shared experiences throughout the Clinical Scholars Program. A detailed protocol was developed by the Evaluation team to guide data collection through semi-structured interviews, data analysis using a grounded theory approach, and dissemination [25].

The semi-structured interviews focus on participants' experiences and reflection in four main areas:

1. Individual leadership changes
2. Organizational leadership changes
3. Community leadership changes
4. Experience since graduating from Clinical Scholars

Themes, examples, and other data obtained through the exit interview process will guide discussions around curriculum needs that may surface, which skills and learning participants may be continuing to use, and how to best connect with program alumni.

3. Outcome evaluation

As discussed above, attribution error is a common concern when evaluating leadership development programs, because the training does not exist in isolation and there is a high likelihood there are additional factors outside of Clinical Scholars impacting participants' actions and behaviors, as well as observed outcomes [11]. We address such challenges by utilizing a multi-level and mixed-method approach, which provides a well-rounded picture of how participants report utilizing the skills learned through the training, what changes participants attribute to the training, and how community partners and stakeholders experience participants' leadership. For the purposes of the Clinical Scholars Program, our outcome evaluation assesses changes and trends that occur during the three-year training program.

3.1 Competency assessment

The competency assessment is designed to measure changes in individual participants' knowledge, attitude, self-efficacy, and use of the 25 Clinical Scholars competencies (see **Figure 1**) over the course of the 3-year program as participants work to implement solutions to wicked problems in their communities. In this survey, we address four measures: knowledge, attitude, self-efficacy, and use [26–32]. Each measure is adapted from previously validated items, and are measured on a 7-point Likert-type scale.

This survey is administered at four time points to model trends in change over time: 0 months, 6 months, 18 months, and 36 months. At the 0- and 6-month time points, items are asked using a retrospective pre/post-test approach, where participants are directed to provide a rating for each item for both 6 months ago and current day. The remaining timepoints, 18 and 36 months, participants are directed to provide only current day ratings for each measure. This data collection timeline provides data for six time points, including 6 months prior to the start of the program, allowing us to compare differences in the magnitude of change before and after the start of the program. After each data collection, reports on the self-efficacy scores for each Participant are provided to individual executive coaches to discuss during coaching meetings. All other data are shared only in the aggregate of each cohort. Data are analyzed with a paired-sample t-test measuring the differences in scores at each time point. Trends in change across time are measured using a generalized linear model.

This longitudinal approach allows us to observe short- and intermediate-term outcomes in competency skill, usage, and self-efficacy - ultimately providing insight into the "stickiness," or sustainability, of the leadership learning and growth experienced by participants during their time in the Clinical Scholars Program.

3.2 Online leadership logs (OLLs)

In order to better understand behavioral changes the Clinical Scholars Program contributes to, participants' submissions to Online Leadership Logs (OLLs) are analyzed. Throughout their three years in the Clinical Scholars Program, participants are asked to describe how they have used each of the 25 Core Competencies in their leadership. This web-based skills inventory self-assesses competence in the Core Competencies of the Clinical Scholars Program utilizing a method known as the Behavioral Event Interview (BEI) [33]. This method provides a means for gathering specific examples of behavior [33]. As part of their personal reflection and development, participants are asked to provide examples of how they are using each of the 25 Core Competencies by submitting "STAR" statements, where they are prompted to describe the Situation, Task, Action, and Results for the event in which they used each specific competency. The OLL gives Clinical Scholars participants practical experience in developing behavioral statements related to performance of the top 25 competencies taught throughout the Clinical Scholars Program curriculum.

As each cohort completes their three-year program, OLLs will be obtained from program staff. Data will be analyzed using a grounded theory approach to identify themes related to how the Core Competencies are operationalized in the real-world settings in which participants exist [25].

3.3 Social network analysis

The networks that participants build within their cohort, across cohorts, and within their home community is an essential component of the Clinical Scholars experience. Collaboration across disciplines and sectors builds social capital in the form of shared knowledge and experience. Social Network Analysis (SNA) is a tool that has been developed over the past century to measure the density and centrality of a component, or individual, to understand how information (or in other settings, behaviors or diseases) are transmitted between individuals [34]. We measure the network that each cohort is building at three time points: 0 months, 24 months, and 48 months. Measuring at these three timepoints, we can track how networks grow and deepen throughout the program. The complexity of the SNA utilized for the Clinical Scholars Program requires specific skills and expertise. As such, we have contracted with an outside agency to conduct the SNA [35].

Our SNA is unbounded, asking about collaboration within each participant's team, the Clinical Scholars cohort, and across the Clinical Scholars Program cohorts, team satisfaction, and social capital in each participant's broader community. Networks are measured by the frequency of interaction, types of activities that participants engage in with identified connections, number of collaborative activities, strength of relationships, and satisfaction with team members. Social capital is measured by asking participants to indicate whether they have helpful contacts with individuals in 14 occupations and, if so, the closeness and length of each relationship. Changes in strength and density of relationships within and across the Clinical Scholars Program cohorts is indicative of network growth.

3.4 Community stakeholder assessment

An essential factor in building equity in a culture of health in a community is the ability to build relationships with community stakeholders [36]. The Community Stakeholder Assessment is intended to explore community engagement between participants and key stakeholders during the Clinical Scholars Program. The Community Stakeholder Assessment seeks to answer six primary questions:

1. To what extent are participants engaging with stakeholders as they implement their Wicked Problem Impact Projects (WPIP)?

2. Is trust being established between participants and stakeholders?

3. To what extent is a sense of collaboration being developed between participants and stakeholders?

4. Are the relationships between participants and stakeholders based on principles of community engagement?

5. Are participants engaging with stakeholders from people whose cultures differ from their own?

6. To what extent do stakeholders agree/disagree with participants' assessment of engagement?

Participants in the Clinical Scholars Program are asked to provide names and contact information for their community stakeholders 12 months and 36 months into the program. Community stakeholders are defined as:

- Anybody outside the Clinical Scholars participant team who is actively contributing to, has contributed, or is integral to their team's WPIP
- A community partner who has been involved in the WPIP above and beyond a phone conversation or meeting to serve in an advisory role or who meaningfully contributes to a tangible component of the planning, development, implementation, dissemination, or marketing of the WPIP (ex. school council member)
- Someone who the Clinical Scholars participant team has partnered with explicitly for the purposes of the WPIP.

A survey is sent to each identified community partner or stakeholder at 12 and 37 months. The instrument asks respondents to use a Likert-type scale to respond to items in the following domains. Each of these domains are derived from validated evaluation measures [37, 38].

1. Collaboration (how collaboration impacts the program and community)
2. Resources (how resources impact the program and community)
3. Bridging (how members of the community and the members of the Clinical Scholars Project Team interact)
4. Alignment with Community Engagement Principles (learning how the WPIP aligns with principles for community-engagement)
5. Trust[1] (trust between team members and the community stakeholders)
6. Health Outcomes (how the WPIP is improving health outcomes in the community)
7. Demographics[1]
8. General Feedback[1]

Measures of community engagement are analyzed to look for trends in the above identified community engagement domains from 12 months to 36 months. Given the evolving nature of WPIPs and often high turnover at small community-based organizations, we cannot expect to survey the same individual community partners at each time point. Rather, by surveying more than one partner from each team and examining trends, we aim to observe any differences in how community engagement principles play out in these relationships.

[1] These domains include items with open-ended or measure specific response options.

3.5 Most significant change

In order to gather data regarding changes experienced and observed by participants as a result of their participation in Clinical Scholars, we utilize the Most Significant Change (MSC) methodology [39, 40]. Additionally, data gathered through the MSC process will serve to illustrate the operationalization of the concepts participants identified in the Concept Mapping project (see below).

MSC is a form of participatory monitoring and evaluation. In short, the approach collects change stories directly from participants, and then goes through a systematic process to select and present the stories that indicate the greatest impact [39]. This approach is best utilized in programs with diverse and emerging outcomes, that contain programmatic elements focused on social change, and that do not have defined outcomes against which to evaluate [39]. Because of the Clinical Scholars Program's unique, multi-level approach to leadership development toward cultural shifts in approaching health, such an approach is appropriate to integrate with our additional evaluative efforts.

MSC includes multiple steps to gather and analyze results. The Clinical Scholars Program evaluation utilizes the following components:

- *Obtaining Most Significant Change stories from participants in Clinical Scholars.* As part of their final program report, Clinical Scholars participants are asked to submit at least one story responding to this prompt: "Please describe in one or two paragraphs the most significant change that has resulted from your involvement with the Clinical Scholars Program. Think about this like telling a story. Please describe the situation, task, actions, results, or other details you can that are related to the change."

  Participants receive detailed instructions on how to answer the question, and are asked to select whether the impact occurred on an individual leadership, organizational, or community level.

- *Selection of MSC stories.* The evaluation team recruits a selection committee of Clinical Scholars Program staff, stakeholders, and participants to engage in a systematic process of selecting the stories that represent the most significant changes at each level (individual, organizational, or community).

- *Analysis.* Multi-level analysis is conducted with the data obtained through the stories. Qualitative analysis uses ATLAS.ti to code and identify themes utilizing a grounded theory approach [41]. In addition, secondary analyses are conducted on the data to identify any additional insights (i.e. differences between disciplines, demographic groups, cohort, etc....)

4. Impact evaluation

RWJF's mission to build a Culture of Health in the United States includes many lofty and important goals to address health equity and ensure good health is available to all [36]. Such goals that create impact in culture and institutions are difficult to evaluate and largely beyond the scope of the Clinical Scholars Program evaluation plan. In addition, as with measuring outcomes, attribution is a large concern [2–5]. To address such challenges, we implement two evaluation activities – Concept Mapping and an Alumni Survey – to obtain data about how the Clinical Scholars

Program trainings may be contributing to eventually achieving a Culture of Health, and how participants continue to report activities and changes they are engaged in across multiple levels of the Social Ecological Model [8, 9].

4.1 Concept mapping

In order to determine participants' conceptual understanding of what it means to build a Culture of Health, we conduct a Concept Mapping project during the third training year of each cohort. Concept Mapping is "a structured process, focused on a topic or construct of interest, involving input from one or more participants, that produces an interpretable pictorial view (concept map) of their ideas and concepts and how these are interrelated [42]." For the purposes of the Clinical Scholars Program, the results from the concept mapping process illustrate participants' perceptions of various concepts represented in the Culture of Health (COH) Action Framework [41]. Understanding participants' perceptions of building health can give us insight into what they value and are committed to in their work. Because building a Culture of Health is ultimately about creating cultural shifts in how people perceive health, values and commitment are important factors to explore [36].

During each cohort's third year, we initiate the concept mapping project. The concept mapping process consists of six specific steps. More detailed descriptions of Concept Mapping methodology is widely available. What follows is the Clinical Scholars Program's specific implementation of this methodology:

1. Preparation – Evaluation staff and partners determine the main aims of the project and develop a protocol and timeline.

2. Generation - Participants are asked to complete an online brainstorming activity where they provide as many statements as come to mind to complete a specific focal prompt. Each cohort focuses on a different topic. For example, Cohort 1 focused on components that are essential to building a Culture of Health. Cohort 2 focused on a specific topic within the COH Action Area ("Making Health a Shared Value") [43].

3. Structuring – Participants are asked to complete two additional online activities: sorting and rating. For the sorting activity they will be asked to sort the statements into groupings that make sense to them, based on similar meanings or themes. They are then asked to name each of the groups. For the rating activity, participants rate each statement on each of three Likert-type scales that are developed based on each year's topic.

4. Representation – Multi-level analysis is then conducted with the sorting and rating activity data using statistical software [44]. These analyses generate a cluster map to visually communicate the relationships between the statements provided.

5. Interpretation – At an onsite retreat during each cohort's third year, an in-person group discussion develops an understanding of the meaning of the cluster maps. During this discussion, the group comes to consensus on names for each of the clusters on the map and provides insight into how these clusters relate to and impact various aspects of participants' experience in building a Culture of Health.

6. Utilization –The findings from this project will contribute to increasing the understanding of how participants' perceptions relate to the overall conceptualization of building a Culture of Health. Findings will not only be used to identify possible perceptual outcomes of the Clinical Scholars curriculum, but will also be used to inform the Clinical Scholars Program of any potential program improvements that may be needed to better align with the COH Action Framework.

4.2 Alumni evaluation

Our Alumni Evaluation is evolving over time and is developing in partnership with other programs funded by RWJF as part of their Leadership for Better Health initiative [45]. At the time of writing, the Clinical Scholars Program had just graduated its first cohort, and we are in data gathering stages of the internal and Initiative-wide alumni evaluation. In addition, we plan to work with RWJF partners to develop methods to obtain and analyze long-term impacts related to expansion of a Culture of Health and improved health outcomes. Specific to the Clinical Scholars Program, we plan to continue monitoring the following topics in order to understand participants' future activities and influence:

- Individual leadership practice and growth;
- Network development and expansion;
- Leadership within organizations; and
- Leadership within home communities.

5. Conclusion

It is our ultimate aim that the results of each of the evaluation approaches listed in this chapter be used for two purposes: 1) to inform and improve the implementation of the Clinical Scholars Program and 2) to better understand how leadership development training can best equip health practitioners to build a Culture of Health – to expand health equity and ensure that good health is available to all. Results are disseminated to all stakeholders, including Clinical Scholars program staff, RWJF staff and the participants of Clinical Scholars themselves. It is our hope that our findings will also be of benefit to the broader field of leader and leadership development and, as such, we will focus on disseminating these results via a variety of methods, including academic publication, professional conferences, media outlets, and widely available web-based platforms, among others.

In addition, it is our goal to learn as the program and evaluation unfolds. Owing to the novel nature of RWJF's mission to build a Culture of Health, the Clinical Scholars Program's innovative approach to combining leadership and equity, diversity, and inclusion training, and our developmental evaluation approach, we anticipate changes and modifications to occur. Part of our internal evaluation is to document the rationale behind such changes and continue to refine our approach in order to ensure the best, and ultimately, most useful data is available to assist the Clinical Scholars Program to reach its goal of equipping clinicians to influence their communities in order to build a Culture of Health.

Appendix A: clinical scholars program logic model

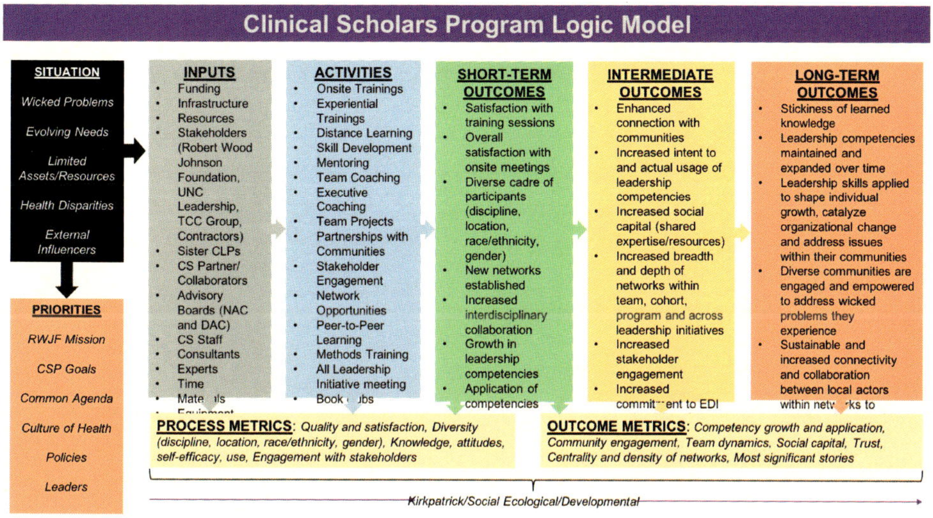

Author details

Gaurav Dave[1], Cheryl Noble[2]*, Caroline Chandler[3]†, Giselle Corbie-Smith[1] and Claudia S.P. Fernandez[3]

1 University of North Carolina at Chapel Hill School of Medicine, North Carolina, United States

2 Independent Evaluation Consultant, California, United States

3 Gillings School of Global Public Health, University of North Carolina at Chapel Hill, North Carolina, United States

*Address all correspondence to: cnobleconsulting@gmail.com

† Ms. Chandler was supported in part by a training grant from the National Institute of Child Health and Development (T32 HD007376).

References

[1] Robert Wood Johnson Foundation. About a Culture of Health [Internet]. 2020. Available from: https://www.rwjf.org/en/cultureofhealth/about.html

[2] Dvir T, Eden D, Avolio BJ, Shamir B. Impact of transformational leadership on follower development and performance: A field experiment. *Acad Manag J*. 2002;45(4):735-744. doi:10.2307/3069307

[3] Malling B, Mortensen L, Bonderup T, Scherpbier A, Ringsted C. Combining a leadership course and multi-source feedback has no effect on leadership skills of leaders in postgraduate medical education. An intervention study with a control group. *BMC Med Educ*. 2009 ;9(1):1-7. doi:10.1186/1472-6920-9-72

[4] Frese M, Beimel S, Schoenborn S. Action Training for Charismatic Leadership: Two Evaluations of Studies of a Commercial Training Module on Inspirational Communication of a Vision. *Pers Psychol*. 2006;56(3):671-698. doi:10.1111/j.1744-6570.2003.tb00754.x

[5] Packard T, Jones L. An outcomes evaluation of a leadership development initiative. *J Manag Dev*. 2015;34(2):153-168. doi:10.1108/JMD-05-2013-0063

[6] Measuring The Impact Of Leadership Development: Getting Back To Basics - Harvard Business Publishing. https://www.harvardbusiness.org/measuring-the-impact-of-leadership-development-getting-back-to-basics/. Accessed March 8, 2020.

[7] The State of Leadership Development Report - Harvard Business Publishing. https://www.harvardbusiness.org/insight/the-state-of-leadership-development-report/. Accessed March 8, 2020.

[8] Social Ecological Model. In: *Encyclopedia of Behavioral Medicine*. ; 2013. doi:10.1007/978-1-4419-1005-9_101634

[9] Mcleroy KR, Bibeau D, Steckler A, Glanz K. An Ecological Perspective on Health Promotion Programs. *Heal Educ Behav*. 1988. doi:10.1177/109019818801500401

[10] Robert Wood Johnson Foundation. What Drives Health. http://www.commissiononhealth.org/WhatDrivesHealth.aspx. Published 2016. Accessed September 24, 2018.

[11] Kirkpatrick DL, Kirkpatrick JD. *Evaluating Training Programs*. 3rd ed. San Francisco: Berrett-Koehler Publishers; 2006. https://www.bkconnection.com/static/Evaluating_Training_Programs_EXCERPT.pdf.

[12] Kirkpatrick DL, Kirkpatrick JD. *Implementing the Four Levels: A Practical Guide for Effective Evaluation of Training Programs*. San Francisco: Berrett-Koehler Publishers; 2007. https://www.bkconnection.com/static/Implementing-the-Four-Levels-EXCERPT.pdf.

[13] Patton MQ. *Developmental Evaluation: Applying Complexity Concepts to Enhance Innovation and Use*.; 2011.

[14] Curnan S, LaCava L, Sharpsteen D, Lelle M, Reece M. W.K. Kellogg Foundation evaluation handbook. *Evaluation*. 1998. doi:10.1007/s13398-014-0173-7.2

[15] Fernandez CSP, Noble CC, Jensen E, Steffen D. Moving the Needle: A Retrospective Pre- and Post-analysis of Improving Perceived Abilities Across 20 Leadership Skills. *Matern Child Health J*. 2014. doi:10.1007/s10995-014-1573-1

[16] Lam TCM, Bengo P. A comparison of three retrospective self-reporting methods of measuring change in instructional practice. *Am J Eval*. 2003. doi:10.1016/S1098-2140(02)00273-4

[17] Pratt CC, Mcguigan WM, Katzev AR. Measuring program outcomes: Using

retrospective pretest methodology. *Am J Eval*. 2000. doi:10.1177/109821400002100305

[18] Rockwell SK, Kohn H. Post-Then-Pre Evaluation. *J Ext*. 1989.

[19] Rohs FR. Response Shift Bias: A Problem In Evaluating Leadership Development With Self-Report Pretest-Posttest Measures. *J Agric Educ*. 1999. doi:10.5032/jae.1999.04028

[20] Saleh SS, Williams D, Balougan M. Evaluating the effectiveness of public health leadership training: The NEPHLI experience. *Am J Public Health*. 2004. doi:10.2105/AJPH.94.7.1245

[21] Sprangers M, Hoogstraten J. Pretesting Effects in Retrospective Pretest-Posttest Designs. *J Appl Psychol*. 1989. doi:10.1037/0021-9010.74.2.265

[22] Fernandez CSP, Noble CC, Jensen ET, Chapin J. Improving Leadership Skills in Physicians: A 6-Month Retrospective Study. *J Leadersh Stud*. 2016. doi:10.1002/jls.21420

[23] Moustakas C. *Phenomenological Research Methods*.; 2011. doi:10.4135/9781412995658

[24] Creswell JW. *Qualitative Inquiry and Research Design*.; 2013.

[25] Strauss A, Corbin JM. *Grounded Theory in Practice*. SAGE Publications; 1997.

[26] Schnall R, Stone P, Currie L, Desjardins K, John RM, Bakken S. Development of a self-report instrument to measure patient safety attitudes, skills, and knowledge. *J Nurs Scholarsh*. 2008. doi:10.1111/j.1547-5069.2008.00256.x

[27] University of Oregon. Discussion of 7-point Expertise Scale [Internet]. Available from: http://pages.uoregon.edu/moursund/ICT-planning/discussion_of_7-point.htm

[28] Vagias W. Likert-type scale response anchors. *Clemson Int Inst Tour ....* 2006. doi:10.1525/auk.2008.125.1.225

[29] Bandura A. Guide for constructing self-efficacy scales. *Self-efficacy beliefs Adolesc*. 2006. doi:10.1017/CBO9781107415324.004

[30] Mencl J, Tay L, Schwoerer CE, Drasgow F. Evaluating Quantitative and Qualitative Types of Change: An Analysis of the Malleability of General and Specific Self-Efficacy Constructs and Measures. *J Leadersh Organ Stud*. 2012. doi:10.1177/1548051812442968

[31] Schwoerer CE, May DR, Hollensbe EC, Mencl J. General and specific self-efficacy in the context of a training intervention to enhance performance expectancy. *Hum Resour Dev Q*. 2005. doi:10.1002/hrdq.1126

[32] Russo D. Competency Measurement Model. In: *European Conference on Quality in Official Statistics*. ; 2016.

[33] McClelland DC. Identifying Behavioral-Event Interviews. *Psychol Sci*. 1998;9(5):331-339.

[34] Valente TW, Palinkas LA, Czaja S, Chu KH, Hendricks Brown C. Social network analysis for program implementation. *PLoS One*. 2015;10(6):1-18. doi:10.1371/journal.pone.0131712

[35] Duke Network Analysis Center. About: The Duke Network Analysis Center [Internet]. Available from: https://dnac.ssri.duke.edu/about.php.

[36] Robert Wood Johnson Foundation. Taking Action [Internet]. 2020. Available from: https://www.rwjf.org/en/cultureofhealth/taking-action.html

[37] Oetzel JG, Zhou C, Duran B, et al. Establishing the psychometric properties of constructs in a community-based participatory research conceptual model. *Am J Heal Promot*. 2015. doi:10.4278/ajhp.130731-QUAN-398

[38] Arora PG, Krumholz LS, Guerra T, Leff SS. Measuring community-based participatory research partnerships: The initial development of an assessment instrument. *Prog Community Heal Partnerships Res Educ Action*. 2015. doi:10.1353/cpr.2015.0077

[39] Davies R, Davies R, Dart J, Dart J. *The 'Most Significant Change' (MSC) Technique, a Guide to Its Use.*; 2005. doi:10.1104/pp.110.159269

[40] Choy S, Lidstone J. Evaluating leadership development using the Most Significant Change technique. *Stud Educ Eval*. 2013. doi:10.1016/j.stueduc.2013.09.001

[41] Strauss A, Corbin J. *Basics of Qualitative Research: Grounded Theory Procedures and Techniques (2nd Ed).*; 1998. doi:10.4135/9781452230153

[42] Trochim WMK. An introduction to concept mapping for planning and evaluation. *Eval Program Plann*. 1989. doi:10.1016/0149-7189(89)90016-5

[43] Robert Wood Johnson Foundation. Making Health a Shared Value [Internet]. 2020. Available from: https://www.rwjf.org/en/cultureofhealth/taking-action/making-health-a-shared-value.html

[44] The Concept System® groupwisdom™. Build 2019.24.01. Web-based Platform. Concept Systems, Incorporated, 2019. Browser based statistical platform, Available from: https://www.groupwisdom.tech.

[45] Robert Wood Johnson Foundation. Leadership for Better Health [Internet]. 2020. Available from: https://www.rwjf.org/en/our-focus-areas/focus-areas/health-leadership.html

Chapter 4

Culture of Health Leaders: Building a Diverse Network to Advance Health Equity

Natalie S. Burke, Gail C. Christopher, Tara S. Hacker, Jeffrey Moy and Andrea Williams

Abstract

The Culture of Health Leaders Program takes a holistic approach to leadership development, having participants work through a three-year process centered around four Areas of Mastery (self, relationships, environment, and change). Applying an equity lens to their leadership style and systems-level change work, a focus on the inner world, and network activation are some of the unique approaches the program uses that have resulted in advancing equitable leadership and a culture of health around the country. Use of rapid cycle learning and participant-led activities has allowed program staff to build upon lessons learned and adapt to participant needs in order to evolve the programming and participant experience since its inception in 2016.

Keywords: Leadership development, Culture of Health, health equity, rapid cycle learning, equitable leadership, inner world, systems change, perspective transformation, peer-to-peer learning, networks

1. Introduction

The Culture of Health Leaders Program is funded by the Robert Wood Johnson Foundation and is offered through a collaboration of the National Collaborative for Health Equity (https://www.nationalcollaborative.org/) and CommonHealth Action (https://commonhealthaction.org/). The Center for Creative Leadership (https://www.ccl.org) is a key partner and provides leadership development content, faculty expertise, and coaching to program participants and staff. This program is designed to engage and support a strong and diverse network of leaders as they build a culture of health and health equity within communities. The program attracts visionary individuals who are sparking changes in their communities, organizations, and sectors to overcome injustice and promote opportunity, allowing everyone access to what they need to thrive. Leaders in the program develop deep relationships with other diverse thinkers and doers, knowing that meaningful change cannot be achieved alone. During the course of the program, leaders undertake a personal and professional journey that broadens their perspectives and approaches, increasing their ability to solve complex health challenges in their communities.

2. Program design & theory of change

Participants of the Culture of Health Leaders (COHL) program work through a three-year process that results in their ability to produce mastery of self, relationships, environment, and change. As depicted in **Figure 1** below, the COHL program model moves beyond the traditional leadership development focus of behavioral adaptation and competencies. Based on the Beyond Competencies Model [1], the COHL program is designed to also address three elements of the inner world – circuitry, conscious engagement, and inner content. With this additional element, the program takes a more holistic approach to leadership by allowing participants to explore how the inner world influences and is influenced by their behaviors and lived experiences. It is through the interplay of the Areas of Mastery ("Nexus of Mastery"), that participants will make decisions, demonstrate behaviors, and take actions that lead to building a culture of health. By applying our approach to equity, diversity, and inclusion (EDI), program participants will apply an equity lens to the development and implementation of policies, programs, and practices that create and support the Culture of Health Action Areas (Shared Value, Cross-Sector Collaboration, Healthier Communities, and Integrated Systems), leading to improved outcomes for population health, wellbeing, and equity.

Self-knowledge is an important element of effective leadership. To increase self-knowledge, leaders participate in an assessment process through multiple forms of feedback in a safe, confidential environment. Throughout the program, participants engage in 360 degree and self-assessments, individual reflection, and peer feedback to better understand their own approaches to leadership, communication, working in diverse teams or partnerships, cultivating, and maintaining relationships, and navigating conflict and change. The 360 assessment was designed specifically for the COHL program and is taken at the beginning, middle, and end of the program to identify individual and cohort-level changes. The COHL 360 assessment provides insights on strengths and gaps in leadership competencies for participants to understand and explore with their executive coaches. The program's sixteen leadership competencies are defined below in **Table 1**.

Throughout the program, coaches partner with Leaders in a thought-provoking, dynamic, and supportive process. The 360 and other assessment results serve as a bridge for participants to better understand their own preferences and leadership style alongside their personal coaches who offer them continuous feedback and space for reflection. Leaders reflect on areas of growth they have identified as

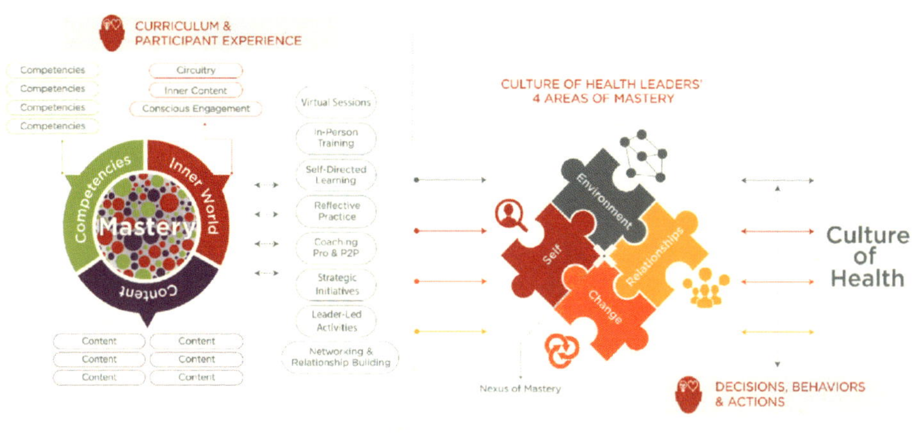

Figure 1.
Culture of Health Leaders Program Model & Theory of change.

Mastery of Self	Mastery of Relationships	Mastery of Environment	Mastery of Change
Self-management; self-insight, self-development Compensates for own weaknesses, capitalizes on own strengths; learns from own experiences and makes needed adjustments in own behavior; takes care of self and is aware of his/her feelings.	**Building Collaborative Relationships** Builds productive working relationships with co-workers and external parties.	**Acts Systemically** Understands the political nature of the organization and works appropriately within it; effectively establishes collaborative relationships and alliances throughout the organization.	**Influencing, Leadership, Power** Good at inspiring and promoting a vision; able to persuade and motivate others; skilled at influencing superiors; delegates effectively.
Handles Disequilibrium Can put stressful experiences into perspective and can handle mistakes, stress, and ambiguity with poise.	**Values Diversity** Avoids prejudging or making assumptions when dealing with others who differ by gender, race, or culture.	**Getting Information, Making Sense of It; Problem Identification** Seeks information and can create order out of large quantities of information. Gets to the heart of the problem.	**Change Management** Uses effective strategies to facilitate organizational change initiatives and overcome resistance to change.
Learns Through Others Values other people's perspectives and input and recognizes limits of own point of view.	**Brings out the Best in People** Has a special talent with people that is evident in his/her ability to pull people together into highly effective teams.	**Sound Judgment** Makes timely decisions; readily understands complex issues; develops solutions that effectively address problems.	**Communicates Effectively** Communicates organization goals and is able to inspire through presentation of information.
Interpersonal Savvy Understands own impact on situations & people; accurately senses when to give and take when negotiating.	**Managing Conflict Negotiation** Negotiates adeptly with individuals and groups; effective at managing conflict and confrontations skillfully.	**Demonstrates Vision** Understands, communicates, and stays focused on the organization's vision.	**Risk-Taking; Innovation** Visionary; seizes new opportunities and consistently generates new ideas; introduces and creates needed change even in the face of opposition.

Table 1.
COHL competencies to develop equitable leadership Behaviors.

critical to effectively leading in their context. Coaches provide an ongoing, supportive relationship designed to help Leaders produce fulfilling results in their personal and professional lives. In addition to the individual coaching relationship, each participant works with two or three other participants in a peer coaching team to support each Leader's development, provide a practice field to explore new leadership behaviors, and provide feedback in a supportive environment. Through this process Leaders develop the critical skill of coaching, one of the most effective tools available to take leadership development to a deeper and more sustainable level.

3. Program curriculum

In addition to a robust learning process through assessments and coaching, the program offers several courses, trainings, and other opportunities for participants to study, discuss, practice and apply content related to change leadership, communications, equitable leadership, health equity, policy, systems change, and social determinants of health. Throughout the program, leaders develop a foundation in equity, diversity, and inclusion (EDI) as a guiding principle in their work to build a culture of health.

Designed for both self-paced and cohort learning, courses are primarily delivered online with a few select trainings or course modules delivered in-person to maximize group learning, interaction, and participation. Included in the program's design are opportunities for current participants and alumni to lead the development and delivery of learning content, peer coaching, and group engagements (e.g., roundtable discussions, topic-based or skill-building workshops, community conversations, networking and relationship-building activities or events, book clubs, affinity groups, etc.) Based on participant feedback and interest over the years, the program has evolved to allow more space for leaders to create personalized learning paths that help shape the development of their program experience as well as the trajectory of their leadership journey.

4. Strategic initiatives

Participants in the Culture of Health Leaders program develop and implement a strategic initiative in their final two years of the program that is expected to produce measurable improvements in leaders' communities. **Strategic initiatives** are designed to catalyze long-lasting, sustainable change that foster a culture of health *and*, importantly, serve as a space for practice and application of what participants are learning through the program. The work done in the program convenings and virtual courses is critical to developing the Leaders, but it's not enough. Seminal research studying how leaders learn, grow, and change revealed an approach for leveraging the power of experiences for leader development [2]. To be truly effective, classroom learning must be directly connected and extended to the leader's context for practical application. Through the strategic initiatives, participants work to deeply understand a real problem, take wise actions, and reflect on and apply what they have learned: integrating knowledge, practicing skills, collaborating with one another, enacting equitable leadership, and using tools and resources from the COHL Program. Building upon their knowledge and skills, leaders support shifts in policies, programs, practices, and environments to advance health equity. Calling upon their networks, they use practices that foster perspective transformation[1] among individuals, communities, organizations, sectors, and societies to bring about change. Leaders work to mobilize stakeholders, increase collaboration between silos, and redistribute power and resources to address systemic inequities.

In their first year, National Program Center staff begin working with each new cohort to establish a shared vision and definition for a culture of health to help ground their work in the collective. Participants also engage in various activities and guided exercises to help them craft their own vision for the change they hope to create. From there they move into an exploration and planning stage to better understand the needs of their community/organization/sector along with the historical context and issues or experiences pertaining to equity. Throughout the development

[1] **Perspective Transformation** is the process of becoming critically aware of how and why our assumptions have come to constrain the way we perceive, understand, and feel about our world; changing these structures of habitual expectation to make possible a more inclusive, discriminating, and integrating perspective; and, finally, making choices or otherwise acting upon these new understandings. Source: Mezirow [3].

of their grant proposals in year two, Leaders are provided technical assistance; guidance, support, and follow-up from program staff; opportunities for mentorship from fellow participants and alumni; and coaching support. The program also began providing access to a shared pool of funding to support community engagement activities starting with Cohort 2 based on feedback from participants and recognition that engagement of community members is critical for the planning and development process and that their time, expertise, and input adds value and should be compensated. Program staff review each strategic initiative grant proposal using an equity lens and provide one-on-one feedback to expand perspectives and/or identify potential connections in the field and from within the program. Our team of reviewers serve as a connector of people and resources throughout the proposal development and implementation processes.

During the implementation phase, each participant receives a $35,000 grant to launch their initiative. Throughout this phase, they receive guided practice, feedback, and thought partnership from program staff, their peers and coaches, and a panel of sustainability experts and technical assistance providers. Given our focus on sustainability, the program provides resources and space for participants to generate additional sources of funding or revenues in support of continuing this work even after they become alumni. Leaders submit regular progress updates to program staff including those specific to their monitoring and evaluation plans. Given the diversity of our participants in terms of their initiative focus, fields/disciplines, experiences and leadership levels, the progress updates keep staff informed and more readily attuned to meet their individual needs. Toward the end of their last year in the program, they are provided with additional communications coaching and video recording and editing support for them to share their COHL work and leadership journey with wider audiences. Many of our leaders go on to conduct media interviews and write publications about this work and its impact.

5. Network-building & activation

Another important element of the program's design is our focus on relationship building among and across cohorts, as well as interactions with alumni and other RWJF Leadership for Better Health (LBH) programs, to develop lasting connections and relationships that are mutually supportive of their leadership and that serve to deepen and strengthen their networks as a collective. This is achieved through the use of diverse networking groups and peer coaching groups; collaboration and support on strategic initiatives during proposal development and implementation (both within and across cohorts); funding for Leaders to contract with alumni and other program participants to provide technical assistance on their strategic initiatives; funding dedicated to bringing in alumni as subject matter experts who design and deliver various content and facilitated sessions with active cohorts; as well as space, logistical support, and limited funding for participants to design their own relationship-building initiatives and activities.

Some examples of network activation from our first cohort of Leaders include the creation of a COHL Alumni nonprofit group working to elevate and support the alumni network; formation of a consulting group, Vertical Strategies (https://www.verticalstrategies.net/), that is dedicated to providing services to elevate nonprofits so they can achieve a culture of health in their respective communities; and the launch of Shift Health Accelerator (http://shifthealthaccelerator.org/) whose mission is to simplify access to money and expertise for peer leaders in communities to increase equity in health outcomes. All of these initiatives include members from multiple cohorts and grow each year as they identify various skills, expertise, and experiences presented among new COHL cohorts. Our second cohort of Leaders self-organized regional community tours and cohort retreats in conjunction with our in-person convenings. They also found opportunities to enter each other's communities via their strategic initiative work to provide on-the ground technical assistance and learning with their fellow cohort members. Cohorts three and four spearheaded the creation of affinity groups and learning circles that are topic- or social identity-based as a means for supporting, learning, and amplifying their participation in the program and their work to advance a culture of health. In response to the Coronavirus pandemic, participants from all of the cohorts came together in 2020 and led the creation of the COHL COVID-19 Task Force – this group of Leaders went on to launch the Coronavirus Support Network (https://coronavirusnetwork.org/) and Project Finish Line (https://covidfinishline.com/), both of which provide communities and leaders with information, resources, tools, and strategies for addressing health inequities exacerbated by the pandemic and in support of vaccine distribution.

Each year we have seen our participants collaborate, ideate, innovate, and shape their individual and collective experience in the program. The National Program Center actively collects participant feedback through multiple methods (e.g., annual participant experience surveys, post-event surveys, focus groups, in-depth interviews, alumni surveys, end of program surveys, one-on-one and cohort-wide feedback sessions, etc.) and applies rapid cycle learning to evolve our program throughout the year(s). Cross-cohort relationship building has been identified as a significant desire among participants, especially as the program grew with each additional cohort. In the Spring of 2021, we will be testing and launching a new online community platform that will serve as the central hub for program participants and alumni to better connect and share resources and continue expanding and deepening their relationships with one another. We have also brought on Community Managers and Mentors who will focus on activating virtual engagement and network building within and across cohorts, train alumni to serve in this role in future years and maintain this focus on remote relationship-building even as we return to in-person convenings. We believe this will further amplify engagement and collaboration and help strengthen and grow their networks.

6. Program goals: Breakdown by year

As outlined in the program snapshot below, each program year builds upon the content, learning, and experience from the year prior. The focus shifts each year to achieve all four areas of mastery by the end of their three-year experience (**Figure 2**).

The goal of the Culture of Health Leaders Program is that by the end of Year 1, successful leaders will have made progress toward achieving mastery in the four areas of mastery of self, relationships, environment, and change in the following ways:

- Gained a heightened self-awareness and understanding of the relationship between self-knowledge and successful leadership to develop their mastery of self.

- Developed an individual leadership development plan.

- Initiated and developed mutually supportive relationships with other Culture of Health Leaders to support cohort cohesion.

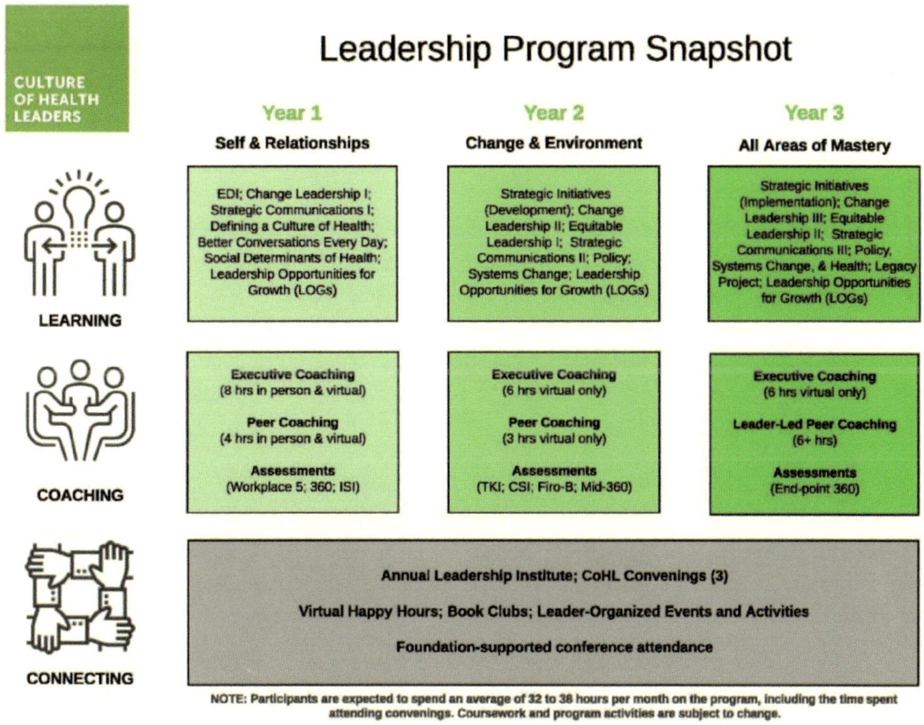

Figure 2.
Note: Based on an annual review of learning and participant feedback, the National Program Center made changes to content, curriculum, and programming each year. The snapshot above was pulled from the September 2019 – August 2020 program year. Significant efforts were made beginning in April 2020 to reduce the overall level of effort to an average of 10–12 hours required per month (down from 32 to 38 hours per month in prior years).

- Developed skills as a peer coach.
- Developed an understanding of the production of health and the factors that drive it to support their mastery of environment.
- Identified the factors within their community, sector, or industry that support or hinder building a culture of health.

By the end of Year 2[2], successful leaders will have made progress toward achieving mastery in the four areas of mastery of self, relationships, environment, and change in the following ways:

- Expanded and deepened relationships across the COHL ecosystem to support participants in the planning, design, and implementation of their Strategic Initiative and Culture of Health work.
- Built or strengthened teams in their home communities, organizations, and/or sectors on which they will be focusing their Culture of Health efforts.

[2] In response to the Coronavirus Pandemic that struck in early 2020, the National Program Center made several changes to the program as a means for reducing overall level of effort, allowing for more flexibility and personalization of coursework, and moving up the timeline for strategic initiative funding and implementation. We also moved the program completely virtual starting in March 2020 to present day (March 2021). It is not yet clear when we will return to hosting in-person convenings.

- Deepened understanding of changing systems and institutions and developed a plan to assess the environments and power structures in building a culture of health in their communities, organizations, and sectors.

- Completed targeted work on Individual Leadership Development Plans (ILDPs) based on Year 1 assessment results and feedback/coaching.

By the end of Year 3, successful leaders will have made progress toward achieving mastery in these four areas of mastery of self, relationships, environment, and change in the following ways:

- Expanded and deepened relationships across the COHL ecosystem to support participants in the ongoing implementation of their Strategic Initiative and Culture of Health work.

- Applied learning from the Program and other Leaders to advance equity in an organization, community, institution, or system.

- Practiced and enhanced their approaches to cultivate, broker, and manage relationships with, between, and among people who can help advance equity.

- Practiced and enhanced their ability and approaches to recognize and manage elements, conditions, and factors within the environment by taking action and/or engaging others appropriately; anticipate windows of opportunity opening and closing; and being in tune with social, political, and cultural landscapes while navigating them effectively.

- Developed heightened self-awareness regarding the inner world and how to leverage it for successful leadership in terms of decisions, behaviors, and actions.

7. Program evaluation strategy

The Culture of Health Leaders National Program Center applies rapid cycle learning by actively collecting quantitative and qualitative data from participants through methods such as surveys and interviews. These evaluation methods are utilized on a regular basis in conjunction with events (in-person or virtual convenings), coursework (completion of a training or course), at the end of each program year, as well as on an as-needed basis, such as recent interviews to inform a virtual engagement strategy. As previously described, these results have helped inform program adjustments to ensure leaders are receiving an experience in keeping with the program model and theory of change previously described. Assessments related to the 16 competencies the program aims to develop provide measurements of participants' progress throughout the program. Additional support from RWJF informs evaluation related to the network aspects of this and the other LBH programs.

8. Conclusion

Five years and nearly 200 leaders later the Culture of Health Leaders Program continues to grow, support, and expand its outreach to leaders from business and tech professionals to artists and community organizers - who have the drive and passion to collaborate in building thriving communities. Early findings from our first two cohorts indicate that over the course of their three years in the program, participants were successful in advancing their equitable leadership behaviors -- growing their effectiveness as individuals and as a collective in their leadership journey. Their innovation helps build a Culture of Health, one in which everyone in America has a fair and just opportunity to achieve the best possible health and wellbeing.

Chapters 10 and 15 have been contributed by members of the first Cohort of the Culture of Health Leaders program and exemplify the typical kinds of leadership projects typical of the program Leaders. In Chapter 10, Dr. Kent Key shares his work in the Flint Youth Public Health Academy, through which he is collaboratively addressing the under-representation of African American researchers in public health. In Chapter 15, Dr. Laurel Berman shares her work in the field of environmental sciences, where toxic sites are transformed back into places that can support a culture of health.

Author details

Natalie S. Burke[1], Gail C. Christopher[2]*, Tara S. Hacker[1], Jeffrey Moy[2] and Andrea Williams[3]

1 CommonHealth ACTION, Washington, D.C., USA

2 National Collaborative for Health Equity, Washington, D.C., USA

3 Center for Creative Leadership, North Carolina, USA

*Address all correspondence to: gchristopher@nationalcollaborative.org

References

[1] Ruderman, M.N., Clerkin, C., Connolly, C. (2014) "Leadership Development Beyond Competencies: Moving to a More Holistic Approach." Center for Creative Leadership. https://www.ccl.org/articles/white-papers/leadership-development-beyond-competencies-moving-to-a-holistic-approach/.

[2] McCall, M. W., Lombardo, M. M., & Morrison, A. M. (1988). The lessons of experience: How successful executives develop on the job. Lexington, Mass: Lexington Books

[3] Mezirow, J. (1978). Perspective Transformation. Adult Education Quarterly, 28(2), 100-110. doi: 10.1177/074171367802800202.

Chapter 5

From Margins to Mainstream: Creating a Rural-Based Center of Excellence in Transgender Health for Upstate, New York

Carolyn Wolf-Gould

Abstract

Transgender people face many barriers to healthcare, especially in rural America. The work to decrease barriers to care and address health care disparities for this population meets criteria for a *wicked problem,* each of which is unique and has no clear solution. The barriers are related to the individual and society and are both formal and informal. The definition for a Center of Excellence in healthcare is loose, but these organizations aspire to serve as specialized programs that offer comprehensive, interdisciplinary expertise and resources within a medical field to improve patient outcomes. With funding and leadership training from the Robert Wood Johnson Clinical Scholars program, a group of medical and mental health clinicians worked for three years with the goal of creating a Rural-Based Center of Excellence in Transgender Health embedded within a family practice to approach the wicked problem of transgender healthcare in their region. The goals of the center were six pronged: the provision of competent and affirming medical, surgical and mental health services, training for healthcare professional students, medical-legal advocacy and patient-centered research. The team created a strategic plan, with five strategic directions, including 1) developing infrastructure and organizational capacity, 2) expanding awareness, knowledge and skills, 3) fulfilling staffing needs, 4) ensuring gender-affirming care, and 5) advancing evidence-based care. I describe our work to bring transgender health from the margins to the mainstream for our region through implementation of this strategic plan.

Keywords: Transgender Health, Center of Excellence, Healthcare Disparities, Rural Healthcare, Barriers to Care, Wicked Problem

1. Introduction

Transgender and gender-nonconforming people face relentless discrimination in employment, family life, education, housing, faith-based settings, and public accommodation, but some of the most appalling discrimination occurs in healthcare settings, when individuals reach out for help [1]. Transgender people are among the most marginalized in our nation and that marginalization extends to healthcare.

A recent survey of transgender people shows minimal improvement in access to affirming healthcare between 2011 and 2015, and many continue to face insurmountable barriers [1, 2]. Of those recently surveyed, 25% reported experiencing a problem with their insurance in the past year related to being transgender; 33% who saw a healthcare clinician reported at least one negative experience related to being transgender; 55% of those who sought coverage for transition-related surgery were denied; and 23% of respondents did not see a doctor when they needed to, due to fear of maltreatment [2].

Barriers to healthcare, visualized in **Figure 1**, include problems related to the *individual* and *society* and are both *formal* and *informal*. *Individual/informal* barriers to care include self-stigma and minority stress, which negatively impact the ability of transgender people to reach out for care. Minority stress refers to the protracted level of stress faced by members of stigmatized, minority populations, leading to the internalization of negative societal mores, shame, or fear of personal harm [3, 4]. This may result in self-stigma, leading to denial or concealment of one's identity in medical settings. *Individual/formal* barriers to care include the absence of affirming services for transgender people, due to the lack of medical training, clinician ignorance and/or implicit bias and transphobia [5–8]. The result is clinician discomfort that is reflected, intentionally or unintentionally, onto transgender patients who, when asking for help, are met instead with confusion, curiosity, hostility and incompetence.

Formal/Institutional barriers to care, in turn, include structural stigma resulting from the lack of protections that ensure a right to affirming care; the problem of structural stigma is further associated with higher mortality in sexual and gender minorities [9]. Causes of structural stigma include the dearth of governmental policy protections; the lack of insurance coverage for transition related care; the exclusion of gender identity/gender expression in antidiscrimination policies; the absence of institutional trainings on cultural responsiveness; and the failure to employ electronic medical records (EMR) to capture the nuanced experience and demographics of gender diverse people [10, 11].

Finally, *societal/informal* stigma, in the form of rejection, abuse, and discrimination, leads to increased rates of depression, suicidality, violence, substance abuse, HIV, unemployment and homelessness, all conditions that impede an individual's ability to access and follow through with healthcare [12–19].

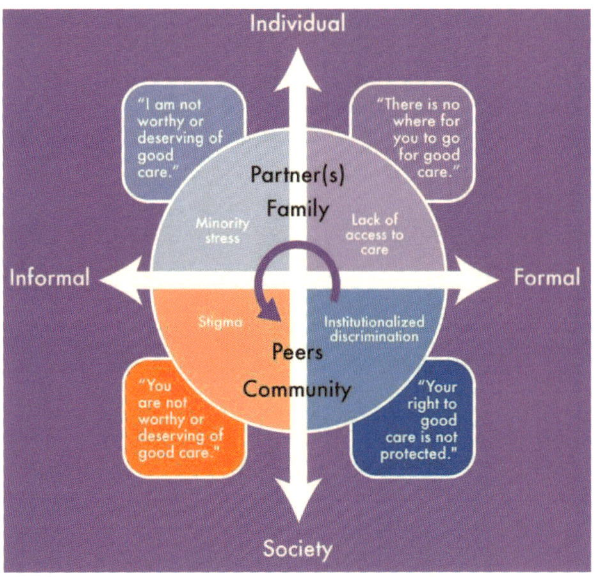

Figure 1.
Barriers to care for transgender patients.

These barriers to care are linked and strengthened by a circular, self-perpetuating energy. The result? Most transgender people face inordinate stress while attempting access to healthcare. Many delay care, presenting only to emergency rooms, in extremis. Others forgo all healthcare, ignore illness, and self-treat their gender dysphoria with unregulated hormones purchased on the internet. Others fear coming out and requesting help from clinicians, presenting instead with a bewildering array of symptoms and behaviors related to minority stress/dysphoria that are not disclosed, acknowledged or addressed. The effects of the resultant healthcare disparities ripple into the wider world where the suffering of transgender people is translated into devastating and expensive societal problems. Individuals, families, peers, healthcare institutions, and communities are all damaged by the costs of poor care.

Place of residency/environmental circumstance is a critical social determinant of health and significant research gaps exist around the experience and needs of rural transgender populations. Limited studies suggest that rural transgender people experience additional barriers to healthcare, including decreased access to trans-competent medical and mental health professionals, social isolation, transportation issues, financial constraints, and concerns about confidentiality [20, 21]. They have less political power, increased visibility, fewer alternatives in the face of discrimination, fewer support structures, and less support from faith organizations and local government [22]. Rural LGBTQ people devote more time to travel for healthcare, a factor associated with higher rates of depression and anxiety [23]. Higher scores on stigma scales for rural transgender people is associated with lower utilization of healthcare services [24]. Rural transgender people express higher Brief Symptom Inventory Somatization Scales, higher rates of depression, unprotected sex and decreased self-esteem compared to their urban counterparts [25]. Rural transgender veterans show increased rates of tobacco use and PTSD compared to urban peers [26]. The ability of transgender men to integrate in a rural environment is limited to those who are not out and who conform to "sameness," "whiteness and enacting appropriate rural working-class heterosexual masculinities" [27].

Population and student surveys estimate the incidence of transgenderism at 0.5% to 2.7% [28, 29]. Over the last few years, the visibility of transgender people across the nation has reached a tipping point, leading to an increase in the numbers of people seeking healthcare and the demand on healthcare facilities to respond to this need [30, 31].

In urban centers, specialized clinics may exist to provide LGBTQ affirming healthcare services, but clinicians in rural areas lack a replicable model for healthcare delivery. In the Northeast United States, clinics offering gender-affirming care are usually urban, federally qualified health centers [32–34]. These centers are designed to address identified healthcare disparities for LGBTQ individuals in communities with high need. They advertise well, offer a sense of community and expertise regarding LGBTQ health, and hire staff who represent and are committed to serving this population. In rural areas, most LGBTQ people receive services in primary care offices from clinicians who offer LGBTQ specific services from within a general practice [35]. This embedded model for care provides anonymity to patients who prefer not to self-identify. However, these settings may be staffed by clinicians with limited training in LGBTQ health who have a narrow scope of practice and cannot provide services for social support and education.

The complex, interdisciplinary nature of transgender healthcare and the inability of most medical systems to offer competent trans-specific and gender-affirming healthcare meets criteria for a *wicked problem* [36]. Wicked problems are systemic, malignant, persistent and inflict incalculable pain and suffering onto individuals and communities. By definition, a wicked problem is one "for which each attempt to create a solution changes the understanding of the problem" [36]. The usual linear approach to problem solving with planning and implementation only creates additional work. Every small solution to a piece of the puzzle leads to an entirely new set of wicked problems, each with its own muddy set of expensive consequences, requiring urgent and consuming attention. The larger problem is "ill structured, an evolving set of interlocking issues and constraints" [37]. Each wicked problem is unique and has no clear solution. Efforts to solve them must use novel approaches that are hard to measure, rarely finished, and usually limited by dwindling resources.

To address the wicked problem of transgender healthcare, clinicians and staff may take deliberate steps to create welcoming environments for transgender patients by constructing appropriate visual cues, providing cultural responsiveness training, capturing appropriate demographic information, updating policies and procedures, and mastering clinical skills [35, 38]. But most clinicians and staff have neither the interest, time, nor resources for these tasks and require organizational mandates and support. Effecting organizational change to create welcoming clinic/hospital networks is a larger wicked problem, requiring institutional leadership to recognize the barriers to care, perform honest assessments, and commit to cultural change.

One organizational change model to promote inclusion and reduce disparities for LGBTQ people identifies a need for both *elements* (organizational resources) and *processes* (dynamic strategies) to effect change [39]. Six *elements* identified as critical for success are: organizational champions, organizational priority, depth of mission, commitment to continuous learning, commitment to diversity and inclusion, and organizational resources. The six *processes* required for success include: management of change, information exchange, action research, relationship building, putting values into action, and leveraging resources. While effecting organizational change requires a daunting multi-dimensional transformation within the entire Culture of Health, this process is often sparked when one person recognizes the barriers to care for an individual patient.

Rural and urban healthcare systems develop Centers of Excellence (COE) to tackle the complex needs of specific populations. These organizations aspire to serve as specialized programs that offer comprehensive, interdisciplinary care and resources within a medical field to improve patient outcomes [40]. COEs are developed to create cultures that put patients first and keep people healthier and out of the hospital [41]. Clinicians in COEs provide leadership, demonstrate best practices, measure quality, conduct research, and offer support and training for a focus area. However, no strict criteria exist for programs to achieve the designation of a COE, and institutions demonstrate uneven success in ensuring that the term is used to reflect quality, rather than used as a marketing ploy [42]. Institutions have started creating quality-based Centers of Excellence to address the wicked problem of transgender health in a few urban settings, but not in rural healthcare institutions [43, 44].

This chapter describes how clinicians within a family practice addressed the wicked problem of access to healthcare for their region by working toward the creation of a Rural-Based Center of Excellence in Transgender Health. This story began with a request for care from a transgender patient in 2007 to the author, a family physician with no experience in the field. Using the embedded model for care, the practice has evolved and in 2019, exists as an interdisciplinary center that has provided medical, surgical, and mental health services to over 1000 transgender patients and their families. This paper describes our journey. It is our hope that our embedded care model will be replicated in rural-based primary care clinics across the nation, ensuring that transgender healthcare is brought from margins to mainstream medical practice in the United States.

2. Wicked problem impact project (WPIP) description

The creation of the rural-based Gender Wellness Center (GWC) began in 2007, when a transgender man asked the author to provide continuation of his testosterone therapy. Uncertain of how to proceed but unwilling to turn the patient away, she agreed to self-train to manage the patient's hormone regimen. Over time, more patients presented for care, necessitating the addition of additional services. A clinical social worker began providing mental health services and local surgeons began providing some basic gender-affirming surgeries (chest reconstruction, breast augmentation, hysterectomy and orchiectomy). In December 2014, Governor Andrew Cuomo mandated that all New York State public and private insurance cover medical and surgical treatment for transgender patients which in turn led to a sharp uptick in patient volume at our clinic. In 2015, to recognize this development in specialized care, we established the GWC as part of the family practice by hanging a new office sign for The Gender Wellness Center/Susquehanna Family Practice and creating a website (www.genderwellnesscenter.com).

By 2016, over 350 transgender patients had received services at the GWC and problems around the delivery of care began to surface. Due to complex

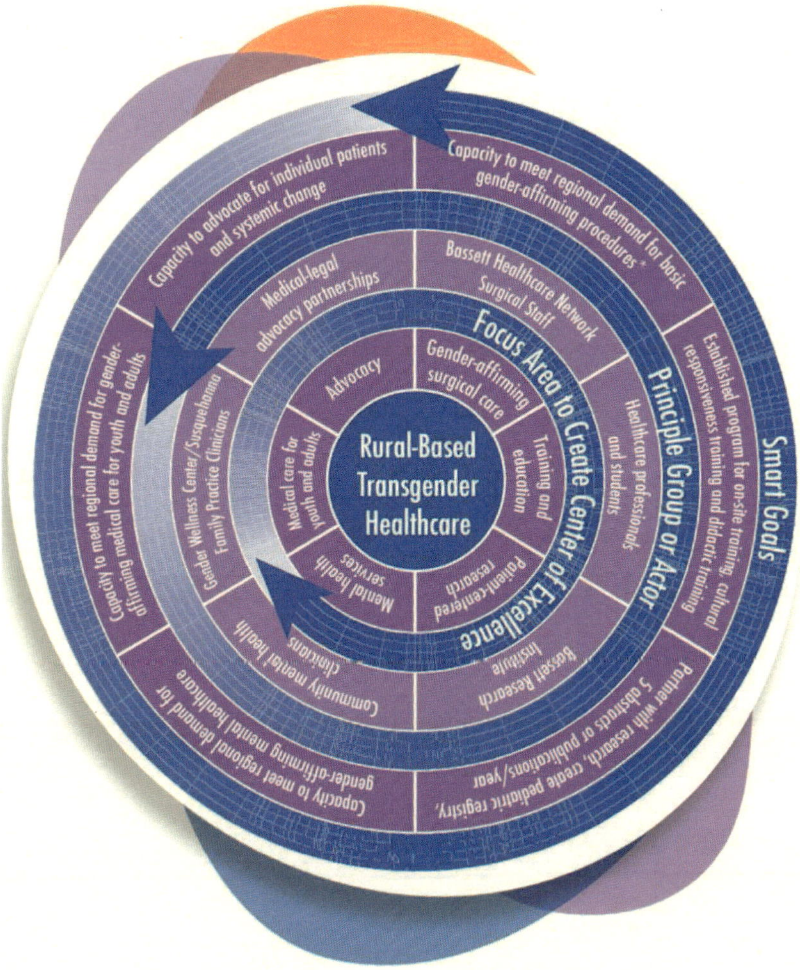
Smart Goals
Principle Group or Actor
Focus Area to Create Center of Excellence
Rural-Based Transgender Healthcare
Capacity to advocate for individual patients and systemic change
Capacity to meet regional demand for basic gender-affirming procedures*
Established program for on-site training, cultural responsiveness training and didactic training
Partner with research, create pediatric registry, 5 abstracts or publications/year
Capacity to meet regional demand for gender-affirming mental healthcare
Capacity to meet regional demand for gender-affirming medical care for youth and adults
Medical-legal advocacy partnerships
Bassett Healthcare Network Surgical Staff
Healthcare professionals and students
Bassett Research Institute
Community mental health clinicians
Gender Wellness Center/Susquehanna Family Practice Clinicians
Advocacy
Gender-affirming surgical care
Training and education
Patient-centered research
Mental health services
Medical care for youth and adults

Figure 2.
The wicked wheel: creating a rural-based center of excellence for transgender health.

biopsychosocial needs, the patients often required extra time and support from staff and clinicians, including the provision of medical-legal advocacy, staff training, and coordination of care with interdisciplinary services, community-based organizations, schools and employers. Though proud of the quality of services offered, we were aware that the GWC had been hastily cobbled together to meet the immediate needs of desperate patients and lacked institutional support and a sustainable organizational structure. Although the hospital administration had offered tentative support, they had not helped to identify and address the changing needs of the practice and, like all rural hospitals in upstate New York, faced financial challenges and a multitude of competing priorities. Many of the patients required complex care coordination with service organizations and specialists who lacked basic education about transgender people. A transgender man was denied hysterectomy at a network hospital due to gender identity issues, indicating a critical need for organizational education.

In 2016, as the author began looking for funding to expand and improve services, she assembled an interdisciplinary team (two family practice physicians, an OB/GYN surgeon, and a clinical social worker) to meet the complex medical, mental health and surgical needs of this population. The team applied for and was awarded a Robert Wood Johnson Foundation (RWJF) Clinical Scholars Grant to explore the possibility of creating a Center of Excellence in transgender health for the Bassett Healthcare Network.

The focus in creating a COE was six pronged, and included specific goals around 1) the provision of gender-affirming healthcare for transgender and gender nonconforming youth and adults, 2) the provision of gender-affirming mental health services, 3) the provision of gender-affirming surgical care, 4) effective medical-legal advocacy, 5) training and education, and 6) patient-centered research. **Figure 2** depicts the wicked problems around transgender healthcare and the team's six identified SMART goals.

3. Methods

The Gender Wellness Center (GWC) is embedded within Susquehanna Family Practice (SQFP), one of several primary care practices affiliated with A.O. Fox Hospital, a small community hospital in Oneonta, New York (**Figure 3**). A college town, with a population of 14,000, Oneonta is located within 1–2 hours of the urban centers of Albany, Syracuse and Binghamton. A.O [45]. Fox Hospital recently merged with The Bassett Healthcare Network (BHN), a collection of rural based hospitals and outpatient clinics serving a large swath of upstate, NY. In this chapter the "team" refers to the group of seven mental health, medical, nursing and surgical clinicians who worked closely together from within the GWC at SQFP on this project.

Our team's first step was to create a mission, vision, and values statement. We intentionally aligned our statement with the mission of our healthcare network, embracing the tenets of excellence in patient care, health research and healthcare education [46]. Additionally, our vision statement included the intent to "bring transgender healthcare from the margins to the mainstream" by creating a model for rural-based comprehensive care (**Figure 4**).

To advance exploration around creating a COE, our team met frequently with a research team from the Center for Evaluating Rural Interventions (CERI) at the Bassett Research Institute (BRI). CERI and the GWC clinicians conducted focus groups to assess community need and created logic models to explore project goals and the steps required to achieve them. Our team developed project evaluation tools, including Social Network Analysis, pre and post testing for trainings, and quality assurance chart audits, and a plan to create a pediatric patient registry.

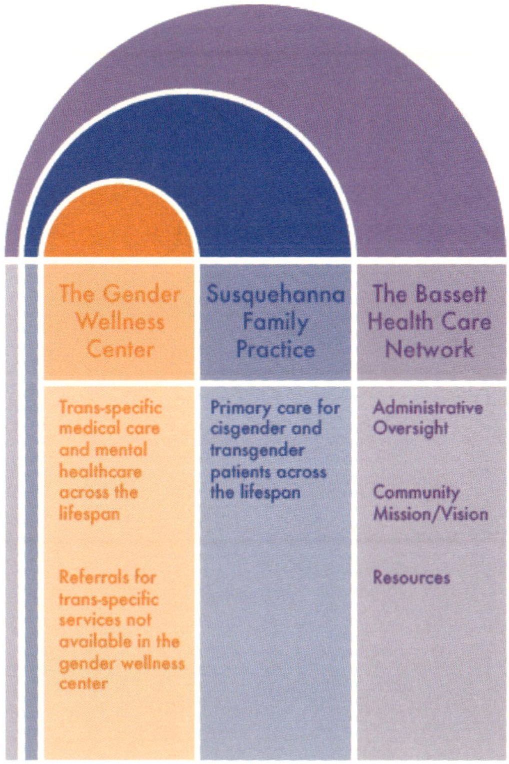

Figure 3.
The embedded model of care for the gender wellness center.

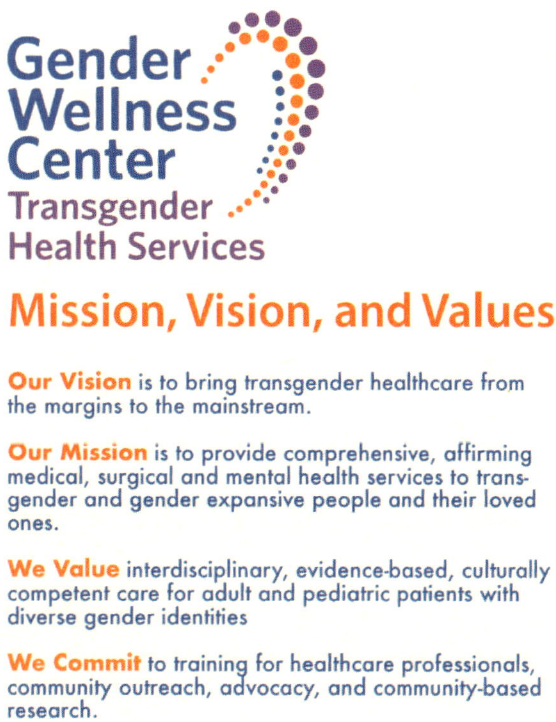
Gender Wellness Center
Transgender Health Services
Mission, Vision, and Values
Our Vision is to bring transgender healthcare from the margins to the mainstream.
Our Mission is to provide comprehensive, affirming medical, surgical and mental health services to transgender and gender expansive people and their loved ones.
We Value interdisciplinary, evidence-based, culturally competent care for adult and pediatric patients with diverse gender identities
We Commit to training for healthcare professionals, community outreach, advocacy, and community-based research.

Figure 4.
The Mission, vision and values of the gender wellness center.

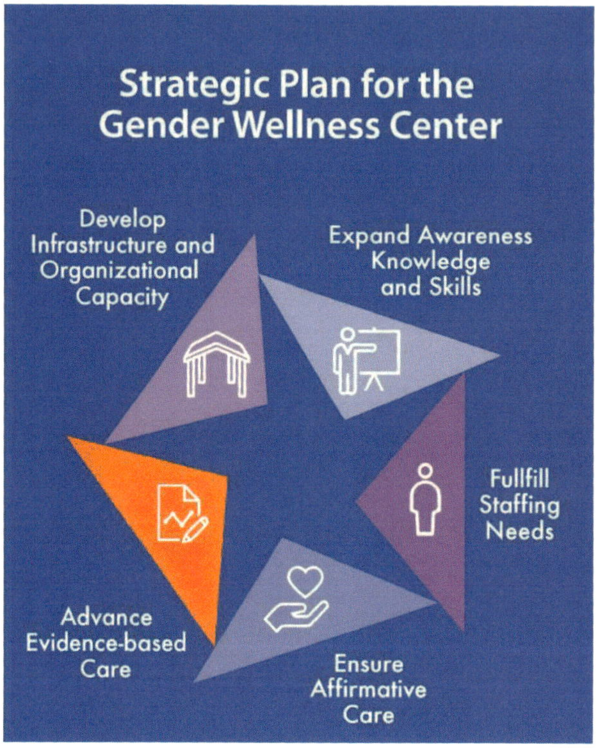
Strategic Plan for the Gender Wellness Center
Develop Infrastructure and Organizational Capacity
Expand Awareness Knowledge and Skills
Fullfill Staffing Needs
Ensure Affirmative Care
Advance Evidence-based Care

Figure 5.
The gender wellness center strategic plan: five strategic directions.

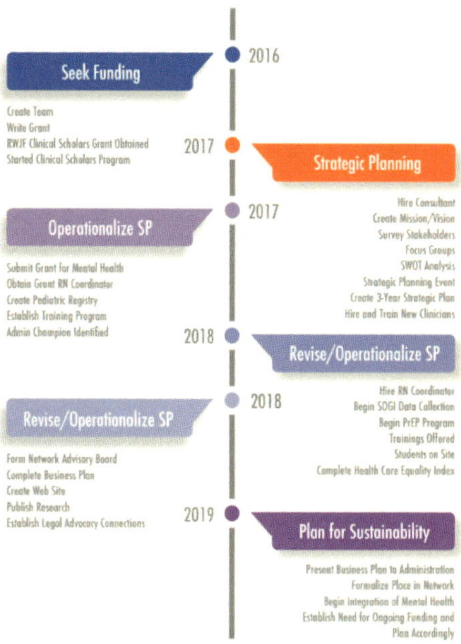
2016
Seek Funding
Create Team
Write Grant
RWJF Clinical Scholars Grant Obtained
Started Clinical Scholars Program
2017
Strategic Planning
2017
Hire Consultant
Create Mission/Vision
Survey Stakeholders
Focus Groups
SWOT Analysis
Strategic Planning Event
Create 3-Year Strategic Plan
Hire and Train New Clinicians
Operationalize SP
Submit Grant for Mental Health
Obtain Grant RN Coordinator
Create Pediatric Registry
Establish Training Program
Admin Champion Identified
2018
Revise/Operationalize SP
2018
Hire RN Coordinator
Begin SOGI Data Collection
Begin PrEP Program
Trainings Offered
Students on Site
Complete Health Care Equality Index
Revise/Operationalize SP
Form Network Advisory Board
Complete Business Plan
Create Web Site
Publish Research
Establish Legal Advocacy Connections
2019
Plan for Sustainability
Present Business Plan to Administration
Formalize Place in Network
Begin Integration of Mental Health
Establish Need for Ongoing Funding and Plan Accordingly

Figure 6.
Timeline for the gender wellness center strategic plan.

July 2017 saw the start of the strategic planning process. We conducted individual stakeholder interviews, a network/community survey, a student survey, and a patient satisfaction survey. In October 2017, stakeholders, including patients, employees from regional Community Based Organizations (CBOs), network administrators, employees, and community members participated in two forums to review data from the surveys, and identify strengths, weaknesses, opportunities and threats to the evolving program. Our team then developed a 2-year strategic plan with five strategic directions, and specific goals for each direction. The five strategic directions included 1) Developing infrastructure and organizational capacity, 2) Expanding awareness, knowledge and skills, 3) Fulfilling staffing needs, 4) Ensuring gender-affirming care, and 5) Advancing evidence-based care (**Figure 5**). The plan was distributed to all stakeholders.

The remainder of the grant funding period was devoted to operationalizing the strategic plan. During this time, the team met quarterly to assign projects, review the status of projects, and then update the strategic plan, including identifying and addressing a number of specific projects and goals for each strategic initiative. We met weekly to discuss project implementation at a granular level by assessing, planning, executing, and evaluating. **Figure 6** depicts the timeline for project development and implementation.

4. Outcomes/results

The numbers of patients served at the GWC grew significantly during the three-year period of the RWJF Clinical Scholars program, as demonstrated in **Figure 7**. To date, we have served over 750 medical patients and 300 mental health patients. On average, patients travel 60 miles to be seen at the GWC but the catchment area for

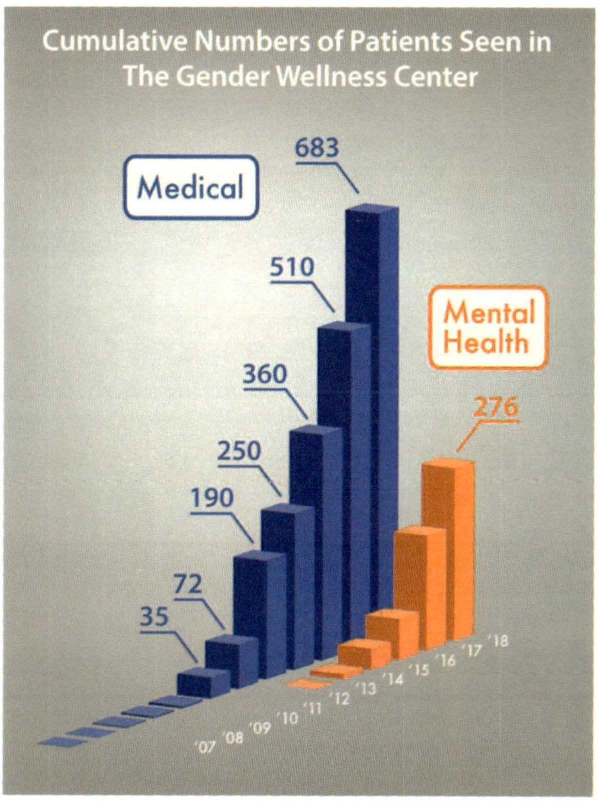

Figure 7.
Cumulative numbers of patients seen in the gender wellness center 2007–2018.

adults includes many counties across New York state as well as neighboring states [47]. **Figure 8** depicts the catchment area for GWC pediatric patients, as captured in the GWC Pediatric Registry with rural–urban distribution by zip code [48]. Transgender patients currently represent approximately 25% of the total number of patients seen at Susquehanna Family Practice [47].

4.1 Developing infrastructure and organizational capacity

Due to the interdisciplinary nature of transgender healthcare, our team identified the need to employ an interdisciplinary approach to organization and administrative oversight, in addition to patient care. To this end, we formed a Network Advisory Board (NAB) comprised of leaders in the network administration; members of the surgical, mental health and medical divisions; and transgender community members. This group served as a sounding board as our team developed and presented our business plan and explored a place for the GWC within the network organizational structure.

We also developed organizational structure within our office and A.O. Fox Hospital. We established monthly, peer protected, interdisciplinary rounds for case review and care coordination. We created quality measures, based on

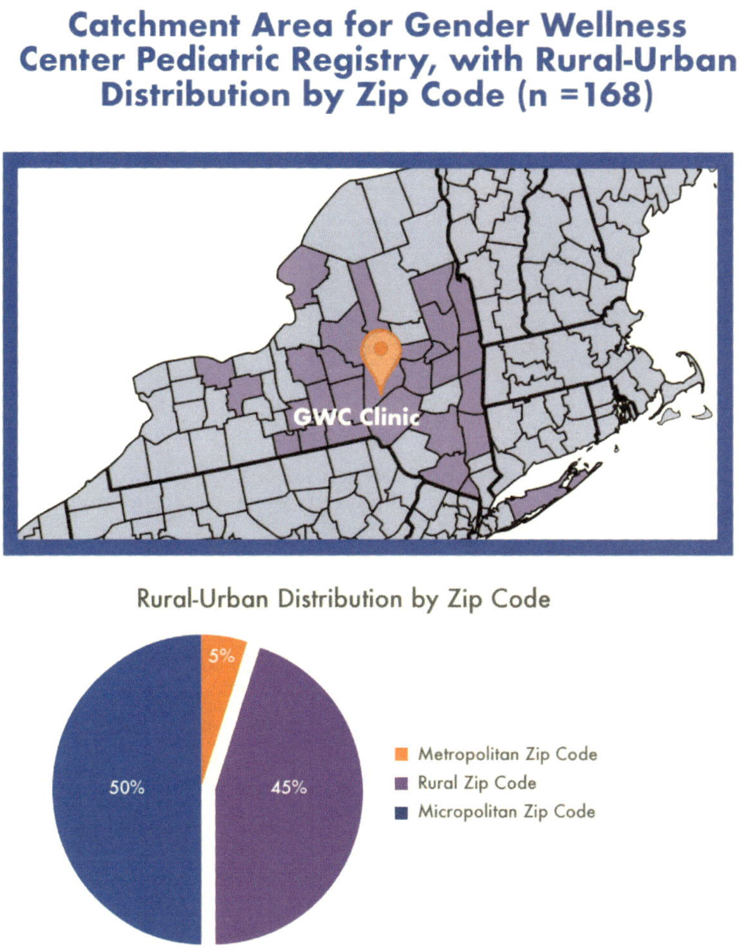

Figure 8.
Catchment area for gender wellness center pediatric registry.

recommendations from the World Professional Association's Standards of Care and Endocrine Society Clinical Practice Guidelines and performed quarterly chart audits [49, 50], and designed practices to ensure smooth entry to appropriate services within the GWC and referrals between disciplines.

Team members worked with A.O. Fox Hospital staff to achieve certification as a "Leader in LGBTQ Health" from the Healthcare Equality Index (HEI). This benchmarking tool, offered by the Human Rights Campaign, ensures LGBTQ affirming hospital policies, procedures and services [51].

Developing ties to a number of regional LGBTQ-affirming CBOs, including Planned Parenthood, the AIDS Institute, the NYS LGBTQ Network, community centers, counseling centers, government programs, and legal agencies, created partnership opportunities for meaningful connection to others doing similar work as well as important patient services.

4.2 Expanding awareness, knowledge and skills

The team identified the need to train ourselves, our staff, our network, healthcare professional students, and our wider community. Three of the clinicians served as coordinators for educational initiatives and all clinicians assisted with training. Several of our clinicians were new to transgender health and intentionally developed clinical skills through training and mentoring. Our office staff required cultural responsiveness training and forums to discuss ethical concerns around the care of trans youth. We developed onboarding procedures for new hires. We partnered with a professional trainer to offer trans-led cultural responsiveness education within the network and community. These trainings were filmed and will soon be included in orientation for all network hires. We offered didactic trainings at professional conferences, for specific organizations and via webinar. The physicians developed on-site clinical rotations to train professionals and students and established formal training connections with Yale and Columbia-Bassett Medical School.

4.3 Fulfilling staffing needs

To meet the growing demand for services, we recruited new clinicians and developed specialized roles within the team. Assigning job titles and creating job descriptions for team members contributed to the business plan (i.e. Director of Training, Coordinator for Surgical Services, Liaison to Research Team, etc.). The organizational chart is continually reviewed and adjusted as the COE evolves and there is ongoing discussion with network administrators about how to fit our chart within the larger network organizational structure.

We identified a senior network administrator to serve as our champion. Our team liaison met with him regularly to review plans and solicit advice. Our team met frequently with local and network administrators to address specific healthcare disparities faced by our patients and to advocate for improved services.

Our office was appointed an experienced office manager who ensured that staff were appropriately trained and monitored around the provision of culturally responsive care for all patients. We created a job description for the position of RN Coordinator for the GWC, which includes patient care coordination, project development, training and assisting with research, applied for funding and were awarded a two-year grant for this position.

As common in rural areas, we have struggled with limited access to adult and pediatric psychiatric care. In year two of our grant, the network hired a psychiatric clinician with an interest in transgender health. During his stay, we developed an effective collaborative process.

Our team identified the need to develop a sustainable model for mental health services as a key strategic initiative. Until 2019, our mental health clinicians worked with a private practice model and low sliding scale fee, a system that was not sustainable. In 2019, the New York State Department of Health awarded our team a 5-year grant to establish salaried positions for mental health clinicians within the BHN and offer mental health services for free.

We developed legal advocacy services through years of collaboration with regional CBOs who assist with problems around Medicaid law, insurance denials, discrimination, family law, and document changes, but patient need has continually exceeded capacity. We met with a community partner to assess need, envision a plan, and seek funding. This partner then also received a 5-year grant to develop formal medical-legal partnerships with the GWC and other regional transgender health providers.

The phrase "nothing about us without us" reflects the need for inclusive hiring to create welcoming communities. Our office included a transgender person to serve on our clinical team.

The need to ensure community participation in review of ethical concerns related to trans healthcare led our team to ask that a member of the transgender community be appointed to the hospital ethics committee. This request was readily adopted by our hospital administration.

4.4 Ensuring gender-affirming care

Placing visual cues, including welcoming signs, patient education materials, and notices about local LGBTQ services in the office waiting room, coupled with displaying our hospital's revised non-discrimination policy, which now includes gender identity/expression, became useful strategies. We designated all single stall restrooms in the office as gender neutral and updated forms to ensure inclusivity for diverse gender identities and family structures. All staff were trained in cultural responsiveness. We worked with our network public relations team to develop branding, update our website and develop an affirming marketing plan.

To ensure appropriate collection of demographic data, we worked with information technology from the BHN to include a collection tool for data on sexual orientation/gender identity (SOGI) in the EMR. The medical clinicians collect SOGI data on all patients in the family practice. A subsequent network-wide upgrade to our EMR and accompanying educational campaign soon ensures that SOGI data is collected in all clinical settings.

The medical clinicians sought training in the provision of Pre and Post-Exposure Prophylaxis for HIV (PrEP and PEP) and Medication Assisted Therapy (MAT) for the treatment of substance abuse so that these critical services can be accessed by all patient at the GWC/SQFP. Our team works closely with network surgeons who offer basic gender-affirming surgical services, including breast augmentation, chest reconstruction, orchiectomy, and hysterectomy. We developed educational materials and practices to assist patients with referrals for specialized gender surgery services not available in network and for postoperative care. Two of the GWC physicians volunteer at a community based free clinic in Oneonta to offer care to transgender people without insurance.

To advance evidence-based care, our team recreated a Community Research Advisory Team (CREATE) of transgender community members to assist us in ensuring that our research efforts are affirming and appropriate to community need. This group meets quarterly and has recently also begun to serve as a Community Advisory Board (CAB) to advise our team around the provision of affirming services.

4.5 Advancing evidence-based care

We developed close collaboration with members of the Bassett Research Institute with the goal of creating a patient registry and producing five publications/abstracts per year. This larger team created the first rural-based patient registry for gender-expansive pediatric patients in the country and we have begun publishing our data. Team members also contribute to the field with abstracts, case reports and book chapters [48, 52–60].

We identified a need to develop quality assessment measures. With the assistance of the A.O. Fox Quality Management Services, our team developed a tool for quarterly audit of medical charts, based on published care guidelines [49, 50]. We formed our Interdisciplinary Rounds based on these same published guidelines, a venue for peer protected, team review of complex cases and for youth receiving medical interventions [50].

5. Project evaluation

Our team employed seven different evaluation methods to track program implementation. Recording the cumulative growth of patients seen by medical

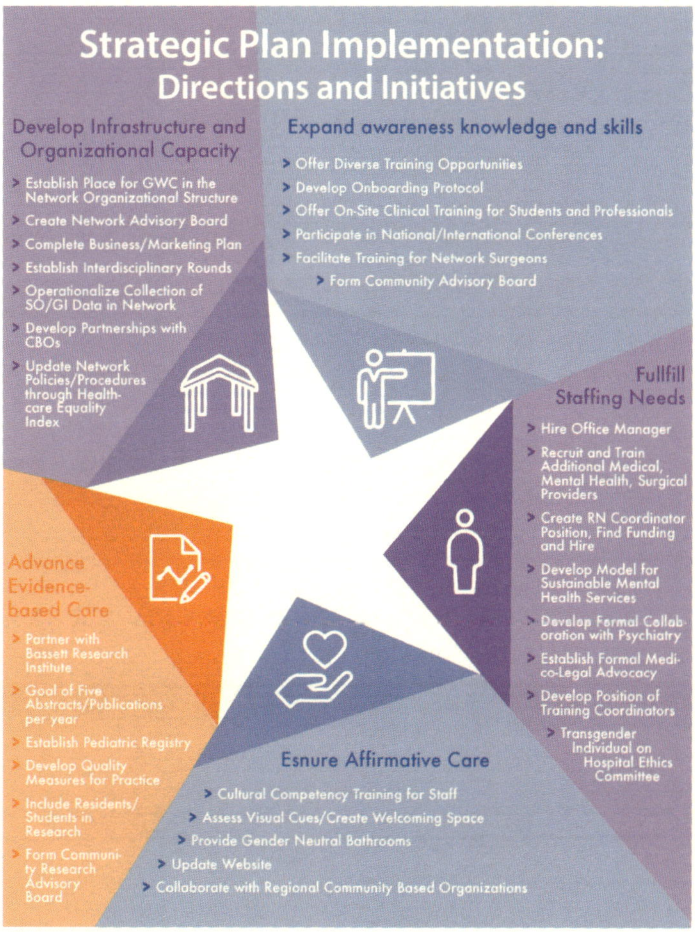
Strategic Plan Implementation:
Directions and Initiatives
Develop Infrastructure and Organizational Capacity
> Establish Place for GWC in the Network Organizational Structure
> Create Network Advisory Board
> Complete Business/Marketing Plan
> Establish Interdisciplinary Rounds
> Operationalize Collection of SO/GI Data in Network
> Develop Partnerships with CBOs
> Update Network Policies/Procedures through Healthcare Equality Index
Expand awareness knowledge and skills
> Offer Diverse Training Opportunities
> Develop Onboarding Protocol
> Offer On-Site Clinical Training for Students and Professionals
> Participate in National/International Conferences
> Facilitate Training for Network Surgeons
> Form Community Advisory Board
Fullfill Staffing Needs
> Hire Office Manager
> Recruit and Train Additional Medical, Mental Health, Surgical Providers
> Create RN Coordinator Position, Find Funding and Hire
> Develop Model for Sustainable Mental Health Services
> Develop Formal Collaboration with Psychiatry
> Establish Formal Medico-Legal Advocacy
> Develop Position of Training Coordinators
> Transgender Individual on Hospital Ethics Committee
Advance Evidence-based Care
> Partner with Bassett Research Institute
> Goal of Five Abstracts/Publications per year
> Establish Pediatric Registry
> Develop Quality Measures for Practice
> Include Residents/Students in Research
> Form Community Research Advisory Board
Esnure Affirmative Care
> Cultural Competency Training for Staff
> Assess Visual Cues/Create Welcoming Space
> Provide Gender Neutral Bathrooms
> Update Website
> Collaborate with Regional Community Based Organizations

Figure 9.
Strategic plan implementation: direction and initiatives.

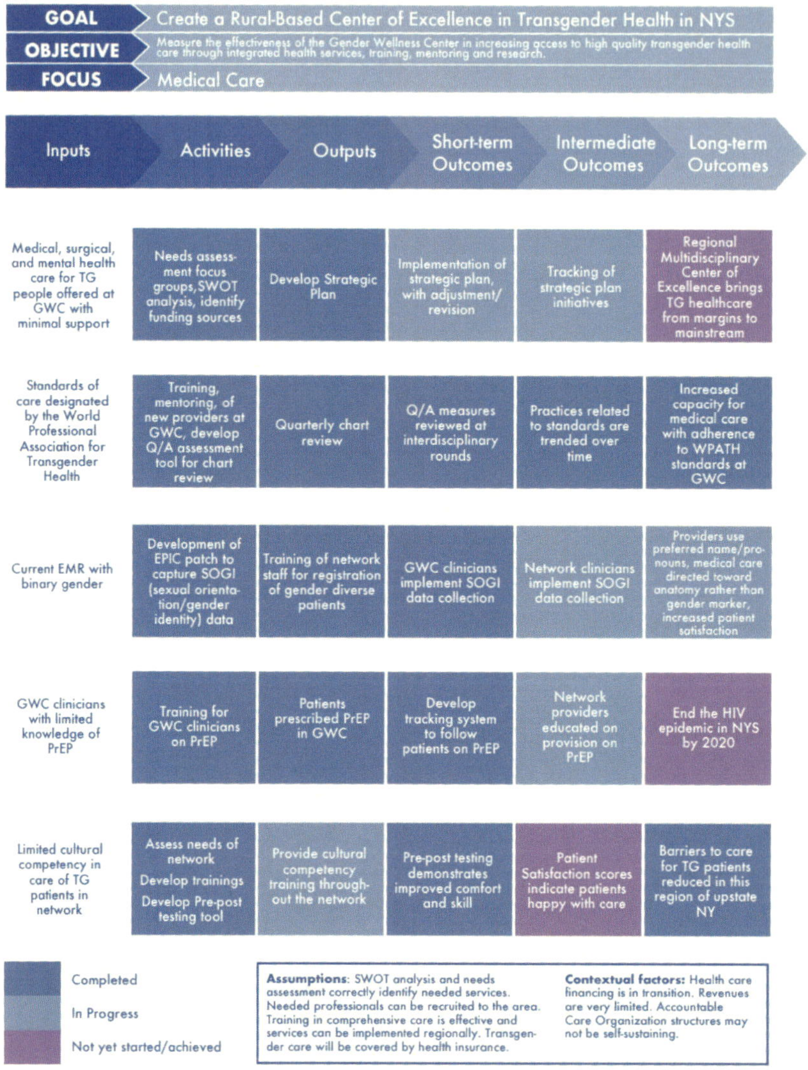

Figure 10.
Logic model: creating a center of excellence in transgender health.

and mental health clinicians was a process that started with the first patient in 2007 (**Figure 7**). We developed a chart to track strategic plan implementation (**Figure 9** depicts strategic directions and initiatives) and updated our logic models to demonstrate progression of projects over time (**Figure 10**). We recorded all publications, including abstracts, book chapters and articles and tracked didactic and on-site clinical trainings and obtained pre- and post- testing to illustrate how training "moved the needle" around staff/clinician comfort in the provision of care. We performed Social Network Analysis (SNA) to measure engagement and map the relationships of the GWC clinicians with others, locally and outside the BHN. **Figure 11** is the SNA map for a three-year grant period, demonstrating an increasingly denser network (more ties) with a rounder shape, (increasing connection within and external to the BHN) for our clinicians. It demonstrates improvements in networks/communications and cosmopolitanism over time. Our medical team reviewed all quarterly quality assurance reports with appropriate administrators

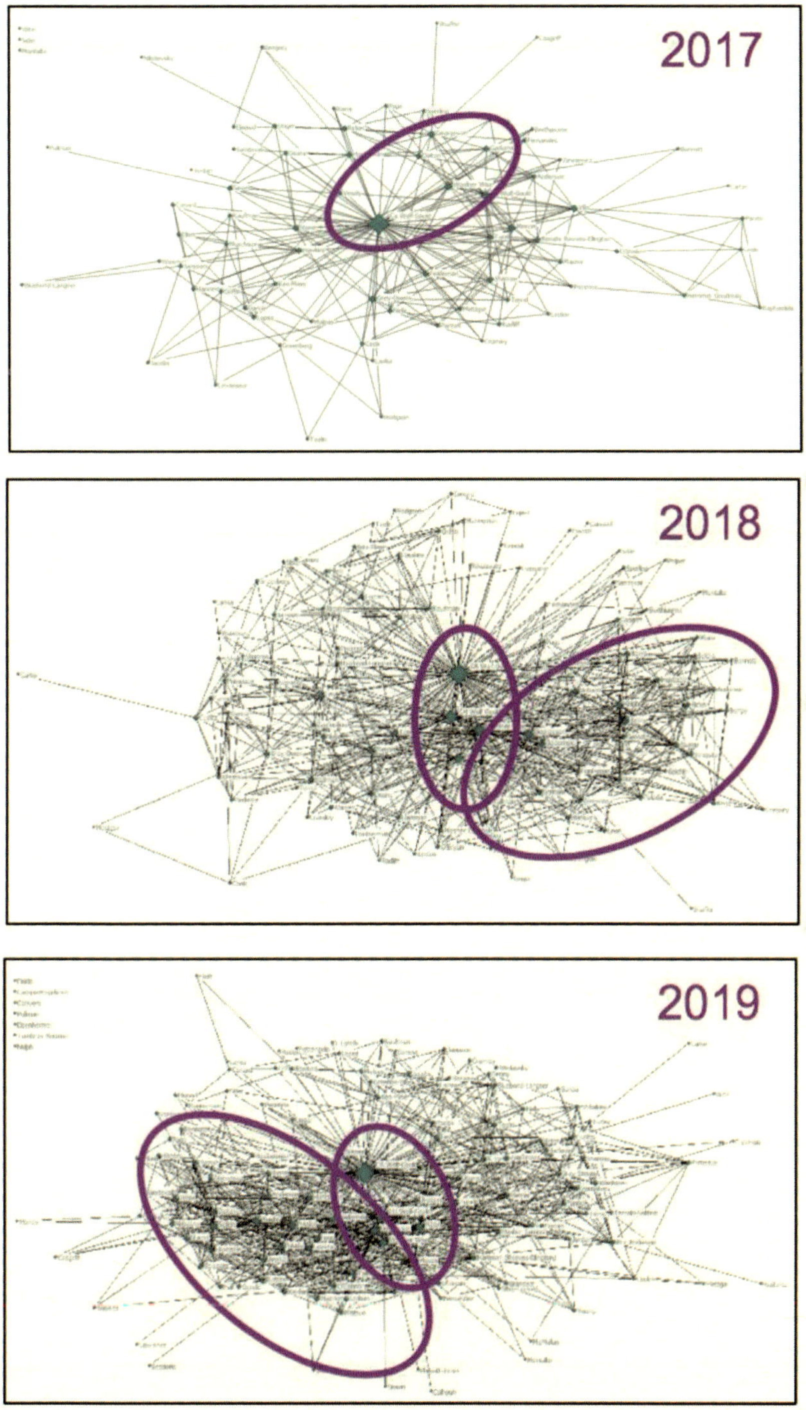

Figure 11.
SNA mapping to measure social capital and network formation.

within the BHN. We worked with the Bassett Research Institute to employ the Consolidated Framework for Implementation Research to evaluate project implementation (**Figure 12**) [61–63]. This system assesses results through a wide lens that includes the formative successes and limitations of project performance at various levels (i.e. level of patient, clinician team, organizational and market/policy level), within our specific setting, with our unique leadership, culture and team [64].

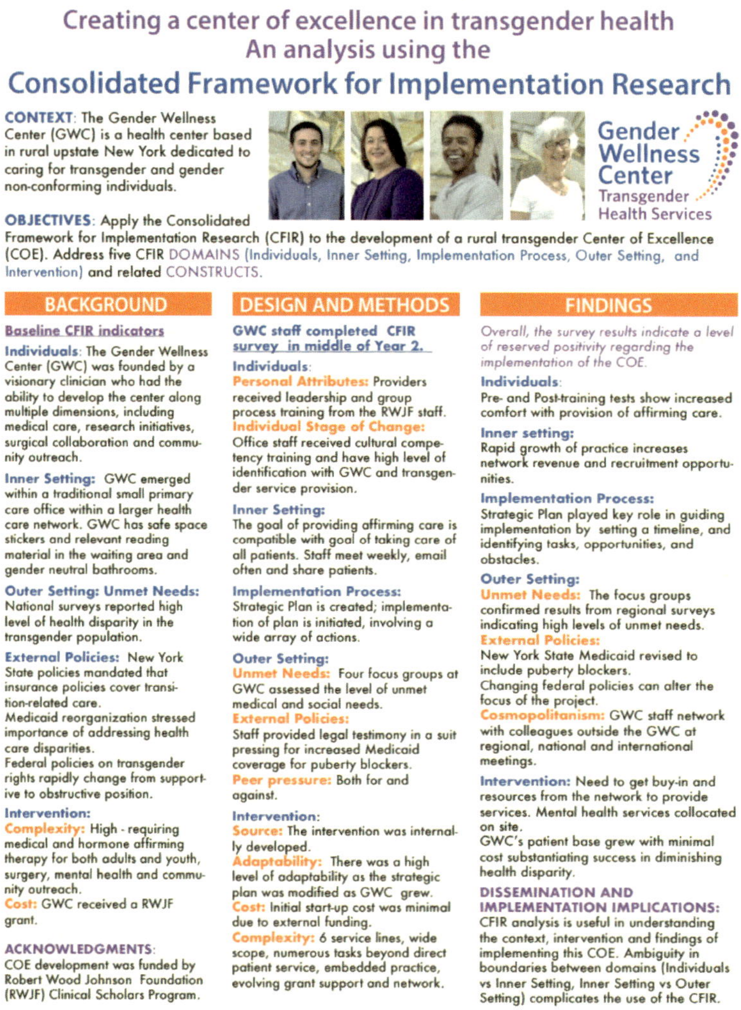
Creating a center of excellence in transgender health
An analysis using the
Consolidated Framework for Implementation Research
CONTEXT: The Gender Wellness Center (GWC) is a health center based in rural upstate New York dedicated to caring for transgender and gender non-conforming individuals.
Gender Wellness Center
Transgender Health Services
OBJECTIVES: Apply the Consolidated Framework for Implementation Research (CFIR) to the development of a rural transgender Center of Excellence (COE). Address five CFIR DOMAINS (Individuals, Inner Setting, Implementation Process, Outer Setting, and Intervention) and related CONSTRUCTS.
BACKGROUND
Baseline CFIR indicators
Individuals: The Gender Wellness Center (GWC) was founded by a visionary clinician who had the ability to develop the center along multiple dimensions, including medical care, research initiatives, surgical collaboration and community outreach.
Inner Setting: GWC emerged within a traditional small primary care office within a larger health care network. GWC has safe space stickers and relevant reading material in the waiting area and gender neutral bathrooms.
Outer Setting: Unmet Needs: National surveys reported high level of health disparity in the transgender population.
External Policies: New York State policies mandated that insurance policies cover transition-related care.
Medicaid reorganization stressed importance of addressing health care disparities.
Federal policies on transgender rights rapidly change from supportive to obstructive position.
Intervention:
Complexity: High - requiring medical and hormone affirming therapy for both adults and youth, surgery, mental health and community outreach.
Cost: GWC received a RWJF grant.
ACKNOWLEDGMENTS:
COE development was funded by Robert Wood Johnson Foundation (RWJF) Clinical Scholars Program.
DESIGN AND METHODS
GWC staff completed CFIR survey in middle of Year 2.
Individuals:
Personal Attributes: Providers received leadership and group process training from the RWJF staff.
Individual Stage of Change: Office staff received cultural competency training and have high level of identification with GWC and transgender service provision.
Inner Setting:
The goal of providing affirming care is compatible with goal of taking care of all patients. Staff meet weekly, email often and share patients.
Implementation Process:
Strategic Plan is created; implementation of plan is initiated, involving a wide array of actions.
Outer Setting:
Unmet Needs: Four focus groups at GWC assessed the level of unmet medical and social needs.
External Policies:
Staff provided legal testimony in a suit pressing for increased Medicaid coverage for puberty blockers.
Peer pressure: Both for and against.
Intervention:
Source: The intervention was internally developed.
Adaptability: There was a high level of adaptability as the strategic plan was modified as GWC grew.
Cost: Initial start-up cost was minimal due to external funding.
Complexity: 6 service lines, wide scope, numerous tasks beyond direct patient service, embedded practice, evolving grant support and network.
FINDINGS
Overall, the survey results indicate a level of reserved positivity regarding the implementation of the COE.
Individuals:
Pre- and Post-training tests show increased comfort with provision of affirming care.
Inner setting:
Rapid growth of practice increases network revenue and recruitment opportunities.
Implementation Process:
Strategic Plan played key role in guiding implementation by setting a timeline, and identifying tasks, opportunities, and obstacles.
Outer Setting:
Unmet Needs: The focus groups confirmed results from regional surveys indicating high levels of unmet needs.
External Policies:
New York State Medicaid revised to include puberty blockers.
Changing federal policies can alter the focus of the project.
Cosmopolitanism: GWC staff network with colleagues outside the GWC at regional, national and international meetings.
Intervention: Need to get buy-in and resources from the network to provide services. Mental health services collocated on site.
GWC's patient base grew with minimal cost substantiating success in diminishing health disparity.
DISSEMINATION AND IMPLEMENTATION IMPLICATIONS:
CFIR analysis is useful in understanding the context, intervention and findings of implementing this COE. Ambiguity in boundaries between domains (Individuals vs Inner Setting, Inner Setting vs Outer Setting) complicates the use of the CFIR.

Figure 12.
Consolidated framework for implementation research.

6. Discussion

Approaching the conclusion of the RWJF Clinical Scholars grant period, our team reflected on the following: 1) Is the GWC a Center of Excellence yet? 2) What have been our biggest successes and challenges? 3) Have we moved transgender healthcare from the margins to mainstream? 4) How have we benefited from the leadership training of the Clinical Scholars program? 5) And, what legacy do we leave behind from our work?

Is the Gender Wellness Center a Center of Excellence yet? Loose definitions for COEs leave room for generous interpretation and tempt us to premature claims of success. As the first to attempt to create a Rural-Based COE in Transgender Health, we have had to draw our own road map and create our own measures for success. After discussion among our team members, we conclude that **we have not yet arrived**. This effort still lacks key components of sustainability, including a clear place in our network organizational structure, a plan for succession, adequate financial resources and assistance with project administration. Our team needs new clinicians, and an infusion of energy. We remain uncertain if the GWC will live beyond our new New York State Department of Health grant funding and the careers of the current clinicians. We have seen that the process of 1) stating our intention and then 2) working toward the creation of a Center of Excellence has allowed us to employ both change *elements* (organizational resources) and *processes* (dynamic strategies) to promote inclusion and reduce health care disparities in our region [39]. But changing the Culture of Health is slow work. Although our team has not yet attained our goal of creating a Center of Excellence, we believe that we have created a **Center for Exceptional Care in Transgender Health (CFECTH).**

The nature of the *wicked problem* of transgender healthcare led to significant challenges around program implementation. Like all *wicked problems*, ours has evolved, not been solved. Every small solution to a piece of our puzzle has led to an entirely new set of *wicked problems*, requiring ongoing attention. While the logic model depicts an organized approach to problem identification and solving, **Figure 13**. more accurately reflects the chaos and complexity we experienced while addressing our *wicked problem*.

For example, as we devoted time and energy to addressing health care disparities for transgender patients, we were criticized by some hospital personnel and community members for "discriminating against cisgender patients." Staff turnover/resistance and the loss of some cisgender patients who objected our changing focus presented obstacles as well. We struggled to "change this narrative" through education on health equity and by continuing to provide primary care for cisgender patients (roughly 75% of total patient care). Other staff left because we were not progressive enough, the pay was too low, and the demands of the office too high. We are challenged by the fact that the stigma and erasure faced by our patients extends, to a lesser degree, to us as clinicians. Historically, physicians in this field have been viewed as quacks or practicing on the fringe. While the members of our team have not been subject to harassment and death threats, as have colleagues in other states, we have received some negative attention from our community and peers.

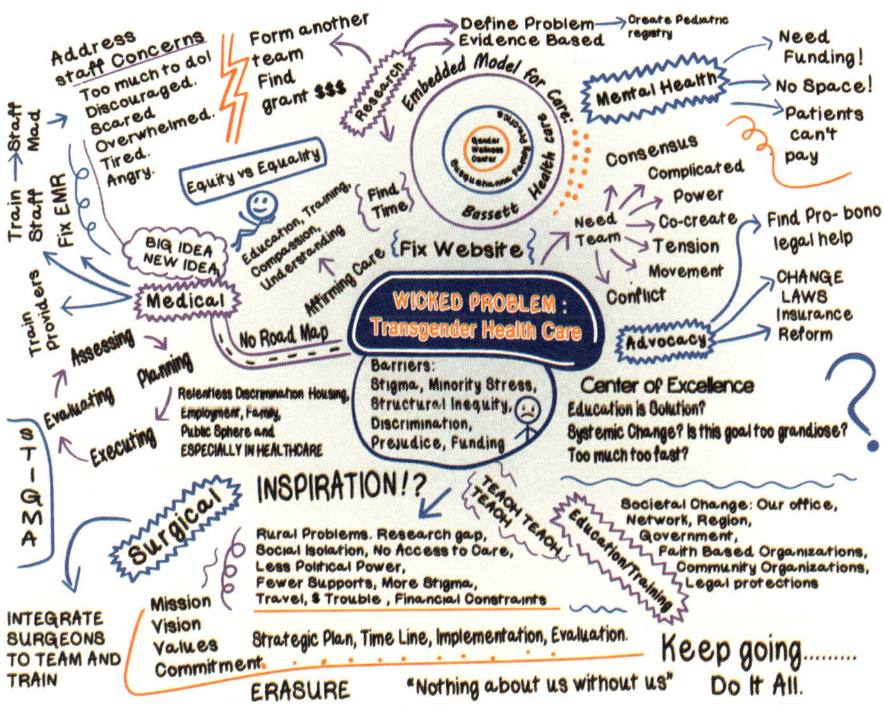

Figure 13.
The wicked problem of transgender healthcare.

Like many rural healthcare systems, our network faces financial challenges, leading to system wide cuts and the need to prioritize profitable programs over those that require funding to flourish. Typically, programs designed to address health care disparities are not money-making ventures. Our surgical program is potentially lucrative, though still small. Our medical practice brings in significant downstream revenue but like all primary care practices, struggles to stay in the black. Our mental health services are grant funded for limited terms [47]. We have come to understand that, by necessity, we will need to rely on grant funding for program sustainability.

Review of data collected through our pediatric registry indicates that our patient population is 89% white, a demographic that reflects our county, but not our larger catchment area. Communities of people of color (POC) in our region face additional barriers to care that our small rural clinic has been unable to address.

Our biggest challenge has been that our *wicked problem* is huge and there is too much to do. Our team members faced personal limitations around time and energy. It has been surprisingly difficult to move past personal differences to work on common goals as a functional team. These problems led to burn-out, a common problem for teams working on *wicked problems*, and one that requires us to reflect on problematic aspects to our personal styles or leadership skills.

Despite the challenges, we are proud to celebrate our program successes. Our team kept up with the increasing demands for services by expanding delivery of trans-competent and culturally responsive medical, mental health and surgical care to youth and adults. Our patients report high satisfaction with our services. We developed a vibrant research partnership to advance evidence-based care and trained numerous staff members, clinicians and healthcare professional students. We developed strong community partnerships with a number of regional CBOs, resulting in improved patient care and transformational personal relationships for ourselves. Our team sought and obtained grant funding to develop our nursing and mental health services and to develop a formal medical-legal advocacy program. Our center receives national recognition for our innovative work to create a new model for rural-based care.

We have also witnessed a significant regional shift toward moving transgender healthcare "from the margins to the mainstream." The shift is, in part, documented through our evaluation tools, but also comes to us in the form of stories from patients, community members and peers. An elderly cisgender man described a meaningful conversation with a young transgender woman in our waiting room. A physician from another network hospital sent us photos of their new gender-neutral bathrooms signs. A patient described being cheered after finding the courage to speak at a human rights rally on Main Street, in Oneonta. The physical therapy department reached out for training in order to better serve our patients. Bassett education arranged a visit with a prominent gender surgeon for a yearly celebratory teaching event and asked us to provide on-site rotations training for residents and medical students. Our network EMR will facilitate system-wide collection of SOGI data. Community mental health clinicians are flocking to our mental health training program. These stories illustrate profound systemic change at many levels in our community.

As individuals and as a group, we have benefited enormously from the RWJF leadership training. We studied how thought diversity and culture influence change and used personal assessment tools to gain a deeper understanding of our personalities and styles, and how these factors affect one another. Our team learned how to assess team roles and assign tasks to our strengths. Learning how to speak truth to power through the creation of a strategic plan, a business plan, and organizational charters proved exceptionally helpful. We learned to pay attention to the soft skills of interpersonal connection and learned to share leadership and responsibility for our work.

And finally, we learned that the process of bearing witness to the struggles and transformative journeys of our transgender patients challenges us to consider our own authenticity as human beings in a complex world. The word *privilege* may be used to describe unjust racial and class-based entitlement, a special birthright, an advantage. In hospitals, clinicians apply for and, if they meet qualifications for training and competency, are granted *privileges* -- the opportunity to practice under the auspices of that institution. This privilege includes how we benefit as individuals from our participation in the clinician-patient relationship. We are privileged to serve as guides through our patients' transformative journeys related to illness or health. We have all been profoundly changed by this work. The process of listening to and serving our patients in this complex world provides us with an extraordinary opportunity to learn, reflect and grow as individuals – an experience that, in small ways, mirrors the transformative change of our patients.

We've been asked by the RWJF Clinical Scholars directors to consider our legacy, a process that requires us to step back from the immediate and consuming project work to take the bird's eye view. Our hope is that, in our quest for excellence around rural-based transgender healthcare, our team has created a model for gender-affirming care that can and will be replicated in other primary care practices across the country. Our work is proof that a single patient asking for help from an uninformed clinician in a broken system can create a spark that drives that system to change. We have individually, as a group, and with our patients and community partners spoken out on the need to serve this at risk/at need population and have watched in awe as our system slowly and often painfully rose to the challenge. This model for care is our legacy and it rests in the collective ruckus raised from this work: the hubbub of direct patient care, the clamor of education and training, the din of legal advocacy and the rumpus of patient-centered research. This hullabaloo has pierced decades of erasure and neglect of transgender people in our region and led to the creation of a **Center for Exceptional Care in Transgender Health**.

It's a start. It's imperfect. We have all kinds of problems and still more to do. We say to you clinicians out there wanting to learn how to offer gender-affirming care from your primary care practice: *Go ahead. Do it. All big things start small. You will be profoundly changed by the trek toward this goal. We stand by you, cheering, as you make change happen too.*

7. Toolkit

To assist other clinicians to offer gender-affirming care using an embedded, primary care model we have created the following tool kit (**https://clinicalscholarsnli.org/community-impact**) of resources.

Acknowledgements

The author wishes to acknowledge the work of her teammates, Justine Woolner-Wise, LMSW, Christopher Wolf-Gould, MD, Diane Georgeson, MD, Patti Noon, LMSW, Susan Turell, PhD, Jackie Kelchlin, FNP, Anne Gadomski, MD, MPH, Nancy Tallman, Melissa Scribani PhD.

Author details

Carolyn Wolf-Gould
The Gender Wellness Center/Susquehanna Family Practice, The Bassett Healthcare Network, New York, United States

*Address all correspondence to: carolyn.wolf-gould@bassett.org

References

[1] Grant J, Mottet L, Tanis J, Harrison J, Herman J, Keisling M. Injustice at Every Turn: A report of the National Transgender Discrimination Survey. 2011.

[2] James SE, Herman JL, Rankin S, Keisling M, Mottet L, Anafi M. The report of the 2015 US Transgender Survey. *Washington: National Center for Transgender Equality*. 2016.

[3] Makadon HJ. *The Fenway Guide to Lesbian, Gay, Bisexual, and Transgender Health*. ACP Press; 2008.

[4] Levitt HM, Ippolito MR. Being Transgender: Navigating Minority Stressors and Developing Authentic Self-Presentation. Psychology of Women Quarterly. 2014;38(1):46-64. doi:10.1177/0361684313501644

[5] Kitts RL. Barriers to optimal care between physicians and lesbian, gay, bisexual, transgender, and questioning adolescent patients. Journal of homosexuality. 2010;57(6):730-747.

[6] Obedin-Maliver J, Goldsmith ES, Stewart L, et al. Lesbian, gay, bisexual, and transgender–related content in undergraduate medical education. Jama. 2011;306(9):971-977.

[7] Rondahl G. Students inadequate knowledge about lesbian, gay, bisexual and transgender persons. *Int J Nurs Educ Scholarsh*. 2009;6:Article11. doi:10.2202/1548-923X.1718

[8] Stotzer RL, Silverschanz P, Wilson A. Gender identity and social services: Barriers to care. Journal of Social Service Research. 2013;39(1):63-77.

[9] Hatzenbuehler ML, Bellatorre A, Lee Y, Finch BK, Muennig P, Fiscella K. Structural stigma and all-cause mortality in sexual minority populations. Social Science & Medicine. 2014;103:33-41.

[10] Gehi PS, Arkles G. Unraveling injustice: Race and class impact of Medicaid exclusions of transition-related health care for transgender people. Sexuality Research & Social Policy. 2007;4(4):7.

[11] Roberts TK, Fantz CR. Barriers to quality health care for the transgender population. Clinical biochemistry. 2014;47(10):983-987.

[12] Claes L, Bouman WP, Witcomb G, Thurston M, Fernandez-Aranda F, Arcelus J. Non-Suicidal Self-Injury in Trans People: Associations with Psychological Symptoms, Victimization, Interpersonal Functioning, and Perceived Social Support. The journal of sexual medicine. 2015;12(1):168-179.

[13] Peterson CM, Matthews A, Copps-Smith E, Conard LA. Suicidality, Self-Harm, and Body Dissatisfaction in Transgender Adolescents and Emerging Adults with Gender Dysphoria. *Suicide and life-threatening behavior*. 2016. http://onlinelibrary.wiley.com/doi/10.1111/sltb.12289/full. Accessed March 5, 2017.

[14] Haas AP, Eliason M, Mays VM, et al. Suicide and suicide risk in lesbian, gay, bisexual, and transgender populations: Review and recommendations. Journal of homosexuality. 2010;58(1):10-51.

[15] Clements-Nolle K, Marx R, Katz M. Attempted suicide among transgender persons: The influence of gender-based discrimination and victimization. Journal of homosexuality. 2006;51(3):53-69.

[16] Poteat T, German D, Kerrigan D. Managing uncertainty: a grounded theory of stigma in transgender health care encounters. Social Science & Medicine. 2013;84:22-29.

[17] Toomey RB, Ryan C, Diaz RM, Russell ST. High School Gay-Straight Alliances (GSAs) and Young Adult

Well-Being: An Examination of GSA Presence, Participation, and Perceived Effectiveness. Appl Dev Sci. 2011;15(4): 175-185. doi:10.1080/10888691.2011.607378

[18] Wyss SE. ERIC - "This Was My Hell": The Violence Experienced by Gender Non-Conforming Youth in US High Schools, International Journal of Qualitative Studies in Education, 200. International Journal of Qualitative Studies in Education. 2004;17(5):709-730.

[19] Roberts AL, Rosario M, Slopen N, Calzo JP, Austin SB. Childhood Gender Nonconformity, Bullying Victimization, and Depressive Symptoms Across Adolescence and Early Adulthood: An 11-Year Longitudinal Study. Journal of the American Academy of Child & Adolescent Psychiatry. 2013;52(2): 143-152. doi:10.1016/j.jaac.2012.11.006

[20] Rosenkrantz D, Black W, Abreu R, Aleshire M, Bennett K. *Health and Health Care of Rural Sexual and Gender Minorities: A Systematic Review.* Vol 2.; 2016. doi:10.1037/sah0000055

[21] Knutson D, Koch JM, Arthur T, Mitchell TA, Martyr MA. "Trans broken arm": Health care stories from transgender people in rural areas. Journal of Research on Women and Gender. 2017;7(0):30-46.

[22] Movement Advancement Project | Mapping Transgender Equality in the United States. http://www.lgbtmap.org/mapping-trans-equality. Accessed May 16, 2019.

[23] Kauth MR, Barrera TL, Denton FN, Latini DM. Health Differences Among Lesbian, Gay, and Transgender Veterans by Rural/Small Town and Suburban/Urban Setting. LGBT health. 2017;4(3): 194-201.

[24] Whitehead J, Shaver J, Stephenson R. Outness, Stigma, and Primary Health Care Utilization among Rural LGBT Populations. PLOS ONE. 2016;11(1):e0146139. doi:10.1371/journal.pone.0146139

[25] Horvath KJ, Iantaffi A, Swinburne-Romine R, Bockting W. A comparison of mental health, substance use, and sexual risk behaviors between rural and non-rural transgender persons. J Homosex. 2014;61(8):1117-1130. doi:10.1080/00918369.2014.872502

[26] Bukowski LA, Blosnich J, Shipherd JC, Kauth MR, Brown GR, Gordon AJ. Exploring Rural Disparities in Medical Diagnoses Among Veterans With Transgender-related Diagnoses Utilizing Veterans Health Administration Care. Medical care. 2017;55:S97–S103.

[27] Abelson MJ. 'You aren't from around here': race, masculinity, and rural transgender men. Gender, Place & Culture. 2016;23(11):1535-1546. doi:10.1080/0966369X.2016.1219324

[28] Flores AR, Herman JL, Gates GJ, Brown TNT. How Many Adults Identify as Transgender in the United States? June 2016. http://williamsinstitute.law.ucla.edu/wp-content/uploads/How-Many-Adults-Identify-as-Transgender-in-the-United-States.pdf. Accessed June 28, 2018.

[29] Rider GN, McMorris BJ, Gower AL, Coleman E, Eisenberg ME. Health and Care Utilization of Transgender and Gender Nonconforming Youth: A Population-Based Study. Pediatrics. 2018;141(3):e20171683. doi:10.1542/peds.2017-1683

[30] Garofalo R. Tipping points in caring for the gender-nonconforming child and adolescent. Pediatr Ann. 2014;43(6):227-229. doi:10.3928/00904481-20140522-06

[31] The tipping point Time magazine - Google Search. https://www.google.com/#q=The%20tipping%20point%20Time%20magazine. Accessed March 8, 2017.

[32] Fenway Health. Fenway Health: Your Care, Your Community. http://fenwayhealth.org/. Accessed March 22, 2017.

[33] Mazzoni Center. Mazzoni Center. https://www.mazzonicenter.org/. Accessed March 22, 2017.

[34] Home - Callen-Lorde. https://callen-lorde.org/. Accessed February 6, 2019.

[35] McClain Z, Hawkins LA, Yehia BR. Creating Welcoming Spaces for Lesbian, Gay, Bisexual, and Transgender (LGBT) Patients: An Evaluation of the Health Care Environment. Journal of homosexuality. 2016;63(3):387-393.

[36] Rittel HWJ, Webber MM. Dilemmas in a general theory of planning. Policy Sci. 1973;4(2):155-169. doi:10.1007/BF01405730

[37] Wicked Problems Summary Handout.pdf. http://www.mncounties.org/document_center/Committees/Wicked%20Problems%20Summary%20Handout.pdf. Accessed December 5, 2018.

[38] Bau I. Building Patient-Centered Medical Homes for Lesbian, Gay, Bisexual, and Transgender Patients and Families. May 2016. https://www.lgbthealtheducation.org/wp-content/uploads/Building-PCMH-for-LGBT-Patients-and-Families.pdf. Accessed March 22, 2017.

[39] Eckstrand KL, Lunn MR, Yehia BR. Applying organizational change to promote lesbian, gay, bisexual, and transgender inclusion and reduce health disparities. LGBT health. 2017;4(3):174-180.

[40] Elrod JK, Fortenberry JL. Centers of excellence in healthcare institutions: what they are and how to assemble them. *BMC Health Serv Res*. 2017;17(Suppl 1). doi:10.1186/s12913-017-2340-y

[41] Why hospitals must become 'centers of excellence.' athenaInsight. https://www.athenahealth.com/insight/why-hospitals-must-become-centers-of-excellence. Published January 4, 2017. Accessed September 26, 2018.

[42] Mehrotra A, Dimick JB. Ensuring excellence in centers of excellence programs. Annals of surgery. 2015;261(2):237-239.

[43] The Center of Excellence for Transgender Health. http://transhealth.ucsf.edu/. Accessed February 16, 2019.

[44] Klein P, Narasimhan S, Safer JD. The Boston Medical Center experience: An achievable model for the delivery of transgender medical care at an academic medical center. Transgender health. 2018;3(1):136-140.

[45] U.S. Census Bureau QuickFacts: Oneonta city, New York. https://www.census.gov/quickfacts/fact/table/oneontacitynewyork/PST045217. Accessed February 20, 2019.

[46] Mission, Vision & Values :: Bassett Healthcare Network. https://www.bassett.org/medical/locations/hospitals/bassett-medical-center/about-us/mission-vision-values. Accessed February 16, 2019.

[47] The Gender Wellness Center Business Plan: Creating a Rural-Based Center of Excellence in Transgender Health for the Bassett Healthcare Network. November 2018.

[48] O'Bryan J, Leon K, Wolf-Gould C, Scribani M, Tallman N, Gadomski A. Building a Pediatric Patient Registry to Study Health Outcomes Among Transgender and Gender Expansive Youth at a Rural Gender Clinic. Transgender health. 2018;3(1):179-189.

[49] Coleman E, Bockting W, Botzer M, et al. Standards of care for the health of transsexual, transgender, and

gender-nonconforming people, version 7. International Journal of Transgenderism. 2012;13(4):165-232.

[50] Hembree WC, Cohen-Kettenis PT, Gooren L, et al. Endocrine Treatment of Gender-Dysphoric/Gender-Incongruent Persons: An Endocrine Society* Clinical Practice Guideline. The Journal of Clinical Endocrinology & Metabolism. 2017;102(11):3869-3903.

[51] Campaign HR. Healthcare Equality Index 2018. Human Rights Campaign. https://www.hrc.org/hei/. Accessed February 24, 2019.

[52] Wolf-Gould CS, Wolf-Gould CH. A transgender woman with testicular cancer: a new twist on an old problem. LGBT health. 2016;3(1):90-95.

[53] Deutsch MB, Green J, Keatley J, et al. Electronic medical records and the transgender patient: recommendations from the World Professional Association for Transgender Health EMR Working Group. J Am Med Inform Assoc. 2013;20(4):700-703. doi:10.1136/amiajnl-2012-001472

[54] Goldberg AE, ed. A History of Transgender Medicine in the United States. In: *The Sage Encyclopedia of LGBTQ Studies*. SAGE Publications, Incorporated; 2016:n.p.

[55] O'Bryan J, Wolf-Gould C, Matsuo Y. Mammary myofibroblastoma in a transgender patient on feminizing hormones: literature review and case report. Transgender health. 2018;3(1):1-9.

[56] Wolf-Gould CS, Riley MR, Carswell JM. A trans-feminine youth with a BRCA1 mutation: Case study. LGBT health. 2018;5(4):270-272.

[57] Wolf-Gould CS, Riley MR, Carswell JM. Complex medical decision-making for a trans-feminine youth with a BRCA1 mutation. LGBT health. 2018;5(4):221-225.

[58] Wolf-Gould C, Wolf-Gould C. Primary and Preventive Care for Transgender Patients. In: *Comprehensive Care of the Transgender Patient*. First. Elsevier; 2019. https://www.elsevier.com/books/comprehensive-care-of-the-transgender-patient/unger/978-0-323-49642-1. Accessed April 28, 2019.

[59] Lev AI, Wolf-Gould C. Collaborative Treatment Across Disciplines: Physician and Mental Health Counselor Coordinating Competent Care. In: *The Gender Affirmative Model: An Interdisciplinary Approach to Supporting Transgender and Gender Expansive Children*. First. APA; 2018. https://www.apa.org/pubs/books/4317487. Accessed April 28, 2019.

[60] Wolf-Gould, C. Family Oriented Medical Care for Gender Nonconforming Children, Adolescents and their Families. In: *Families in Transition, Parenting Gender Diverse Children, Adolescents and Young Adults*. First. New York, NY: Harrington Park Press, LLC; 2019:258-282. http://cup.columbia.edu/book/families-in-transition/9781939594297. Accessed April 28, 2019.

[61] Bauer MS, Damschroder L, Hagedorn H, Smith J, Kilbourne AM. An introduction to implementation science for the non-specialist. BMC psychology. 2015;3(1):32.

[62] Damschroder LJ, Aron DC, Keith RE, Kirsh SR, Alexander JA, Lowery JC. Fostering implementation of health services research findings into practice: a consolidated framework for advancing implementation science. *Implementation Science*. 2009;4(1). doi:10.1186/1748-5908-4-50

[63] The Consolidated Framework for Implementation Research. The Consolidated Framework for

Implementation Research. https://cfirguide.org/. Accessed January 30, 2019.

[64] Improving the Quality of Health Care in the United Kingdom and the United States: A Framework for Change - Ferlie - 2001 - The Milbank Quarterly - Wiley Online Library. https://onlinelibrary.wiley.com/doi/abs/10.1111/1468-0009.00206. Accessed January 30, 2019.

Chapter 6

Building a Dental Home Network for Children with Special Health Care Needs

Mark DeRuiter, Jeffrey Karp and Peter Scal

Abstract

Children with special health care needs (SHCNs) live in all communities. They present with a diverse group of diagnoses including complex chronic conditions and diseases; physical, developmental, and intellectual disabilities; sensory, behavioral, emotional, psychiatric, and social disorders; cleft and craniofacial congenital disabilities, anomalies, and syndromes; and inherited conditions causing abnormal growth, development, and health of the oral tissues, the teeth, the jaws, and the craniofacial skeleton. Tooth decay, gum disease, dental injuries, tooth misalignment, oral infections, and other oral abnormalities are commonly seen or reported in the health history of children with SHCNs. Nationally, dental and oral health care ranks as the second most common unmet health need, according to the most recent National Survey of Children with Special Health Care Needs. The State of Minnesota does not have enough dental professionals prepared to meet the demand for care. As a result, children with SHCNs either go untreated or receive inadequate services resulting in treatment delays, the need for additional appointments, poor management of oral pain and dysfunction, adverse dental treatment outcomes and/or a lack of appropriate referrals to needed specialists. Research suggests children with SHCNs are best served when assigned to dental homes where all aspects of their oral health care are delivered in a comprehensive, interdisciplinary, and family-centered way under the direction of knowledgeable, experienced dental professionals working collaboratively with an array of allied health, medical professionals, and community partners. An interdisciplinary team consisting of a pediatric dentist, pediatric physician, and speech-language pathology innovator collaborated to advance current and future dental providers' knowledge and comfort in providing care for children with SHCNs and was accepted into the Clinical Scholars program. Their interdisciplinary collaborative team project was named MinnieMouths and included the following six methods or critical endeavors to ensure success: 1. Development of a project ECHO site focused on advancing care for children with SHCNs. 2. Creation of a 28-participant web-based professional network of current dental, community health liaisons, family navigators, and medical health providers. 3. Establishment of a 32-participant web-based interface of dental and medical students and residents, including new-to-practice dental providers. 4. Launching an annual conference focused on advancing oral health care for children with SHCN. 5. Build a toolkit aimed at allowing dentists and future leadership teams to launch dental home networks focused on children with SHCN. 6. Building a Dental Homes Network Field Guide for Providers who attended our first in-person conference. Findings from the MinnieMouths project suggest that development of peer networks to advance dental homes for children with SHCNs has merit. Network participants gained skills in collaborating with a range of health care providers, understanding the complexities of working within and among health and dental care systems to coordinate care, and the need to better understand and advocate for a more robust medical and dental reimbursement program when launching dental homes for children with SHCN.

Keywords: health care, special needs, dental, oral, dental home, teleECHO, network, clinics, education, toolkit, telementoring

1. Introduction

Today's literature supports a growing need for specialized care and dental homes for children with special health care needs (SHCN). As the rate of children with SHCNs grows, the number of highly qualified oral health care providers who are available to care for them remains stagnant. As the pool of research grows, many health care providers and health systems' leaders understand more fully that oral health is an integral part of general health and well-being [1]. Creating a network of oral health care providers and professionals who support the advancement of dental homes for children with SHCNs has never been more critical.

1.1 Defining the problem

Based on data from the U.S. Census Bureau, approximately 85.3 million Americans live with a disability, with about two-thirds of those classified with a disability as having a severe disability [2]. Of the 85.3 million living with a disability, 12.5 million individuals are children [3].

The American Academy of Pediatric Dentistry defines special health care needs as "any physical, developmental, mental, sensory, behavioral, cognitive, or emotional impairment or limiting condition that requires medical management, health care intervention, and use of specialized services or programs." Conditions may be developmental, congenital, or acquired through disease, trauma, or environmental causes and may impose limitations in performing daily self-maintenance activities or substantial limitations in a significant life activity. Oral and general care for children with special needs requires specialized knowledge, as well as accommodative measures that are beyond routine, increased awareness and attention to specialized care, and adaptation within the clinical setting [4].

Children with SHCNs are at increased risk for oral diseases throughout their lifetime. Oral diseases have a direct and devastating impact on the health and quality of life of those with specific systemic health problems or conditions [5]. Research suggests children with mental, developmental, or physical disabilities who cannot understand, assume responsibility for, or cooperate with preventive oral health practices are susceptible to lower overall health outcomes, including long-term oral health [6].

SHCNs also include disorders or conditions which manifest only in the orofacial complex. These disorders include amelogenesis imperfecta (unusually small teeth), dentinogenesis imperfecta (a genetic condition causing discolored teeth), cleft lip/palate (incomplete fusion of the lip and/or hard/soft palate), and a range of additional health concerns. While these patients may not exhibit the same physical or cognitive limitations of other patients with SHCN, their needs are unique, impact their overall health, and require oral health care of a specialized nature.

As improvements in medical care afford children with SHCNs a longer, healthier lifespan, many formerly acute and fatal diagnoses have become chronic and manageable conditions. Unfortunately, a subset of healthcare organizations, including dental offices, are not prepared for a large pool of uniquely challenged patients. The Americans with Disabilities Act (ADA) defines the dental office as a place of public accommodation [7] meaning that all individuals must be afforded physical access to care, including wheelchair ramps and designated parking spaces. Failure to accommodate patients with SHCNs is not only discriminatory but also a violation of federal and state law. Thus, oral health professionals and the systems that support care are obligated to be familiar with these regulations to ensure compliance. While dental offices have developed new models to provide care to children with SHCN, the initial education, ongoing training, and financial reimbursement provided to practitioners impacts access to care.

Optimal health of children is more likely to be achieved with access to full health care benefits. Families and those adults caring for children with SHCNs pay greater out of pocket amounts and have higher expenditures in general than those families without special needs children. Research suggests that financial limitations and reimbursement rates are cited as the most common barriers to medically necessary oral health care for children with SHCNs. Insurance plays a vital role for families with children with SHCN, but it still provides incomplete protection [8]. Because of the unmet dental care needs of individuals with SHCN, emphasis on a dental home and comprehensive, coordinated services should be established, including essential insurance coverage and explicit financial support [9].

Limitations in oral health care do not typically end as children with SHCNs reach adulthood. Health insurance and oral care benefits coverage may actually become even more restrictive [10]. Data find that many individuals with SHCNs rely on government funding to pay for medical and dental care. Research also suggests these same individuals lack adequate access to private insurance for general and oral health care services. This lack of preventive and timely therapeutic care may increase the need for costly care and exacerbate systemic health issues later in life [10].

Nonfinancial barriers such as psychosocial, structural, cultural considerations, priorities, and transitions to care as adults have a negative impact on access to oral health care among children with SHCN [11]. Psychosocial factors associated with access for patients with SHCNs include reduced understanding or misguided oral health beliefs and norms, as well as likely negative past dental experiences for patients, caregivers and/or family members. Access to transportation, reduced school attendance thereby affecting absence policies and truancy issues, actual and perceived discriminatory treatment, and limitations in the number of available appointment slots within dental offices for those who have Medicaid coverage are documented structural barriers [10]. Priorities and attitudes also serve as impediments to oral care. Parents and medical providers' limited knowledge may hinder children with SHCNs from securing preventive dental care [12]. Moreover, many families determine that their child's more critical health conditions need to take precedence over oral health [13]. Lastly, in a survey of U.S. and Canadian dental schools, data also revealed that pediatric dentists expressed concerns about decreased access to oral health care and dental homes for patients with SHCNs during their transition to adulthood. Transitioning to a dentist who is knowledgeable and comfortable with adult oral health care among patients with SHCNs is difficult [14].

Findings suggest children and adults with SHCN who have a dental home and consistent care provided by trained oral health professionals are more likely to receive appropriate preventive and routine care. The dental home model allows for individualized preventive oral health practices and reduces the child's risk of preventable dental and oral disease [15]. Building a community network of oral and other health professionals committed to making dental homes for children with SHCN is essential. Given the limited financial resources, known barriers, and concerns regarding care transition to adulthood, there is a demonstrated need for a more extensive body of trained professionals.

2. Wicked problem impact project (WPIP) description

Data clearly show that children with SHCNs would benefit from a dental home where all aspects of their oral health care can be delivered in a comprehensive, continuously accessible (including into adulthood), coordinated, culturally competent, interdisciplinary, and family-centered way under the direction of knowledgeable, experienced dental and associated professionals who are comfortable and competent to address their patients' unique dental and oral health treatment needs [16]. We hypothesize that dental and other health care professionals, along with community health workers and interested family members, will embrace the dental home concept and participate in a community-based effort to not only improve dental care for children with SHCNs but also work to build a sustainable program.

Sadly, Minnesota, like most states, does not have enough dental professionals able and ready to meet the dental and oral health demands of its population. As a result, children with SHCNs either go untreated or are subjected to disorganized handoffs between pediatric healthcare professionals, general dentists, local dental specialists, and regional tertiary dental centers. Handoffs are a source of unnecessary appointments, treatment delays, inadequate management of oral pain and dysfunction, limited or absent referrals to appropriate specialists, and result in negative dental treatment outcomes. The time has come to support and prioritize a dental home across the pediatric life course for all children with SHCNs in Minnesota.

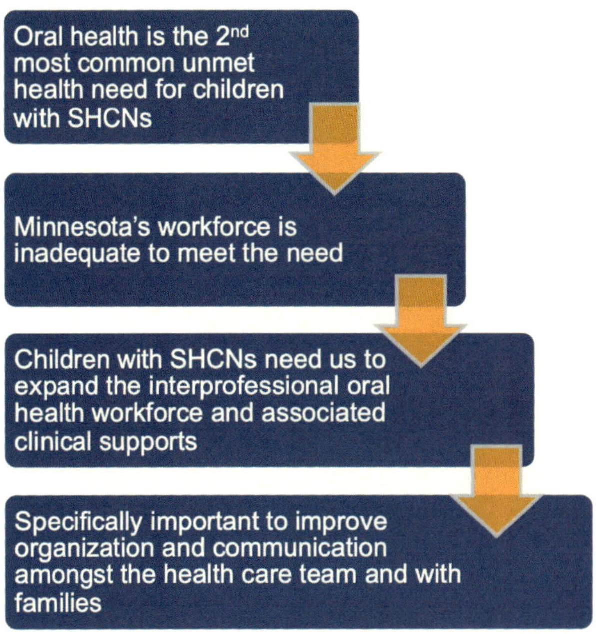

Figure 1.
Visual representation of Oral health wicked problem for children with special health care needs.

Dental care is the second most common unmet need for children with SHCNs [17]. The numbers are alarming. Minnesota has about 180,000 children with SHCNs, and our best estimates are that there are 103 pediatric dentists, with approximately 16 more in training in the state, to care for them.

As altruistic as they may be, oral health care providers often find themselves lacking knowledge, techniques, and networks to simultaneously manage the dental, medical, and behavioral aspects of care for children with SHCNs. Dentists frequently refer pediatric patients and patients with complex conditions to the University of Minnesota's pediatric dental clinic—one of only 3 hospital-based clinics in the state. **Figure 1** provides a graphic description of our wicked problem.

3. Methods

3.1 Background and context

The goal of the MinnieMouths project was to build interdisciplinary dental homes for children with SHCNs to provide quality care within communities where families live and thrive and capture the process so others could replicate our efforts in their communities. Our intervention incorporated principles from Project ECHO (Extension for Community Healthcare Outcomes), a model for lifelong medical learning and collaborative practice that links primary care physicians with specialist care teams to deliver quality treatment to patients with complex chronic conditions. The ECHO model is recognized nationally and internationally and was selected as one of the top solutions in the MacArthur Foundation 100&Change competition. The ECHO Institute at the University of New Mexico has established a process for groups to start or replicate the program and train in methods important to implementing an ECHO project. There is no fee for becoming a replication partner or to start an ECHO program.

Project ECHO breaks down the walls between specialty and primary care. It links expert specialist teams at an academic 'hub' with primary care clinicians in local communities who are the 'spokes' of the model. Together, they participate in regular sessions called clinics, which are like virtual grand rounds, and include mentoring and patient case presentations. The clinics are supported by teleconferencing technology. During the clinics, healthcare providers from multiple sites have educational sessions, share information, present patient cases, discuss new developments relating to their patients, and review treatment options and determine plans. (https://echo.unm.edu/about-echo/model/).

3.1.1 MinnieMouths infrastructure

The University of Minnesota was certified as our ECHO replication site and was also a source for some of our content experts such as pediatric dentists, pediatricians, psychologists, and other professionals with expertise in caring for children with SHCNs. The Minnesota Academy of Pediatric Dentistry facilitated access to Minnesota's pediatric community from which we could draw content experts. As our work unfolded, we also drew upon the expertise of experts across the country.

The MinnieMouths project team consisted of 1) the Clinical Scholars-enrolled leadership team of Peter Scal, MD, MPH (pediatrician); Mark DeRuiter, PhD, MBA (audiologist), and Jeffrey Karp, DMD, MS (pediatric dentist), and non-Clinical Scholars community-based extended team members: 2) a family navigator; family navigators are parents of children with SHCNs trained to partner with health care providers and community leaders, and 3) two Community Health Workers.

Our final piece of infrastructure was the establishment of video capabilities in the communities and practices of core participants, enabling them to participate in teleECHO clinics, not to see actual patients but to have structured educational sessions, receive information on forming community-based dental homes for children with SHCNs, discuss barriers and ways to overcome them, present and learn from case studies, and discuss best and emerging practices among all participants.

3.1.2 Approach

We pursued several methods in four phases to build a dental home network within Minnesota and beyond.

3.1.2.1 Start-up phase

Our initial step in planning the development of a dental homes network focused on children with SHCNs was to meet with diverse stakeholders across Minnesota and throughout the country to understand gaps in care, community knowledge, and provider confidence in providing care to children with SHCNs. Our formative meetings consisted of open-ended discussions with parents of children with SHCNs, family advocacy and health non-profits, pediatric healthcare providers, state-appointed leaders in developmental and physical disabilities, dental professionals (including many pediatric dentists), private dental insurance and government-supported Medicaid plan administrators, academicians working in interdisciplinary health team environments, and leaders of health professional associations. The team analyzed findings from our stakeholder conversations and developed a Driver Diagram, available in the Toolkit for Building a Dental Home Network for Children with Special Health Care Needs.

One of our early actions was to establish a Project ECHO replication site at the University of Minnesota's School of Dentistry. To our knowledge, this was the first Project ECHO site focused on dental care needs of children with SHCNs. In keeping with the Project ECHO model, the MinnieMouths project did not provide direct care to patients but instead provided front-line clinicians with the knowledge and support they needed to manage patients with complex conditions within the patients' communities, dramatically increasing access to the specialized dental care required by children with SHCNs. The leadership team also partnered with the University of Minnesota Continuing Dental Education (CDE) program who supported our efforts by drafting an online and social media presence, providing outreach materials, and planning network events that introduced the MinnieMouths project to a range of oral health professionals, and managing providing continuing education credits to participants and speakers.

We analyzed the current status of dental homes capacity within Minnesota and nationally, conducted a literature review, and refocused our project hypothesis. To ensure we understood the concepts of Project ECHO, the leadership team completed Project ECHO training and patient tracking management through the American Academy of Pediatrics. Next we determined suitable partners for our long-term project. We selected and contracted with Family Voices of Minnesota for our Family Navigators and the Minnesota Community Health Worker Alliance for Community Health Workers.

We extended invitations to 10,000 licensed professionals throughout Minnesota via LinkedIn, Facebook, personal connections, and a MailChimp email campaign to establish a viable group of core participants at the community level. Our goal was to recruit a minimum of 25 professionals who were interested in improving oral health care services for children with SHCNs and could/would attend monthly teleECHO clinics via videoconference links. Simultaneously, we prepared curricula, lined up content experts for the teleECHO clinics, and invited interested healthcare providers and stakeholders to participate as guest attendees and presenters.

3.1.2.2 Phase 1: practicing clinicians

In Phase 1, we targeted practicing providers to participate in a pilot Peer Telementoring Network using the teleECHO clinics model from Project ECHO. We launched an interdisciplinary telementoring and case-based learning network with monthly teleECHO clinics to educate dental professionals and health care providers about establishing dental homes for children with SHCNs within their communities. We integrated community health workers (CHWs) and family navigators into the network to provide insights on cultural competency, family communications, and unique approaches to delivering care within underserved communities. A typical teleECHO clinic included a guest presentation related to barriers in providing care and dental homes for children with SHCN, two case studies, a robust discussion among the attendees regarding the cases and barriers presented, and a conversation regarding resources available to mitigate common obstacles. Once we completed the series of monthly teleECHO clinics, we evaluated the results and began planning for Phase 2.

Figure 2 shows the interdisciplinary network of health care providers who engaged in Phase 1. Note that Phase I had a higher percentage of dental providers, seasoned practitioners who gave informal input on the structure of the ECHO sessions and telementoring in general.

3.1.2.3 Phase 2: next generation scholars

Phase 2 was similar to Phase 1 in that we launched a second interdisciplinary Project ECHO telementoring and case-based learning network via monthly teleECHO clinics, this time focused on educating future and new-to-practice dental students and residents, medical students and residents, and new-to-practice dental and medical professionals. The goal of Phase 2 was to expand young scholars' desire and ability to establish dental homes for children with SHCNs within their future or new-care practices. Family navigators were again integrated into the teleECHO clinics to provide insights on cultural competency, family communications, and unique approaches to delivering care within underserved communities. Each clinic included a presentation related to barriers and ideas in providing care and dental homes to children with

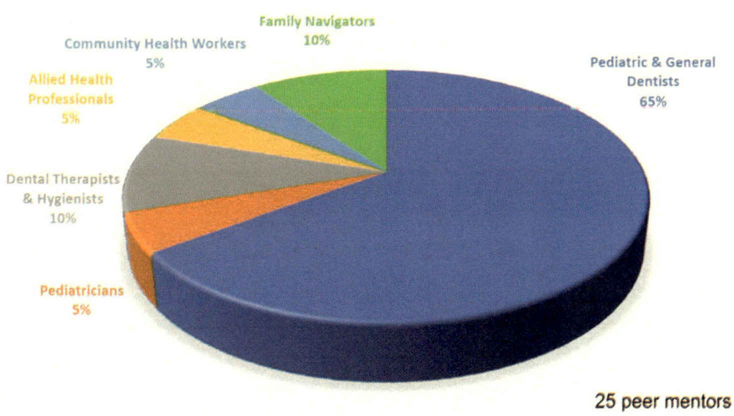

Figure 2.
Interdisciplinary network of healthcare providers (by percent) who engaged in phase I.

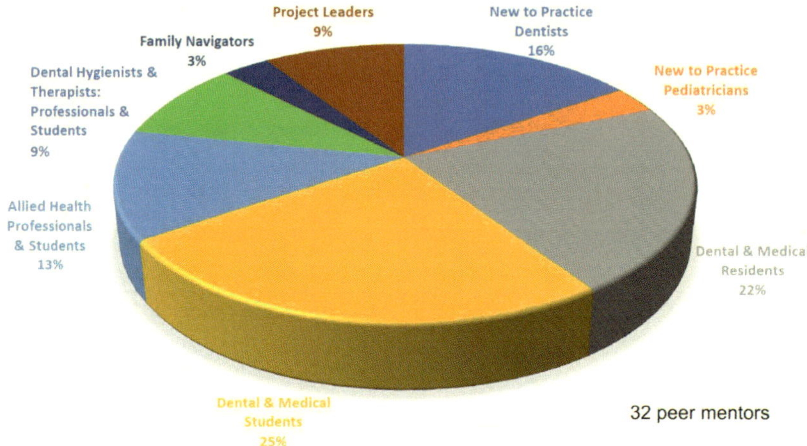

Figure 3.
Percentage of different providers-in-training who attended teleECHO clinics in phase 2.

SHCNs, one case study, a robust discussion among the attendees regarding the cases and barriers presented, and a conversation regarding resources available to mitigate common obstacles. We repeated the cycle of teleECHO clinics, and at the close of the cycle, we again evaluated perceptions of the participants and made plans for the future and for sustainability of the dental homes program.

Figure 3 provides the percentage of different providers-in-training who attended the ECHO sessions.

3.1.2.4 Sustainability phase

Based on findings of the two phases and related research, the leadership team developed a conference focused on building dental homes for children with SHCNs. The conference aimed to expand the network of providers who see the merit in establishing dental homes within their communities, including rural and underserved communities. The meeting included an overview of the national landscape, essentials for expanding the Project ECHO program, critical insights from parents of children with SHCNs, and a presentation of non-profits and organizations that serve children with SHCNs and have the interest in collaborating with providers.

In addition, we built a Dental Homes Network Field Guide for Providers (available to those who attended our in-person conference), a Toolkit for Building a Dental Home Network for Children with Special Health Care needs, disseminated project findings online through professional networks, communicated with the nearly 18,000 professionals who view the Continuing Dental Education website each month, established a Telementoring Study Club, and initiated efforts to update and modernize dental provider directories to enable easy identification of providers who serve children with SHCNs.

4. Results

4.1 Start-up

- Established our team's infrastructure, built the project team, and in conjunction with the ECHO Institute at the University of New Mexico, established the School of Dentistry at the University of Minnesota as a Project ECHO replication, the first project ECHO site focused on oral health care for children with special healthcare needs

- Established continuing dental education credits program for various participants

- Analyzed the current status of dental homes capacity within Minnesota and nationally, conducted a literature review, and refocused our project hypothesis

4.2 Phase 1: practicing clinicians

- Conducted 7 monthly teleECHO clinics involving 28 core participants, parents of children with SHCN, policy influencers, and mentors

- Evaluated treatment, case management infrastructure, and clinical outcomes of ~14 children with SHCNs presented during TeleECHO clinics

- Awarded 180 Continuing Education Units to participants

- Launched a Facebook group to provide a social environment for core participants to meet and engage professionally

- Gauged initial impact of our wicked project idea against the prevailing knowledge found in literature

- Evaluated perceptions of practicing clinicians to assess change in knowledge and comfort in providing oral health services for children with SHCNs

4.3 Phase 2: next generation clinicians

- Launched teleECHO clinic focused on preparing and mentoring new-to-practice providers, and students: dental, dental hygiene, dental therapy, as well as dental and medical residents (Next Generation Scholars) to better understand oral health care for children with SHCNs

- Recruited and trained 32 Next Generation Scholars

- Conducted 11 clinics

- Evaluated treatment, case management infrastructure, and clinical outcomes of ~10 children with SHCNs presented during clinics

- Evaluated perceptions of Next Generation Scholars to assess change in knowledge and comfort in providing oral health services for children with SHCNs

- Initiated planning for May 2019 conference focused on providing oral healthcare for children with SHCNs

4.4 Sustainability phase

- Evaluated project and project participants' perceptions of the ongoing need for dental home engagement efforts

- Re-engaged stakeholders in long-term planning

- Distributed project findings (See below section on outcomes)
- Engaged additional family navigators to expand the reach of oral health educational materials and awareness of dental home network into communities
- Developed learning experiences for Next Generation Scholars to spend time with children with SHCNs in their homes, schools, and during care provider visits
- In April 2019, established the Telementoring Study Club, an optional, informal case-based discussion open to students, residents, and practicing clinicians across health disciplines
- Initiated project to update and modernize dental provider directories in the state, with an emphasis on being able to identify clinicians who provide services for children with SHCNs
- Hosted May 2019 conference focused on providing care for children with SHCNs, including four marquee speakers, scholar presentation posters, a parent panel, and an overview of the next phase of our project
- 193 people attended the 2019 Conference which met our expectations
- Launched toolkit of information focused on expanding dental homes for children with SHCNs, with essentials of reimbursement as one element of this offering; toolkit can be found [https://clinicalscholarsnli.org/community-impact]

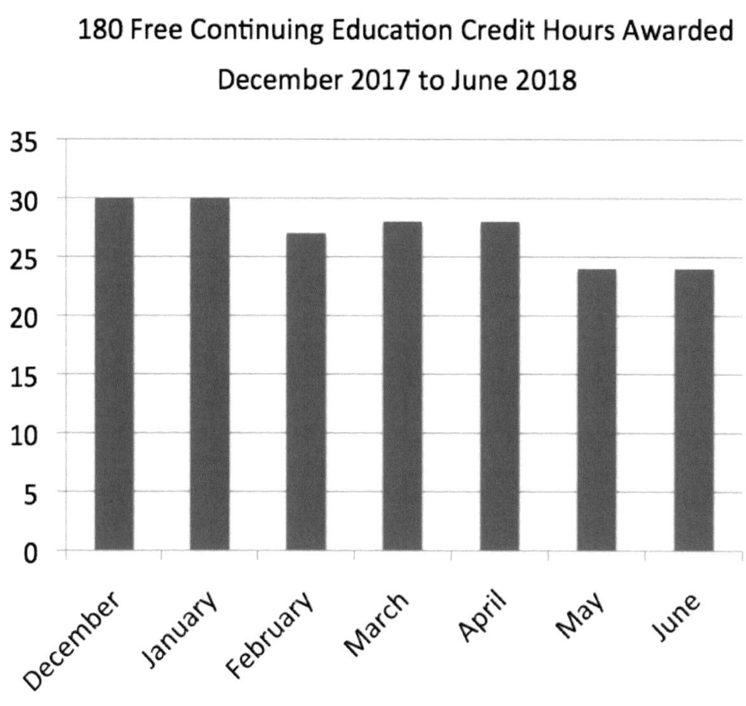

Figure 4.
Number of continuing dental education units awarded by month in phase I of the project.

4.5 Outcomes

Multiple measurable outcomes resulted from our work; here we report on two we consider important: points of contact and continuing dental education units awarded. **Figures 4** and **5** provide information regarding the number of dental CEUs awarded in Phases 1 and 2, respectively.

The more than 1500 credit hours awarded in a span of approximately 18 months demonstrates the strong investment from people who participated in the teleECHO clinics and those who participated face-to-face.

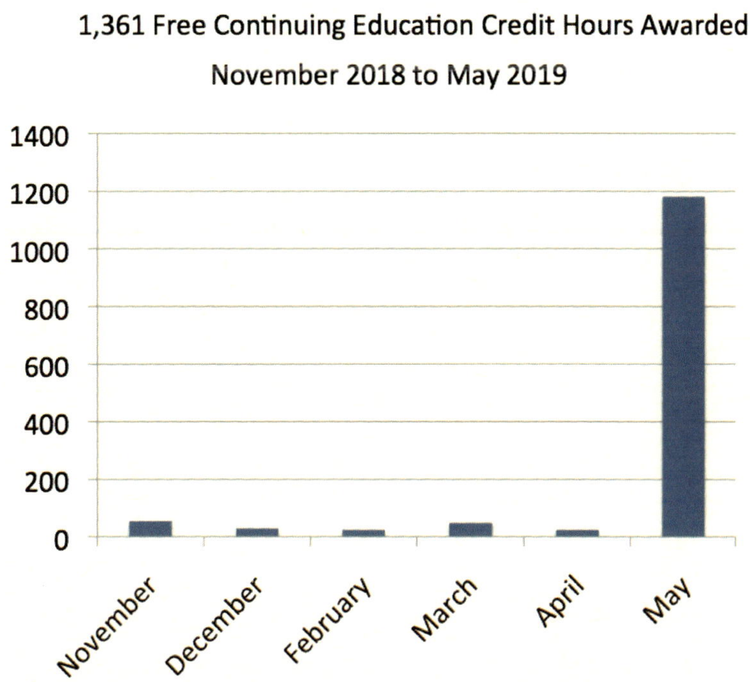

Figure 5.
Number of continuing dental education (CDE) units awarded by month in phase II of the project [note: May 2019 represents CDE units from initial conference].

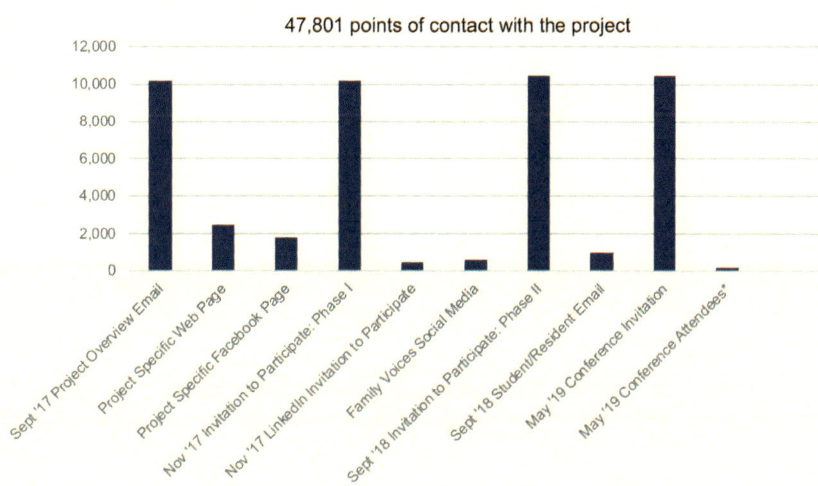

Figure 6.
Points of contact with the project from September 2017 through May 2019.

We measured our overall points of contact in the project during Phases 1 and 2. **Figure 6** provides data on different points of contact we tracked over the time course of the project.

During approximately 18 months, we recorded more than 47,000 different points of contact with the community. Contacts included dental providers, allied health providers, students, and many others. Some of the points of contact were targeted emails, and others were from Facebook followers and web pages designed specifically for the project.

5. Discussion

The wicked problem we chose to address is complex and multi-faceted. The resulting MinnieMouths project had multiple elements and a broad impact. Project team leaders completed their work in a three-year time period, while maintaining clinical positions and engaging in leadership training. Work in this project was specifically designed to be collaborative and interdisciplinary, a way of work that is time consuming but extremely effective and rewarding in the long run.

Our collaboration with a wide range of providers revealed multiple areas that must be addressed to realize the vision of a comprehensive dental home network for children with SHCNs, not only in Minnesota, but also nation-wide.

- Providers who care for children with SHCNs (and those who would if conditions changed) are constrained by limited information on insurance reimbursement codes, time management, allowable payments, and other aspects of the current system of reimbursement.

- Providers have great difficulty in managing the range of co-morbidities and complex cases of children with SHCNs. Training provided to healthcare professionals must include 1) ways to implement the dental homes concept in local communities, 2) simultaneous development of medical homes in underserved and rural communities, and 3) sufficient integration of medical and dental services to allow for comprehensive care across the life span. An expansion of the current project could be an exploration of a combined community-based health care dental and medical home concept for children and adults with special healthcare needs.

- While some oral health and medical care providers have confidence in providing care to children with SHCNs, many do not. Ensuring providers have access to no-cost peer networks where they can ask questions, share concerns, and seek insider tips is essential.

- Families of children with SHCNs often feel negated in their views regarding oral health care, approaches to providing care for their children, and are uncomfortable discussing Medicaid and insurance concerns. Organizations such as Family Voices of Minnesota must continue to work collaboratively with the care community and insurance groups to address ongoing concerns and innovations in care provision.

6. Leader learning

The three program leaders found a range of health equity skills to be imperative when addressing the oral health care of children with SHCNs. Two capabilities that stand out among the three leaders include fostering cross-sector collaboration and strengthening the integration of health services and systems.

The overarching goal of our project was to test whether an interdisciplinary network of oral health care, medical care, allied health, and community partners could begin building sustainable dental homes for children with SHCNs, and to identify aspects that would make the effort successful. Our ability to partner early and receive training on Project ECHO and its telementoring philosophy provided a foundation for what we valued throughout the program. We learned that true cross-sector collaboration occurs only when professionals appreciate each other's ideas and recommendations for care, when families' and community partners' viewpoints are shared at the beginning of programs and threaded throughout experiences, and when young scholars' points of views and desire to develop career-long expertise are regarded as vital.

We learned reimbursement was a common theme and the central challenge among current and well-intentioned future providers. When faced with the reality that Medicaid covers most children with SHCNs, and state and federal funds will, at best, cover 27 to 42 percent of billed costs, the financial solvency of dentists and those who support them quickly comes into question. Many oral health care providers who expressed interest in and have adequate training to provide care to children with SHCNs are limited by their ability to remain financially solvent in the face of current reimbursement systems. We found the future of the project and expanding dental homes for children with special health care needs lies primarily within the purview of policymakers, insurers, and federal funding sources.

We believe fostering cross-sector collaboration and strengthening the integration of health services and systems provides fodder for future projects and grants and requires building relationships with policymakers and funding sources.

7. Toolkit

A comprehensive toolkit can be found at: https://clinicalscholarsnli.org/community-impact.

Author details

Mark DeRuiter[1], Jeffrey Karp[2*] and Peter Scal[2]

1 University of Arizona, Arizona, United States

2 University of Minnesota, Minnesota, United States

*Address all correspondence to: jmkarp@umn.edu

References

[1] U.S. Dept of Health and Human Services. Oral health in America: A report of the Surgeon General. Rockville, Md.: U.S. Dept of Health and Human Services, National Institute of Dental and Craniofacial Research, National Institutes of Health; 2000.

[2] U.S. Census Bureau. Disability Characteristics. 2010 American Community Survey 1-Year Estimates S1810. Available at: "http://factfinder.census.gov/faces/table services/jsf/pages/productview.xhtml?pid=ACS_14_5YR_ DP02&src=pt". Accessed September 24, 2018.

[3] Newacheck PW, McManus M, Fox HB, Hung YY, Halfon N. Access to health care for children with special health care needs. Pediatrics 2000;105 (4 Pt 1):760-766.

[4] American Academy of Pediatric Dentistry. Definition of special health care needs. Pediatr Dent 2016;38(special issue):16.

[5] Thikkurissy S, Lal S. Oral health burden in children with systemic disease. Dent Clin North Am 2009;53(2): 351-357, xi.

[6] Charles JM. Dental care in children with developmental disabilities: attention deficit disorder, intellectual disabilities, and autism. J Dent Child 2010;77(2):84-91.

[7] U.S. Dept of Justice. Americans with Disabilities Act of 1990, as Amended. Available at: "http://www.ada.gov/publicat.htm." Accessed September 4, 2018.

[8] Rouleau T, Harrington A, Brennan M, et al. Receipt of dental care barriers encountered by persons with disabilities. Spec Care Dentist 2011;31(2):63-67.

[9] Lewis C, Robertson AS, Phelps S. Unmet dental care needs among children with special health care needs: Implications for the medical home. Pediatrics 2005;116(3): e426-e431.

[10] Callahan ST, Cooper WO. Continuity of health insurance coverage among young adults with disabilities. Pediatrics 2007;119(6):1175-1180.

[11] Kaiser Family Foundation. Medicaid's role for children with special health care needs: A look at eligibility, services, and spending. Available at: http://files.kff.org/attachment/Medicaid%E2%80%99s-Role-for-Children-with-Special-Health-Care-Needs-A-Look-at-Eligibility,-Services-and-Spending. Accessed December 10, 2019.

[12] Chen AY, Newacheck PW. Insurance coverage and financial burden for families of children with special health care needs. Ambul Pediatr 2006;6(4):204-209.

[13] Shenkin JD, Davis MJ, Corbin SB. The oral health of special needs children: Dentistry's challenge to provide care. J Dent Child 2001;86(3):201-205.

[14] Barnett ML. The oral-systemic disease connection. An update for the practicing dentist. J Am Dent Assoc 2006; 137(suppl 10):5S-6S.

[15] Krause M, Vainio L, Zwetchkenbaum S, Inglehart MR. Dental education about patients with special needs: A survey of US and Canadian dental schools. J Dent Educ 2010;74(11):1179-1189.

[16] American Academy of Pediatric Dentistry. Policy on dental home.

Pediatr Dent 2016;38(special issue):25-26.

[17] U.S. Department of Health and Human Services, Health Resources and Services Administration, Maternal and Child Health Bureau. The National Survey of Children with Special Health Care Needs Chartbook 2009-2010. Rockville, Maryland: U.S. Department of Health and Human Services, 2013.

Chapter 7

Oral Health in Communities and Neighborhoods (OHICAN) Pilot Project: The Burden of Poor Oral Health

Charles E. Moore, Hope Bussenius and David Reznik

Abstract

Poor oral health afflicts many low-income and other vulnerable populations. Lack of access to oral health can lead to unnecessary tooth decay, periodontal disease, pain, and the advancement of oral cancer. The absence of preventive care often leads to unnecessary and expensive visits to hospital-based emergency departments to address the pain of dental disease but not the causal conditions. The consequences on inequitable access to dental care are significant for individuals, families and communities. The OHICAN pilot project looked to address the lack of equitable access to care by creating new points of access, training medical providers to perform oral exams and apply fluoride when indicated, thus increasing the oral health workforce, utilizing technology to bridge clinical practice, education, training and research, educating stakeholders to allow dental hygienists to provide preventive care under general supervision, and creating business models that will assist others who seek to create a dental home for those they serve. Social, political and economic forces all contribute to varying degrees in terms of equity in healthcare. The work of OHICAN was designed to create a blueprint for potential solutions to these issues in order to foster oral health equity. Changes to improve access to dental care can take place in a relatively short period of time when all who care and are impacted by this continued unmet oral health need work together.

Keywords: oral health, business plan, app, marginalized communities, dental, non-traditional provider, school-based clinic

1. Introduction

Poor oral health afflicts many low-income and vulnerable populations with wide disparities in untreated tooth decay, other oral diseases, and days of restricted activity for children [1]. Untreated tooth decay and tooth loss for adults is significantly higher in low-income groups and racial minority populations compared with their higher-income and non-Hispanic white counterparts [1]. The OHICAN pilot project seeks to address the vast inequities in access to oral health care for marginalized, low-resourced, and minority communities by creating a comprehensive oral health network designed to increase access to preventive and restorative dental care in Georgia.

The Centers for Disease Control and Prevention (CDC) reports that one in three children aged 2 through 5 in families with incomes below $10,000 experienced at least one decayed tooth that had not been treated [1]. In contrast, only 1 in 10 preschool children in families with incomes of $35,000 or higher had untreated caries [1]. The CDC indicates this disparity rate is true for teenagers and adults as well.

Oral health is important for many reasons. Untreated caries can lead to problems with eating, speaking, and attending to learning in children, and work attendance in adults [1]. Untreated caries and periodontal (gum) disease will lead to tooth loss. CDC survey data show low-income adults suffer more severe tooth loss than their wealthier counterparts [1, 2]. Adults in families earning less than $15,000 per year were more than 2-1/2 times as likely to have lost six or more teeth from decay or gum disease as adults in families earning $35,000 or more [1].

A 2014 Georgia Department of Public Health report outlines the following dental health disparities in Georgia [3]:

- "The prevalence of tooth decay among children with low socioeconomic status (SES) is 50% higher than the prevalence of tooth decay among children with high SES."
- "The proportion of non-Hispanic Black and Hispanic high school students who visit an emergency room (ER) or urgent care center for oral or dental problems (10.3% each) is twice the proportion of non-Hispanic white high school students who visit an ER for the same problems (4.9%)."
- "Adults earning $50,000 or more per year are significantly more likely to visit a dentist than adults with income less than $15,000 a year (85% vs. 39%)."

These disparities contribute to poor dental health outcomes in the state of Georgia. The Georgia Department of Public Health has identified the following five dental outcomes in Georgia that need to improve [3]:

1. The presence of dental caries in young children age 2-5 years and children in 3rd grade
2. Untreated dental decay
3. Sealant on molars
4. Early detection of oral and pharyngeal cancers
5. Oropharyngeal cancer mortality

Frequently cited barriers to improving the oral health disparities and achieving Georgia's target outcomes include a shortage of dentists in areas of the state, unwillingness of dentists to participate in Medicaid due to low reimbursement rates and perceived high no-show rates, limited adult Medicaid dental benefits, cost of care, and unresolved patient education issues. These barriers contribute to a lack of access to oral health care in low income communities throughout the state.

Beyond the public health consequences of poor oral health are outcomes that affect the financial, educational, and workforce aspects of families and communities. This can lead to a self-reinforcing cycle that prevents families from improving their socioeconomic status and overall quality of life.

1. Studies have found that toothaches are the number one reason for school absence. Toothaches are given as a reason for school absence seven times more than asthma [4, 5]. Missed school days limit a student's access to education and education outcomes are essential to moving out of low-income status.

2. Parents miss work when their child cannot attend school due to toothaches, which limits their ability to earn income on those days [6]. Missed productivity of workers also affects the companies and businesses that employ them.

3. The Health Disparities Report 2008 indicates that Fulton County, Georgia had 35,292 preventable visits to the Emergency Room (ER).[1] Nine thousand of these visits every year are for non-traumatic dental conditions. ER visits are the most expensive form of oral healthcare. Regretfully, ERs are not set up to provide the dental care needed to address the emergency, and patients leave with prescriptions for pain medications and antibiotics, the appropriateness of which is in question. A reduction in these preventable healthcare costs would greatly improve the financial stability of Grady Hospital and other ERs that see a large percentage of uninsured patients.

Poor oral health can lead to unnecessary tooth decay, periodontal disease, pain, and even the quiet and deadly advancement of oral cancer [7]. It also leads to unnecessary and expensive visits to hospital-based ERs to address the pain of dental disease but not the causal conditions. Finding ways to improve oral health in low-income communities is essential to good health and helps individuals move from poverty to middle class status. Improving oral health requires a collaborative effort of a diverse array of health care workers to ensure equitable outcomes that lead to overall health.

2. Wicked problem impact project (WPIP) description

Poor oral health in low income communities is a wicked problem that inflicts significant burdens on children and adults alike. The communities in which we work continue to have wide disparities in untreated tooth decay and restricted activity days for children. The lack of trained providers who can address these problems from both a definitive treatment approach and a preventive perspective is at the heart of the issue. The need for increased oral health literacy among people of all generations throughout the state adds to the disparity. To help close existing gaps in care, knowledge of oral health and disease needs to be incorporated into the fabric of the healthcare system (ie, healthcare professionals who are not in the dental health field) across the lifespan.

OHICAN is a pilot project in which we seek to increase access to oral health services and improve community knowledge on the importance of preventive oral health care in three low income and minority neighborhoods in Atlanta. Our intent is to work locally to demonstrate what can be done and deploy the successes and products nationally and internationally. The OHICAN program is composed of the following initiatives:

[1] More information on the 2008 Georgia Health Disparities Report can be found here: https://dph.georgia.gov/sites/dph.georgia.gov/files/related_files/site_page/Georgia%20Health%20Equity%20Initiative.pdf.

- increasing community knowledge of preventive oral care
- expanding existing oral health care capacity in local communities (includes training and education initiatives and incorporating oral health into care protocols for medical care providers)
- creating new points of access
- advocating on behalf of evidence-based methods to expand care and lower costs
- rolling out/disseminating results of the OHICAN project and transitioning it to an initiative for deployment nationally and internationally

Several key messages recur throughout this work and in this chapter:

- Individuals cannot be healthy without good oral health.
- Technology can be used to bridge clinical practice, education and training, research, and health policy.
- Integrating medical and dental efforts will increase access to preventive care.
- Changes to improve access to dental care can take place in a relatively short period of time when all who care about and are impacted by this continued unmet oral health need work together.

3. Methods

3.1 Context and background

The Oral Health in Communities and Neighborhoods (OHICAN) project is part of the Urban Health Initiative (UHI) at Emory University in Atlanta, Georgia. The geographic area for project development and implementation was three zip codes in Atlanta, Georgia—30311, 30314, and 30318. Leadership for the OHICAN project was provided by an interdisciplinary team from the Robert Wood Johnson Clinical Scholars program and supported by numerous community and academic partners. Our immediate goal was to increase access to oral health services in three target low income and minority neighborhoods in the Atlanta area. Our longer term goal was to develop a blueprint of solutions including documented approaches/ways of work, tools, and resources that could be expanded into a program for addressing poor oral health in communities and neighborhoods outside the project area.

3.2 Approach

Impetus for the OHICAN project came from a 2013 community needs assessment (CNA) done by Dr. Moore and the Emory Rollins School of Public Health faculty, staff and students in a marginalized community of West Atlanta composed of zip codes 30311, 30314 and 30318. According to the West Atlanta Oral Health Community Needs Assessment, lack of equitable access to care was among the top reasons for poor oral health in underserved and other vulnerable populations.

3.2.1 Values guiding our work.

Our values included (1) health equity, (2) cultural sensitivity and relevancy, (3) products we developed would be empowering, easy to use, informative, and self-gratifying, (4) our work would bridge education and training, clinical practice, research, and health policy, and be provided at no cost to users, (5) reflect a desire to serve multiple elements of the healthcare system such as providers and students, patients and families, stakeholders, and partners.

3.2.2 Starting point

Our initial step was to perform a needs assessment in our three target zip codes. We engaged students from the Emory University Rollins School of Public Health to work with our team. Together, we prepared the needs assessment using their expertise combined with information gleaned from interviewing patients, providers, and members of the community we planned to serve. The CNA was based on the OHIP-14 guidelines. The assessments were through in-person interviews using a digital platform. There were also focus groups led by experienced public health professionals that contributed to the knowledge obtained.

In addition to confirming results of the 2013 CNA, our assessments pointed out the need to involve and engage local community members and partner with other individuals and organizations with interests in oral health and whose work aligned with our goals. We formed a community advisory board (CAB) composed of people representing the diversity of the community from faith-based, private and public including non-profit organizations. Additionally, individuals with an interest in oral health that resided in the community were included in this CAB. The age span was from 16 to 74 with primarily female representation.

We expanded our team to include partners from non-profits, public health organizations, business, professional associations, and universities. Our working group included the leadership team of Charles Moore MD, David Reznik DDS, and Hope Bussenius DNP; the Community Advisory Board (CAB); and the partner organizations shown below.

- Georgia Center for Nonprofits
- Emory Rollins School of Public Health
- Emory Business School
- Georgia State School of Public Health
- Emory Urban Health Initiative
- Emory School of Nursing
- NYU – Langone Advanced Education in General Dentistry Residency Program
- Georgia Department of Public Health
- Georgia Dental Hygiene Association
- Georgia Dental Association

3.2.3 Establishing ways of work

Once we had information from community needs assessments, we partnered with the Georgia Center for Nonprofits to develop a strategic plan. We determined who we serve, impacts on those we serve, indicators of success, strategies and key actions, funding strategies, community engagement strategies, key actions, and our next steps.

The strategic plan served as the basis for a monitoring and evaluation plan, which we jointly developed with students from the Emory Rollins School of Public Health. The plan included our program goal, objectives, specific sub-activities, process and output indicators, baseline data, target data, source of data collection and means of verification, frequency of data collection, and responsible team members. In year two of the project, we modified the monitoring and evaluation plan with assistance of the Robert Wood Johnson Foundation Clinical Scholars Evaluation team.

We adopted essentially two modes of work. The first mode was personal contact. Examples of activities included building relationships, delivering hands-on trainings in oral health screening and preventive care, working with the CAB and our partner organizations, collaborating with professional organizations and universities, advocating for and supporting evidence-based methods to expand care and lower its cost, engaging medical care providers in our efforts, serving on boards relevant to our goals, providing lectures and presentations to appropriate audiences, and writing articles and publishing them in peer-reviewed journals.

To expand the reach of our personal contact work, we incorporated technology solutions to broaden the scope of our innovative changes and make them transformative and sustainable. We explored various transformative healthcare models that included technology-based solutions and focused on creating innovative change at the system level, but found none that embraced the values we espoused. Therefore, we decided to incorporate the values stated above in our development of technology-based interventions. We called our approach the 2 Transformative Technology Evaluation and Assessment Model or 2TEAM.

We employed both modes of work (personal contact and technology) in addressing the five OHICAN initiatives:

- increasing community knowledge of preventive oral care
- expanding existing oral health care capacity in local communities (includes training and education initiatives and incorporating oral health into care protocols for medical care providers)
- creating new points of access
- advocating on behalf of evidence-based methods to expand care and lower costs
- rolling out/disseminating results, outcomes, and accomplishments of the OHICAN project and transitioning it to an initiative for deployment nationally and internationally

3.2.4 Increasing community knowledge of preventive oral health care

Personal contact work in this area included (1) educating our CAB of the importance of oral healthcare; (2) developing and conducting a dental provider needs assessment; (3) engaging our CAB in discussions regarding best ways to increase community knowledge and seeking their input and feedback on plans, activities, and educational brochures; (4) work with local medical providers to increase their willingness and capability to incorporate basic dental preventive education into their patient encounters, and learn the appropriateness of knowing when more extensive dental care was needed; (5) developing a brochure called OHICAN in which we introduced ourselves and the OHICAN program, listed service locations, services available, contact information, defined who was eligible to access the services, and provided facts and information about oral healthcare. We had 750 copies of the OHICAN brochure printed and distributed to schools and community organizations in the target area. At these events, we measured the baseline level of knowledge of the respondents then had a brief educational intervention followed by a post survey. These educational interventions to raise community awareness were done in-person. Additional information was provided to the participants through a brochure that also directed the reader to the OHICAN website discussed below.

We developed two technology-based solutions that contribute to increasing community knowledge of preventive oral care. One was a culturally sensitive website (https://ohican.org/) to improve communication and provide information on free resources and local opportunities for dental care. The brochure discussed above is on the website.

The second technology-based solution is a smartphone app (OH-I-CAN) available for download on the website. The phone app has two questionnaires, the OHIP (Oral Health Impact Profile) and the ECOHIS (Early Childhood Oral Health Impact Scale). The OHIP measures people's perceptions of the impact of oral health disorders on their well-being and includes questions regarding dysfunction, discomfort, disability, and handicap resulting from oral health conditions. The ECOHIS measures the quality of oral health-related quality-of-life of preschool children and their families. Both questionnaires are culturally sensitive, easy to use, and self-gratifying because they provide immediate results to improve the health of the individual(s) entering data.

3.2.5 Expanding existing oral health care capacity in local communities

Addressing the need for increased literacy about the importance of oral health is only part of a comprehensive solution. Once people are aware, they need places to go to obtain dental care. Lack of adequate capacity to care for populations in low income and minority areas is a major issue [7, 8]. Personal contact work we did to expand dental health care capacity included (1) identifying, engaging, and training non-traditional dental care providers to perform oral exams and apply fluoride when indicated; (2) training providers to be aware of the requisite steps to address oral health issues and enhance preventive oral health measures in communities (approximately 1000 non-dental healthcare professionals were educated and trained in this area); (3) educating hygienists of recent changes in licensing laws that allow their profession to provide preventive care under general supervision; (4) educating stakeholders (primarily dentists) of the implications of the changes in dental hygienists' practice laws (approximately 325 dentists were educated in this area); (5) supporting implementation efforts for the expanded role for hygienists; and (6) integrating medical and dental efforts to increase access to preventive care.

We used technology to extend the reach of our in-person intervention efforts, primarily through the development of the OHICAN website. The website has educational tools for providers, training modules, provider protocols, videos, a toolkit and other resources, and connects to a metadata repository that gathers information from the quality of life questionnaires on the smartphone app. Using the repository database, providers can examine the oral health-related quality of life of individual patients at discrete points or review an individual patient's status over time. As the repository builds and appropriate safeguards are put in place, providers can compare results with others on national and international levels. The repository will enable providers and researchers to uncover information including hidden patterns, unknown correlations, and customer/patient preferences that can help providers make better-informed clinical decisions. The app, repository, and database will also allow for population-based studies revealing need(s) based on zip code, age, illness, and other parameters.

3.2.6 Creating new points of access

Another way to increase community capacity for providing dental care is to create new points of access. To this end, we (1) partnered with dental residency programs to expand the number of residents at existing sites and establish new ones; (2) worked to establish and support new dental clinics in marginalized neighborhoods; (3) supported the establishment of oral health programs at school-based health centers; and (4) supported efforts to attract dental practices and practitioners to areas with high unmet needs.

Establishing oral health practices can be quite expensive. To aid practitioners and stakeholders in determining financial requirements for establishing new points of access in underserved areas of Georgia, we engaged the Office of Business Practice Improvement, Emory University's Internal Consulting Group, to develop an oral health business plan. The model includes specific service and staffing costs, unreimbursed costs (time for client education, team meetings, referral coordination, training of staff), and supply and technology costs. Any new program or practice must be fiscally sound, therefore our model allows the consideration of costs, identification of payment opportunities, and development of cost containment strategies. The business model allows for an individual or practice to accurately apply the conditions of their unique environment and elicit the costs of running a program within that environment. The financial model also includes cost projections based on volumes and projected revenue, and can provide pro-forma financial statements to give an idea of how the actual statement would look if the underlying assumptions hold true. The interactive business plan is available on the OHICAN website.

3.2.7 Advocating on behalf of evidence-based methods to expand care and lower costs

Throughout our team's project, we personally engaged in advocacy efforts at the individual, regional, state, and national levels to build support for our program. One example was our work in supporting the Dental Hygiene General Supervision for Preventive Care Bill. It was passed into law on January 1, 2018 with the goal of increasing access to preventive oral health care for children and adults in under-resourced areas. In collaboration with the Georgia Dental hygiene Association, Georgia Dental Association, and Eunice Chay, DMD, MPH from the Grady Health System Advance Education in General Dentistry Residency (AEGD) program, we created an implementation toolkit to assist providers in both public and private sectors implement the law. Dr. Reznik from the OHICAN team continues to serve as chair of the general supervision implementation subcommittee, and all three of the OHICAN team leaders are board members of the Georgia Oral Health Coalition.

On the OHICAN website, we included a tab specifically for advocacy in which we post relevant articles, white papers, and other items of interest to advocates. Additionally, the Toolkit for Incorporating General Supervision in Dental Private Practice and Safety Net Settings in Georgia, a product of our collaboration with Dr. Chay, is available on the website.

3.2.8 Rolling out/disseminating results of the OHICAN pilot project and transitioning it to an initiative for deployment nationally and internationally

We employed both in-person and technological methods in rolling out and disseminating the results of the OHICAN project. We designed and implemented a social media roll out (Facebook, Twitter, Instagram) to share information about OHICAN and its purpose and uses, results, and tools. A critical part of dissemination included educating medical providers (physicians, nurse practitioners, physician assistants, nurses) and oral health professionals about the website and its learning opportunities, specifically additional training and education modules, toolkits, videos, and further information on the OH-I-CAN app available on the website. Attendees were instructed through presentations, seminars, and skills workshops. Included in educational sessions was an introduction to the OHICAN website, www.OHICAN.org, and the downloadable app and its purposes and uses. Additional dissemination efforts were accomplished through publication of aspects of this work in peer reviewed journals and via radio and other media appearances, and we plan additional publications for the immediate future. We also incorporated concepts of the OHICAN project in an inter-professional course titled Social Determinants of Health and Health Equity, developed in collaboration with Emory University.

4. Outcomes/accomplishments/results

Oral health is an essential component of good health. Not only is the oral system the primary way we take nutrients into our bodies through the food we consume, the health of that system is critically associated with other health outcomes. Appropriate oral health care and taking preventative measures to protect against diseases of the oral cavity, craniofacial diseases, and cancer are critical elements of good health. However, poor oral health and lack of access to care among low-income, minority, and other vulnerable populations is a significant contributor to health disparities for this population. The OHICAN project developed and implemented multiple approaches using both personal contact and technology to address the lack of equitable access to care. Results, accomplishments, and outcomes of the project are summarized below.

4.1 Starting point and ways of work

- Performed 3 dental Community Needs Assessments (CAN) with Rollins School of Public Health (completed in urban setting; pending in rural settings)

- Performed dental provider needs assessment

- Developed Strategic Plan and Monitoring/Evaluation Plan

4.2 Increasing community knowledge of preventive oral health care

- OHICAN website with educational materials
- Distributed 750 copies of informational brochure; brochure available on website
- Educated 12 CAB members on the importance of preventive oral health care
- Delivered 52 presentations to more than 1700 individuals in the target communities
- Baseline and follow-up assessments of community knowledge of preventive oral health care, demonstrated a greater than 95% increase in knowledge and best practice for oral health care

4.3 Expanding oral health care capacity in local communities

- Completed OHICAN education and training of 300 BSN, ABSN, MSN and AMSN students
- Provided oral health education to inter-professional group of 65 medical providers and support staff
- Gave 2 lectures to more than 250 dental hygienists to inform them of a new law (Dental Hygiene General Supervision for Preventive Care Bill) allowing them to perform oral care preventive services under general supervision and to discuss best practices

4.4 Creating new points of access

- Established a clinic to provide oral health services (Neighborhood Union) in a vulnerable neighborhood
- Provided access to dental screening and other services at Hollis Academy, a Science, Technology, Engineering, and Mathematics (STEM) school in the Atlanta Public School System serving pre-kindergarten through eighth grade students
- Created oral health programs at two additional school-based health centers
- Worked with NYU-Langone AEGD residency program in Georgia, Grady Health System, Ben Massell Dental Clinic, HEALing Community Center and Good Samaritan Atlanta, to increase the number of dental residents to be trained from 4 to 6 providers
- Extended the reach of the residency program to Albany, Georgia by securing a residency site with two residents beginning in the summer of 2020
- Developed the Oral Health Business Plan Interactive Resource in conjunction with the Emory University School of Business

4.5 Advocating on behalf of evidence-based methods to expand care and lower costs

- Supported and advocated for the Dental Hygiene General Supervision for Preventive Care Bill that passed and became law on January 1, 2018

- Created an implementation toolkit to assist dentists and dental hygienists in implementing the new law in both the public and private sectors (toolkit available on website)

- Continued work with Georgia Dental Hygiene Association, Georgia Dental Association and Dr. Chay from the Grady Health System Advance Education in General Dentistry Residency (AEGD) program

- The three members of the OHICAN leadership team are board members of the Georgia Oral Health Coalition

- Dr. Reznik (leadership team) serves as chair of the general supervision implementation sub-committee

- Included a tab on website to post updated information regarding advocacy efforts and posted two articles of interest

4.6 Rolling out/disseminating results of the OHICAN project and transitioning it to an initiative for deployment nationally and internationally

- Designed and completed social media rollout

- Educated physicians, nurse practitioners, physician assistants, and nurses on available learning opportunities of OHICAN initiative

- OHICAN app and website launched in local and global areas, back to school programs in Georgia, a Federally Qualified Health Center (FQHC) dental practice, and is included in the Georgia Department of Public Health State Oral Health Plan

- Through connections of a member of the OHICAN leadership team, launched the website and smartphone app in mobile clinics in Haiti

4.7 Website and app

- Completed OHICAN Smartphone application and connected metadata repository

- Established OHICAN website, www.ohican.org

- Developed OHICAN app with registry for patient needs assessment via the Oral Health Impact Profile 14 (OHIP 14) and the ECOHIS for assessing oral health-related quality-of-life for children

- Launch of OHICAN smartphone application locally and globally

- More than 25,000 users of OHICAN initiative

4.8 Tangible products

- Publications
- Presentations
- Educational software (see www.OHICAN.org)
- Trainings on oral health screening and preventive care such as application of fluoride varnish or fluoride rinses (see www.OHICAN.org)
- Extramural funding
- OHICAN Smartphone App (see www.OHICAN.org)
- OHICAN Website (see www.OHICAN.org)
- OHICAN healthcare provider protocol (see www.OHICAN.org)
- OHICAN Toolkit (see www.OHICAN.org)
- Oral Health Business Plan Interactive Resource (see www.OHICAN.org)

5. Discussion

The OHICAN pilot project was designed to address the burden of poor oral health in marginalized communities. A myriad of factors contribute to poor oral health and include access to and cost of care. Lack of dental insurance and/or transportation to a dental facility both impact an individual's ability to obtain oral healthcare. Factors such as proximity to fresh fruits and vegetables and grocery stores impact the ability to make healthy choices. Social, political and economic forces all contribute to varying degrees to the lack of equity in healthcare. The work of OHICAN was designed to create a blueprint for some potential solutions to these issues. Most training programs for healthcare professionals have neither an exposure to identifying oral health issues, nor do they have educational opportunities for learners to develop the ability to identify and definitively treat oral health issues. Development of training videos in conjunction with specific algorithms for providers should provide healthcare workers, and in particular non-dental healthcare workers, with tools to assist in the treatment of their patients with oral health issues. Likewise, providing in-person trainings in nursing schools, physician assistant schools, and other medical healthcare training programs should help equip future providers to be more adept in addressing dental-related problems in their patients.

While addressing the educational exposure of non-traditional dental care providers, it is also important to increase the level of oral health literacy of the general public across the lifespan. In an ideal setting, oral health would be initiated at the stage of infancy. Training parents or caretakers on the expected oral health milestones and appropriate methods of care in a similar manner as is done with the stages of crawling to walking from infancy to toddler stage, to the teenage years, young adult, to senior years would be an excellent start. Oral health messages and healthy practices can also be reinforced through the creation of new access points that will allow more people to receive care.

A significant part of increasing oral health in marginalized communities includes advocacy efforts to change legislation that in turn creates opportunities for providers to perform at the top of their licenses. Additionally, advocacy efforts are needed to create funding sources for seniors to receive required care such as inclusion of dental benefits for Medicare recipients.

Data are required to provide evidence-based methods for expanding care and lowering costs. The authors are optimistic that data gleaned as a result of the OHICAN App and connected repository will assist in this process. Through the collection of quality of life data which can be compared on a global platform, similarities and differences in patients' experiences can be compared and contrasted across differing age groups, sex, geographic location, and other parameters. Examinations of this type should help provide the basis for evidenced-based work to effectively address the burden of poor oral health in low-resourced communities.

In addition to improving access to oral health services and increasing widespread community prevention efforts, services provided by insurance and public programs must be expanded. For instance in Georgia, adult Medicaid recipients have access only to emergency care and extractions. The disparity between the privately insured and uninsured populations is even larger for children and older adults. Unmet dental care needs continue to be highest among individuals without insurance.

The OHICAN team has worked to train non-traditional providers but there remains the issue that a limited supply of dental providers are willing to work with underserved populations. This shortage is even more pronounced in more rural parts of the state. Additionally, racial and ethnic minorities are under-represented in the dental profession. Minority dentists are more likely to practice in communities that have larger minority populations. Also, African-American and Hispanic-American dentists disproportionately serve African-Americans and Hispanic Americans, respectively, in their private practices and patients are more likely to seek health care from professionals of a similar culture or background. As the population continues to have significant increases in ethnic and racial minorities, there will be an ever increasing need for a more diverse dental workforce, which has been a focus of the American Dental Education Association.

Future efforts by the OHICAN team will include expanding the pool of dental providers and non-traditional dental providers in conjunction with increasing the number of access points and enhancing the oral health literacy of communities and neighborhoods.

6. Leader learning

Through this work, our OHICAN team employed several health equity skills which can be grouped into six categories: communications, cultural competency, program planning and development, analytic assessment, community practice, leadership, and systems thinking. Cultural competence is the ability to understand, communicate with and effectively interact with people across cultures. Program planning and development grow from the base of having appropriate communications in conjunction with cultural competency. This then allows for the repeated analysis of the work at hand with appropriate planning for the community of practice. The group of people who share these common concerns are able to come together in a more effective and efficient manner to fulfill both individual and group goals. Throughout the process, we have been able to identify opportunities to implement multiple leadership styles and identify ways to impact the issue from a systems perspective. By strategically combining health tools and effective communication processes, we have an opportunity to improve healthcare quality and safety.

As with all projects, there are always hurdles to overcome. We faced time limitations establishing effective partnerships. Working to educate key players involved in a legislative process to help increase equitable access to dental care was time intensive as well. Not only did we need to educate key legislators on the human toll of unmet dental need, we had to moderate between the two main constituents in the legislative process: the Georgia Dental Association and the Georgia Dental Hygiene Association. Even after the governor signed the legislation into law, implementation of a new legislative change is taking a significant amount of time to take hold and make a difference in access. We had a 2nd year dental resident put together an implementation toolkit for the new legislation. In over a year and a half since the legislation granting dental hygienists the ability to perform preventive dental care under general supervision was signed into law, only a handful of practices have taken advantage of this new program. Team OHICAN leaders are members of the Georgia Oral Health Coalition and are involved in the implementation of the program.

One of the main barriers to expanding access to oral health care is the expense of starting a dental practice. Dental equipment and supplies are very expensive. Whether you build a two operatory or four operatory clinic, you will still need to purchase basic equipment such as a compressor, suction, autoclaves, X-ray units, developing equipment, an assortment of hand pieces, and an electronic dental record. Staffing is a substantial expense. Building a new program does not mean the patients will automatically show up for care. Time and effort are needed to market the program to those most in need. Salaries for dentists and dental hygienists are expensive. Even with exceptional outside assistance from Emory University's Goizueta School of Business, developing a working business model was time intensive.

Initiating a school-based program involves numerous steps including working with school leadership and families. Establishing relationships and gaining approval for a new service in a school requires a lot of time. As one of our consultant colleagues said, a lot of spaghetti dinners are involved to gain acceptance from families and school leadership.

Our initial plan assumed if you build a new oral health program in an area of high unmet need, patients will be lining up for the service. Regretfully, this was not the case. Oral health literacy for most Americans is lacking. Education and marketing must occur early and often in the process. While this is time intensive, the benefits outweigh the use of education and marketing resources to ensure equitable access to dental care.

Dental students are graduating with enormous educational debt. Corporate dental service organizations, many backed by hedge funds or other sources of investment, are actively recruiting new graduates and even residents before the end of their residency programs. The combination of economic pressure and promises of very high salaries from corporate dentistry makes it difficult to recruit dentists to serve in public health settings.

6.1 Recommendations

If tackling this oral health issue in your community, you should:

- Secure extramural funding
- Expand training opportunities for learners
- Ensure you have community buy-in

- Be prepared to increase the number of dentists in residency programs and Federally Qualified Health Centers (FQHC) or FQHC look-alike dental programs
- Secure site-specific data analyses
- Map out potential sites for expansion of new access points for care
- Explore social media rollout resources

We would not recommend you proceed without community input/needs assessment(s), or too broad of a pilot phase. Instead keep your initial activities confined to local efforts for quality improvement before initiating next steps. If your initiative is intended to open new points of access, we suggest avoiding opening too many sites at the same time. Ensure the systems you have created are functioning well and then develop a detailed plan before expanding.

6.2 Best practices

A project like this will consume much more time than you might anticipate with additional job responsibilities. Accomplishing your goals might take much longer than you expected, so ensure your local institution/employer supports the needed effort for your project. You should also expect your initial plan to change many times, so be open to new opportunities. Ensure all components of the effort and participants are on the same page throughout the project. Wicked problems take a lot of time and effort to address and take many twists and turns. Communication from the highest levels to those on the ground remains vital.

6.3 Our best pieces of advice

- Keep communicating throughout both high and low moments. Also, do not forget to laugh because it is an amazing opportunity to share and help those who cannot help themselves.
- Working toward a goal to address a wicked problem can be hard work. Know it is good work, and work worth doing!

7. Toolkit

A full description of the toolkit can be found at www.ohican.org. The toolkit provides educational and training materials as well as the capability for research endeavors through an online repository. The OH-I-CAN app, downloadable from the website, contains the Oral Health Impact Profile (OHIP-14), questions on blood pressure and head and neck cancer screening, and the ECOHIS applicable to children. The OHIP-14 is a measure of oral health related quality of life. This tool can be used to study specific populations (i.e. zip code, medical conditions including HIV, head and neck cancer, diabetes) in a very easy to use interface that connects to the online repository. The ECOHIS is designed to measure the quality of oral health-related quality-of-life for preschool children and their families. Below is a list of the technology solutions developed by the OHICAN project team.

- Website: OHICAN.org
- Smartphone App: OH-I-CAN for iOS and Android phones
- Online OHICAN Repository
- Twitter: @OHICAN1

A more comprehensive toolkit can be found at https://clinicalscholarsnli.org/community-impact

Author details

Charles E. Moore[1,2,3*], Hope Bussenius[4,5] and David Reznik[3,6]

1 Emory University, Georgia, United States

2 Healing Community Center, Georgia, United States

3 Grady Health System, Georgia, United States

4 Nell Hodgson Woodruff School of Nursing, Emory University, Georgia, United States

5 Take2Heart Initiative, Inc, Georgia, United States

6 NYU-Langone, Georgia, United States

*Address all correspondence to: cemoore@emory.edu

References

[1] United States General Accounting Office. Oral health: Dental disease is a chronic problem among low-income populations [Internet]. 2000. Available from: https://www.gao.gov/new.items/he00072.pdf [Accessed: 2020-01-01].

[2] National Institutes of Health. Dental caries (tooth decay) in children age 2 to 11 [Internet]. 2018. Available from : https://www.nidcr.nih.gov/research/data-statistics/dental-caries/children#dental-caries-in-permanent-adult-teeth [Accessed: 2020-01-01].

[3] Kabore HJ, Smith C, Bernal J, Parker D, Csukas S, Chapple-McGruder T. The Burden of Oral Health in Georgia. Georgia Department of Public Health, Maternal and Child Health, Office of MCH Epidemiology, Georgia Oral Health Program.

[4] Jackson SL, Vann WF, Kotch JB, Pahel BT, and Lee JY. Impact of poor oral health. American Journal of Public Health. 2011;101(10)1900-1906. DOI: 10.2105/AJPH.2010.200915.

[5] U.S. Department of Health and Human Services. Oral Health in America: A Report of the Surgeon General. 2000. Rockville, MD: U.S. Department of Health and Human Services, National Institute of Dental and Craniofacial Research, National Institutes of Health.

[6] Seirawan h, Faust S, and Mulligan R. the impact of oral health on the academic performance of disadvantaged children. American Journal of Public Health. 2012;102(9):1729-1734. DOI: 10.2105/AJPH.2011.300478.

[7] Bussenius H, Reznik D, and Moore c. Building a culture of oral health care. The Journal of Nurse Practitioners. 2017;13(9):623-627. DOI: 10.1016/j.nurpra.2017.07.019.

[8] Moore CE, Reznik DA, Conboy L, Giwa J, Aslam F,5, Bussenius H, Aidman C, and Warren RC. Achieving equity in oral health: A data-driven approach for informing policy changes. Journal of Community Medicine and Health Education 2017;7:511. DOI: 10.4172/2161-0711.1000511.

Chapter 8

underdog DREAMS: Improving Long-Term Quality of Life Outcomes for Florida's Foster Youth and Families

Annette Bell, Slyving Bourdeau, Asha Davis, Amanda Stanec and Derrick Stephens

Abstract

Children and youth in the foster care system face significant and continuing barriers to both physical and mental health, including lack of a medical home, disruptions in primary care providers, frequent moves to new homes, excessive caseloads for oversight providers, and at times continuing exposure to the risk factors that are considered Adverse Childhood Experiences (ACEs). The underdog DREAMS project sought to alter the course of the foster youth experience via a tri-part model that focused on clinical, research, and advocacy interventions for foster youth and the development of the workforce that supports them through training on the impacts of trauma and poverty.

Keywords: Foster youth, Health, Physical, Mental, Adverse Childhood Experiences

1. Introduction

The purpose of the foster care system in the United States is to provide for the well-being of children and youth who have been removed from their family of origin due to abuse, neglect, and/or other reasons: exposures collectively referred to as Adverse Childhood Experiences (ACEs) [1]. Meeting the physical and mental health needs of this population is an acute challenge, as children and youth typically enter the system with an array of significant social and medical issues and factors within the system, such as lack of access to care, compound the problem. Roughly 40% of children (ages 3–9) and youth (ages 10–17) in foster care have a serious mental health disorder, including PTSD; alcohol, nicotine, and other drug abuse; depression and anxiety; eating disorders; and social phobia [2]. They are also more likely to require treatment for physical conditions such as asthma, obesity, chronic pain, and other problems that may interfere with physical activity [3–5]. Unfortunately, national long-term health outcomes associated with foster care include high rates of chronic mental (54%) and physical (30%) health disorders among young adults exiting the foster care system [6].

As of 2017, 443,000 children and youth live in foster care in the United States. The average age of entry is 7, and the average duration in care is 20.1 months [7].

According to 2014 data, Florida is fifth in the nation in the number of children investigated per 1,000 children in the general population (70.6%) [8]. Since October 2013, the number of children and youth in out-of-home care statewide in Florida has risen from just over 17,000 to now almost 24,000 [9].

By 2005, the state of Florida had transitioned to a privatized system. Recent reviews have found this system to be in disarray, and despite some positive signs [10, 11], the state is failing to implement many recommendations related to the physical and mental healthcare needs of children and youth in the foster care system [10, 11]. While the percentage of children and youth in foster care who received some medical care over the previous 12 months has risen from 80% in 2011 to over 95% in 2017, the level of care available continues to fall short of demand **Figure 1** [12]. Shows that less than 75% of foster children and youth are getting their mental, behavioral, physical, and dental needs met.

The information currently available indicates that children and youth with ACEs who remain untreated are at significant risk of suffering a 20-year difference in lifespan compared to their peers who are unaffected by ACEs, as well as increased risk for unemployment, poverty, homelessness, and more [13, 14]. Programs that provide these young people with skills and strategies to improve their health and well-being can mitigate the risk of chronic physical and mental illness [15].

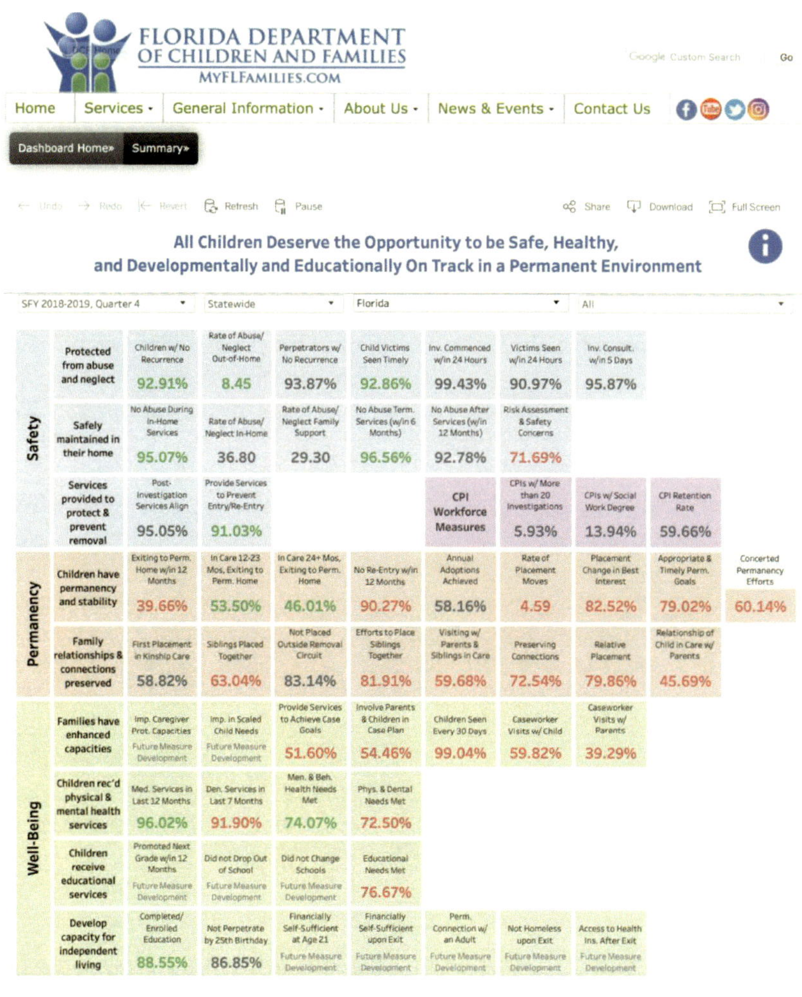
FLORIDA DEPARTMENT OF CHILDREN AND FAMILIES
MYFLFAMILIES.COM
Home
Services
General Information
About Us
News & Events
Contact Us
Dashboard Home»
Summary»
All Children Deserve the Opportunity to be Safe, Healthy, and Developmentally and Educationally On Track in a Permanent Environment
SFY 2018-2019, Quarter 4
Statewide
Florida
All
Safety
Protected from abuse and neglect
Children w/ No Recurrence 92.91%
Rate of Abuse/ Neglect Out-of-Home 8.45
Perpetrators w/ No Recurrence 93.87%
Child Victims Seen Timely 92.86%
Inv. Commenced w/in 24 Hours 99.43%
Victims Seen w/in 24 Hours 90.97%
Inv. Consult. w/in 5 Days 95.87%
Safely maintained in their home
No Abuse During In-Home Services 95.07%
Rate of Abuse/ Neglect In-Home 36.80
Rate of Abuse/ Neglect Family Support 29.30
No Abuse Term. Services (w/in 6 Months) 96.56%
No Abuse After Services (w/in 12 Months) 92.78%
Risk Assessment & Safety Concerns 71.69%
Services provided to protect & prevent removal
Post-Investigation Services Align 95.05%
Provide Services to Prevent Entry/Re-Entry 91.03%
CPI Workforce Measures
CPIs w/ More than 20 Investigations 5.93%
CPIs w/ Social Work Degree 13.94%
CPI Retention Rate 59.66%
Permanency
Children have permanency and stability
Exiting to Perm. Home w/in 12 Months 39.66%
In Care 12-23 Mos, Exiting to Perm. Home 53.50%
In Care 24+ Mos, Exiting to Perm. Home 46.01%
No Re-Entry w/in 12 Months 90.27%
Annual Adoptions Achieved 58.16%
Rate of Placement Moves 4.59
Placement Change in Best Interest 82.52%
Appropriate & Timely Perm. Goals 79.02%
Concerted Permanency Efforts 60.14%
Family relationships & connections preserved
First Placement in Kinship Care 58.82%
Siblings Placed Together 63.04%
Not Placed Outside Removal Circuit 83.14%
Efforts to Place Siblings Together 81.91%
Visiting w/ Parents & Siblings in Care 59.68%
Preserving Connections 72.54%
Relative Placement 79.86%
Relationship of Child in Care w/ Parents 45.69%
Well-Being
Families have enhanced capacities
Imp. Caregiver Prot. Capacities Future Measure Development
Imp. in Scaled Child Needs Future Measure Development
Provide Services to Achieve Case Goals 51.60%
Involve Parents & Children in Case Plan 54.46%
Children Seen Every 30 Days 99.04%
Caseworker Visits w/ Child 59.82%
Caseworker Visits w/ Parents 39.29%
Children rec'd physical & mental health services
Med. Services in Last 12 Months 96.02%
Den. Services in Last 7 Months 91.90%
Men. & Beh. Health Needs Met 74.07%
Phys. & Dental Needs Met 72.50%
Children receive educational services
Promoted Next Grade w/in 12 Months Future Measure Development
Did not Drop Out of School Future Measure Development
Did not Change Schools Future Measure Development
Educational Needs Met 76.67%
Develop capacity for independent living
Completed/ Enrolled Education 88.55%
Not Perpetrate by 25th Birthday 86.85%
Financially Self-Sufficient at Age 21 Future Measure Development
Financially Self-Sufficient upon Exit Future Measure Development
Perm. Connection w/ an Adult Future Measure Development
Not Homeless upon Exit Future Measure Development
Access to Health Ins. After Exit Future Measure Development

Figure 1.
MyFLFamiles dashboard summary.

DOI: http://dx.doi.org/10.5772/intechopen.98457

2. Wicked Problem Impact Project (WPIP) description

Florida's fractured and privatized child welfare system leads to significant deficits in foster child and youth education and physical and mental healthcare. These deficits directly translate to poor quality of life outcomes for Florida's foster children and youth. The Wicked Problem Impact Project of underdog DREAMS was to identify strategies to improve the quality of life and well-being for Florida foster youth. Our work identified three key strategies essential for helping youth in foster care reach their potential:

1. Education

2. Mental and physical wellness

3. Access to innovative technology

3. Approach

The underdog Dreams team participating in the Clinical Scholars program consists of two clinical social workers (DS, SB), a family physician (AB), an adolescent psychiatrist (AD), and a clinical psychologist. The underdog DREAMS project engaged in a multi-faceted approach to support foster youth as well as the healthcare providers who play a role in the foster care system infrastructure. Thus, the team focused on clinical, research, and advocacy interventions for foster youth and on the development of the workforce that supports them through training on the impacts of trauma and poverty. The initial goals for the project were adjusted based on our research and investigative findings, particularly during phase one: *Look, Listen and Learn*.

Phase two concentrated on *Engagement Strategies*, including creating a *Child Welfare Standard of Care Protocol* and developing critical partnerships with the communities served. In phase three, the *Implementation Phase*, the project used rapid-cycle innovation strategies to test youth-intervention protocols and ideas.

Figure 2 is a visual timeline representing the underdog DREAMS team's approach and accomplishments and the next steps to be implemented.

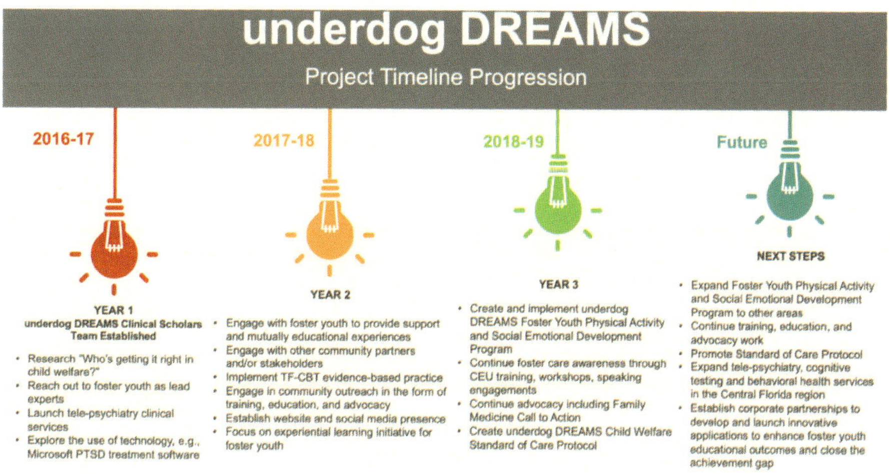

Figure 2.
underdog DREAMS Timeline.

4. Activities and outcomes

4.1 Phase I: look, listen, and learn

Capitalizing on best practices in community-based engagement principles, our team partnered with foster youth so that their perspective served as a foundation for all later actions. Youth sources included foster youth enrolled in the First Star Central Florida Academy, the Job Readiness and Leadership Bootcamp, and other Central Florida area youth. Simultaneously the team conducted an in-depth literature review on this topic, including researching the current foster care environment in the State of Florida. The goal of this exercise was to figure out what had been or was being done in this arena and (more importantly) who seemed to be doing it effectively.

4.2 Phase II: engagement strategies

Team underdog DREAMS executed several engagement strategies which included:

- An active partnership with foster care youth and other community partners;
- A physical activity-based life skills intervention and collaboration entitled underdog DREAMS Foster Youth Physical Activity and Social Emotional Development Program with an organization called Move + Live + Learn;
- Education to promote community awareness and advocacy;
- Education directly tailored for foster youth and advocacy;
- Foster youth mental and physical wellness; and
- Technology solutions to support youth in foster care.

4.2.1 Active partnership with foster care youth and other community partners

Youth in foster care are the most critical community partners, and thus the team emphasized building trust and engaging with them to build a positive and trusting relationship and to identify their physical, social, and emotional needs.

4.2.2 underdog DREAMS foster youth physical activity and social emotional development program

Team underdog DREAMS collaborated with Move + Live + Learn to develop, deliver, monitor, and evaluate an 8-week physical activity-based life skills program. The ongoing collaboration helped underdog DREAMS develop our three strategic categories for maximum impact on the lives of foster youth in Florida: education, mental and physical wellness, and technology. This program was designed to increase:

- Physical activity levels;
- Understanding of healthy eating behaviors;

- Proficiency in practical life skills;
- Proficiency in social–emotional skills such as emotional regulation, communication, and decision making; and
- Understanding of how to make choices that enhance wellness.

4.2.3 Education to promote community awareness and advocacy

- Led or participated in outreach experiences including training and ongoing reflective supervision to professionals, facilitating simulations, and presenting at conferences
- Represented youth voices at Florida Baker Act Task Force for Adolescents
- Served on Florida Child Welfare Advisory Board as an advocate for foster youth
- Hosted the underdog DREAMS Foster Care Month Celebration and Fundraiser Event held at Topgolf Orlando, highlighting underdog DREAMS' $42,000 sponsorship of First Star Central Florida Academy
- Submitted an opinion piece to the American Academy of Family Physicians that included a call to action to create a formal initiative for Family Medicine around the child welfare system
- Created underdog DREAMS Child Welfare Standard of Care Protocol

4.2.4 Education directly tailored for foster youth and advocacy

- First Star Central Florida Academy: underdog DREAMS participated in the academy's onsite summer program and monthly at their Saturday sessions.
- underdog DREAMS Job Readiness and Leadership Boot Camp: The team created and facilitated a preparatory program for 18 Central Florida foster youth ages 16–17.
- Experiential Learning Experiences: The team sponsored trips to North Carolina; Washington, DC; and Puerto Rico.
- Student-led video development: Participants created a video to pitch concepts on how the Microsoft HoloLens can innovate the child welfare system and improve long-term outcomes.

4.2.5 Foster youth mental and physical wellness

4.2.5.1 Clinical care

In an effort to deliver continuity of mental healthcare and address the frequent turnover of medical providers foster youth must endure, we implemented evidence-based treatment rooted in Trauma-Focused Cognitive Behavioral Therapy (TF-CBT), utilizing telepsychiatry to ensure continuity of care and access to child and adolescent psychiatry.

4.2.5.2 Research

We partnered with MOVE + LIVE + LEARN to create the underdog DREAMS Foster Youth Physical Activity and Social Emotional Development Program and evaluate a pilot intervention entitled underdog DREAMS: A physical activity program focused on life skills and social emotional health for deserving youth in foster care. Results of this mixed-methods research project are presented in the Notable Findings section of this chapter.

4.2.6 Telepsychiatry and other modalities

Telepsychiatry and our presence on-line and in social media contributed to the effectiveness of this project. We partnered with remote professionals to deliver innovative and engaging curriculum for youth in our underdog DREAMS Job Readiness and Leadership Boot Camp.

4.3 Phase III: implementation phase

Notable Findings.

4.3.1 underdog DREAMS Child Welfare Standard of Care Protocol

To support a more unifying approach to foster youth across the state, Team underdog DREAMS developed an evidence-based standard of care protocol outlining the necessary services that should be provided to every child entering the child welfare system. Ideally, this protocol would be legally mandated and utilized by the Community-Based Care (CBC) system to ensure all children and youth receive equal access and the highest caliber of treatment across the state.

There are 4 components to this protocol: Access, Assessment, Assistance, & Advocacy (see **Figure 3**).

4.3.2 underdog DREAMS Job Readiness and Leadership Boot Camp

At the end of year 2, underdog DREAMS implemented the underdog DREAMS Job Readiness and Leadership Boot Camp, a preparatory program for CBC Central

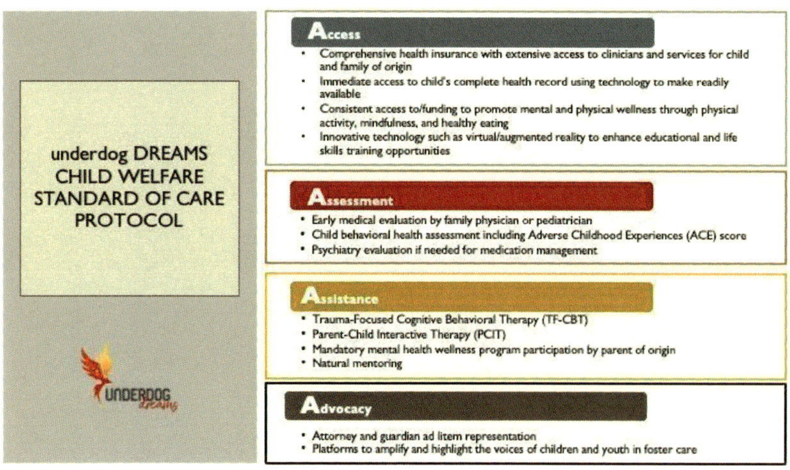

Figure 3.
underdog DREAMS Child Welfare Standard of Care Protocol.

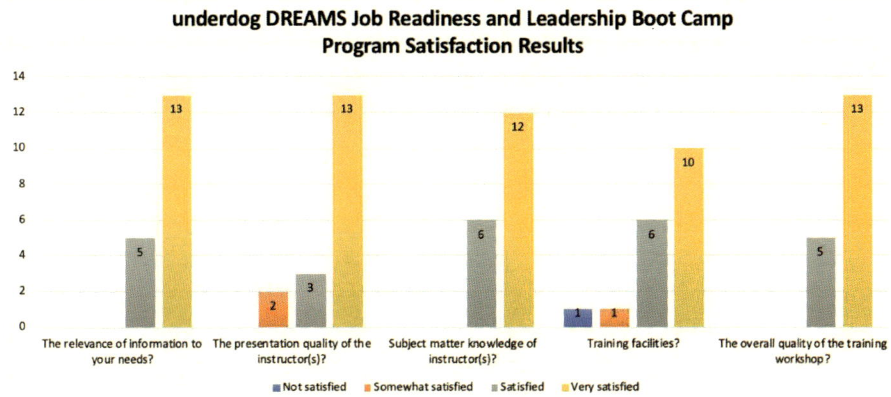

Figure 4.
underdog DREAMS Job Readiness and Leadership Boot Camp Program Results.

Florida foster youth ages 16–17 who were embarking on summer employment opportunities. There were 18 participants who attended the 4-day program that included psychosocial education, life skill training, and experiential learning.

On the final day of the camp, the participants completed a survey that asked for in-depth feedback on different aspects of the program. One set of questions focused on satisfaction, specifically with the presentations, the training facilities, and the overall quality of the workshop. The results of these questions are illustrated in **Figure 4**.

Feedback data was overwhelmingly positive, with 100% of participants being satisfied/very satisfied, stating the program met their expectations, and they would recommend it to others. Results were similar for participants' views about instructional quality. Several youth attendees commented specifically on how much they liked learning with the use of video conference technology.

One theme that stood out among the positive comments from the foster youth was their enjoyment with interacting, hearing others' thoughts, debating, group discussions, and "networking" with one another.

4.3.3 underdog DREAMS Foster Youth Physical Activity and Social Emotional Development Program

In the summer of 2019, Team underdog DREAMS launched an evidence-based youth physical and mental health program consisting of 24 sessions designed to increase physical activity levels and perceptions of physical activity; improve functional life skills (e.g., communication, nutrition education), and improve social emotional learning skills (e.g., coping strategies, decision making). Three group homes were partners in this project and transported youth to a central location for the twice weekly program throughout the summer. Trained coaches facilitated the lessons.

The underdog DREAMS team hypothesized that if the program proved to substantially improve the health (i.e., physical, mental, social, etc.) of youth in residential foster care, the successful elements of the program might be applicable in other residences. A mixed-methodology (quantitative and qualitative) evaluation occurred toward the end of and upon completion of the 8-week program. The quantitative assessments consisted of two previously validated instruments: the Survey (YES) 2.0 and the Life Skills Assessment (LSA) (**Figures 5** and **6**) [16, 17]. The qualitative analysis consisted of an opt-in participation focus group session so that participants' voices could be heard. Program participants also completed an informational questionnaire (Google forms) in a guided opt-in focus group. All program participants completed "exit slips" that indicated the degree to which the learning objectives were met by the session.

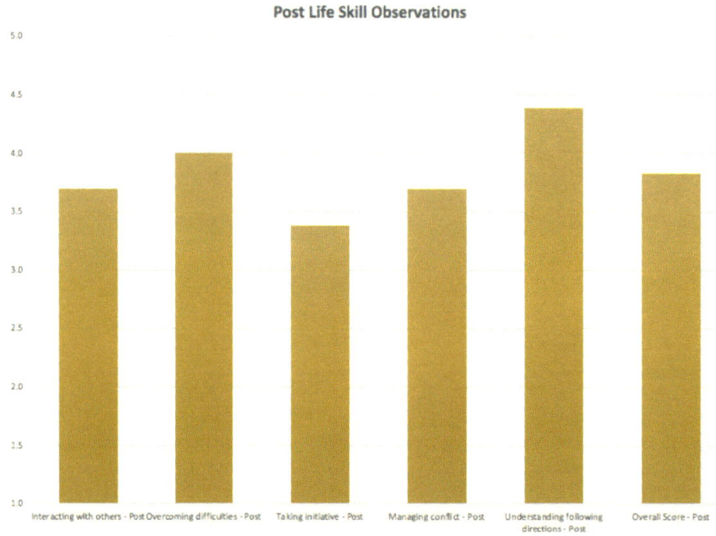

Figure 5.
Life skills assessment (LSA) observation tool findings of program participants, post participation. Legend: 1 = does not yet do; 2 = does with a lot of help; 3 = does with some help; 4 = does with little help; 5 = does independently.

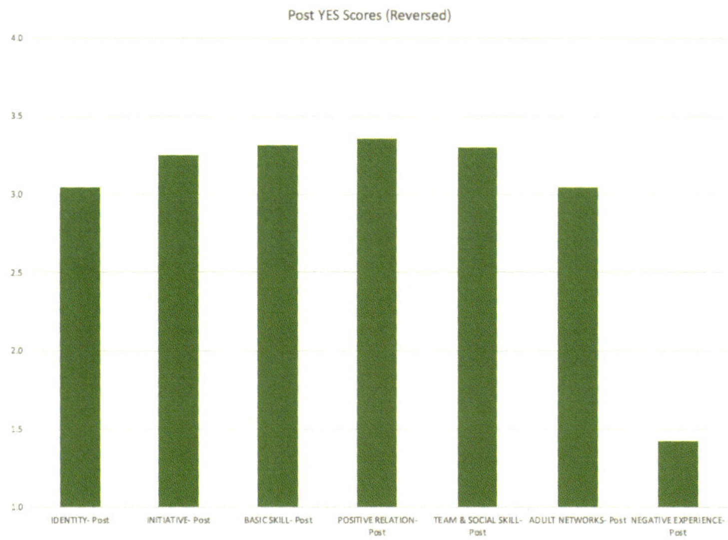

Figure 6.
Youth experience in sport (YES) 2.0 tool findings of program participants, post participation. Legend: 1 = not at all; 2 = a little; 3 = quite a bit; 4 = yes, definitely.

Challenges emerged related to consistency on the part of group home staff to transport youth to the programming. Thus, while underdog DREAMS planned for, recruited, and could accommodate approximately 60 youth for the program, a total of 13 youth attended all 24 sessions. While this reduced expected numbers, it allowed for the intervention to be piloted and points to the key role that transportation plays in intervention planning and design.

4.3.4 Quantitative findings: The Life Skills Assessment

The Life Skills Assessment (LSA) is an observation tool completed by facilitators of the program for each youth who participated in the program. This

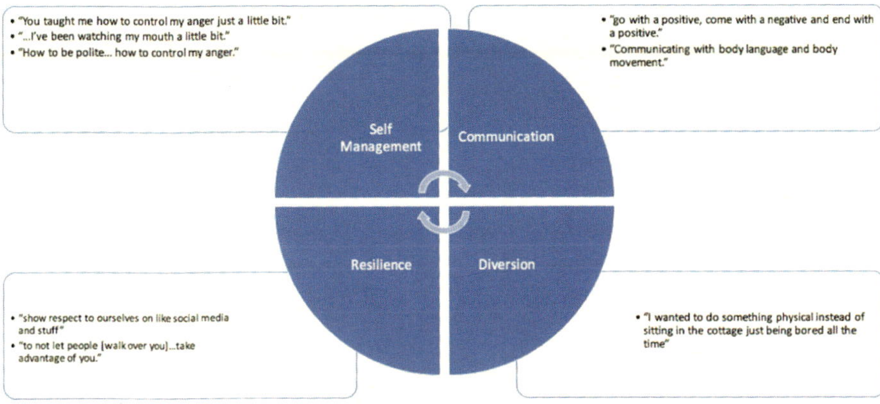

Figure 7.
Focus group themes.

tool provides a sense of where coaches feel youth are in terms of applying the social–emotional skills they were taught in the program. Coaches observed high ratings in the LSA skill areas in youth who had participated in the program.

The YES 2.0 tool was completed by participants following their participation in the program, and specifically referred to the underdog DREAMS physical activity program. Participants of the program stated that overall they had gained helpful skills centered around topics such as goal setting, effort, problem solving, time management, emotional regulation, positive relationships, managing stress, etc. at rates between *quite a bit* and *yes, definitely*.

A stepwise linear regression analysis revealed that positive relationships among youth significantly predicted the observer's overall assessment of the overall life skills of each participant. In other words, the higher someone reported that the program had a positive impact on their relationship with others, the higher the coaches rated their overall use of life skills during the program.

Qualitative data was collected through focus groups with participants. Analysis indicated that youth in the foster care system may respond better in a focus group with one other youth or in a one-on-one setting. Youth had to be continuously directed to refocus and did not share their experiences as much as we anticipated. Four primary themes emerged from the focus groups (**Figure 7**).

Overall, the data suggest that the time and resources designated to teach social emotional skills and functional life skills had a positive impact on those youth in foster care who were able to attend regularly. Participants indicated that the program primarily helped them with self-management and emotional regulation skills (e.g., dealing with conflict, knowing when to step back and walk away).

5. Discussion

Youth in foster care rarely participate in studies on well-being related topics such as physical activity and social emotional skills. There are many reasons for this as highlighted by Quarmby and Pickering, who conducted a scoping review of barriers and policy related to physical activity behaviors of youth in foster care [18]. To illustrate the minimal literature on this topic, only seven research articles qualified for their 2016 review from an original pool of 576 potential articles. The criteria for the authors' broad review included: published in English, published in a peer-reviewed article, published between 1989 and 2014, related to children and youth living in or leaving foster care (including residential homes), and referenced physical activity participation [19]. Thus, drawing comparisons from previous research on physical activity and social emotional learning programs for youth in foster care is difficult; this fact emphasizes the need for work such as our project to determine what types of programming best supports the well-being of youth in the foster care system.

5.1 underdog DREAMS Foster Youth Physical Activity and Social Emotional Development Program

The majority (n = 12) of total participants (n = 13) who participated in all 24 sessions of the physical activity life skills and social emotional program were adolescent girls. According to the 2018 US Report Card on Physical Activity for Children and Youth, only 18% of adolescent girls receive the recommended 60 minutes of moderate to vigorous physical activity daily, compared to 36% of adolescent boys [20]. Given that fact, it was promising to the underdog DREAMS team that something about this particular program kept 12 girls returning to the program. Perhaps it was the social component, the inclusive nature of the evidence-based physical activities provided, and/or the positive relationships established among participants and between participants and facilitators of the program. Choice is highlighted here as a potential motivating factor because previous researchers determined choice in physical activity is a predictor of self-determination [21]. Facilitators of the underdog DREAMS program reported that when participants informally communicated joy from particular activities, they were sure to revisit those activities in future settings, which may have contributed to the girls' continued participation.

While the underdog DREAMS team celebrates that adolescent girl participants increased their physical activity levels and reported learning life skills, one should not assume that local boys in residential homes did not want to participate or that the program is not ideal for adolescent boys in foster care. In this program, two of the three sites with whom we formed partnerships failed to transport youth to the programming location. Decision makers of these group homes were on board for this programming, but group home staff lacked either the capacity or the motivation to transport youth on a consistent basis. Consistent transportation to an off-site venue may have yielded more male participants.

After several weeks of delivering the program to participants from one group home, we changed our program location to their group home property. We did this to reduce transportation needs for that group home and to increase the number of youth from that program participating. This increased participation in the second half of the program implementation.

Youth in this program completed exit slips after some of the sessions as a form of formal, formative assessment. Facilitators analyzed their responses and used them to guide future instruction accordingly. Applying best pedagogical practices to this program was important to the collaborative because this program was not just focused on increasing physical activity behaviors; it was also focused on equipping participants with the necessary social and emotional skills that are often learned from parents. Analyzing these exit slips was extremely promising for the collaborative because participants were able to demonstrate an understanding of the social emotional and life skills taught.

5.2 Methodological Issues in Data Collection on Youth in Foster Care

One particular methodological issue that presented itself during data collection was that participants did not share their experiences in detail during the qualitative focus groups program evaluation portion of the project. Even with qualitative research interview strategies such as probing and prompting, youth seemed reluctant to share information about their experiences in any detail. Fortunately, this evaluation was a mixed-methodology study and included a monitoring phase where participants were welcome to give informal feedback at any time. This informal feedback was critical and contributed to the program's success.

5.3 Replicating underdog DREAMS Foster Youth Physical Activity and Social Emotional Development Program in Other Communities

Our results show a great deal of promise for the underdog DREAMS physical activity program, and communities are encouraged to replicate this program. Key successes of program planning and implementation include the following:

- A **detailed training** is important to make sure all facilitators are on the same page and are prepared to collaborate and help each other work through any issues that may arise. Underdog DREAMS created a day-long training to prepare facilitators on how to deliver the program optimally.

- Program facilitators display **reflective practice and flexibility** throughout the implementation.

- **Informal formative feedback** is gathered from the youth throughout the program.

5.4 Future programming

Future sites that implement this program can learn from our implementation and make every effort to increase participation by minimizing challenges to transportation. While we invested in partnerships with organizations and key decision makers, perhaps more time could have been spent with group home staff (i.e., those directly responsible for transporting the youth).

Future implementation of this program should consider giving youth a choice to record their answers individually rather than in a focus group and/or allowing youth to choose how many and which peers they feel most comfortable sharing their thoughts and experiences within a focus group setting. Youth may also be encouraged to write their responses rather than sharing them verbally.

Future sites should collaborate with the underdog DREAMS team to benefit from the body of research in this area. As the program is replicated it can continuously be monitored to measure the impact. It is critical to contribute to the literature as so few studies examine the influence of physical activity programming for youth in foster care [22].

6. Leader learning

Below are remarks from our team on our crucial leadership insights gained through the experience of serving as a Clinical Scholar.

6.1 Health equity

As defined by the Robert Wood Johnson Foundation, "Health equity means that everyone has a fair and just opportunity to be as healthy as possible. This requires removing obstacles to health such as poverty, discrimination, and their consequences, including powerlessness and lack of access to good jobs with fair pay, quality education and housing, safe environments, and health care" [23]. Belief in this value should be the "north star" for your project and the foundation upon which to build a vision and culture and guide your efforts. In all that our underdog DREAMS team did, we asked ourselves, "does this advance health equity for foster youth?" For example, the underdog DREAMS Child Welfare Standard of Care Protocol is designed to require that *all* foster children and youth receive the same high level of care regardless of geographic location or other factors. Through our awareness and advocacy efforts, we have championed interventions and policies that advance the opportunity for *all* foster children and youth to attain their highest level of health.

6.2 Social determinants of health

Social determinants of health (SDoH) are the conditions in the places where people live, learn, work, and play that affect a wide range of health risks and outcomes [24]. We recommend spending time understanding the SDoH affecting your target population and creating interventions to address them specifically. Foster youth living in group homes have limited accessibility to healthy food choices, are often responsible for making their own meals, and are unable to participate in sports or fitness activities due to lack of transportation. These were the SDoH identified and addressed in our project; other projects and work might address others.

6.3 Visioning

The underdog DREAMS team initially created and were subsequently guided by our vision: Utilizing the value of health equity, create and project a compelling and engaging vision. Our team recommends that others engaging in this work ground their own approach in a strong overarching vision, as indicated in the (**Figure 8**) below.

6.4 Creating effective organizational culture

Assume good intentions: Dr. Brené Brown says, "daring leaders work from the assumption that people are doing the best they can; whereas leaders struggling with

underdog DREAMS Vision Statement

underdog DREAMS exists to provide foster youth opportunities to imagine a future filled with purpose and to live with intention. We do everything we can to meet foster youth where they are - from psychosocial education to experiential learning activities, and from mentorship to group counseling.

Our work is guided by 3 fundamental beliefs:

1. **We believe in the value that every foster child and youth bring to any community.**
2. **We believe that every foster child and youth deserve a thorough and thoughtful approach to their physical and mental healthcare.**
3. **We believe technology is an enabler that allows us to reach children and youth in the 21st century.**

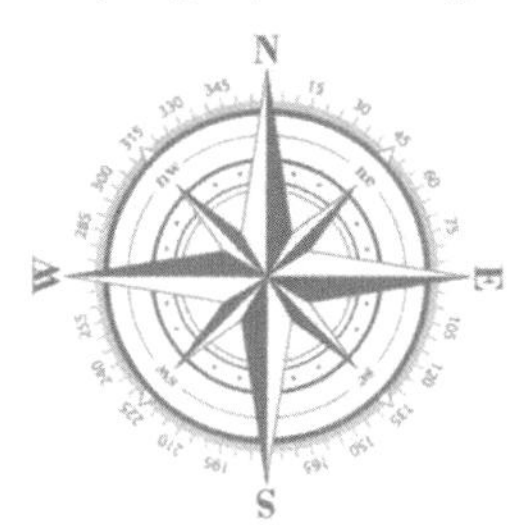

Figure 8.
underdog DREAMS Vision Statement.

ego, armour, and/or lack of skills, do not make that assumption" [25]. We continuously tried to live this truth by allowing team members to express opinions and freely vocalize their thoughts without fear of attack or retribution. By assuming that the person's intent was to be positive, even if someone had an opinion that was a dissension from the group, it was welcome.

Avoid rushing and/or committing to too many initiatives: The excitement of making an impact can lead to a tendency to address several things at once. Continuous reflection from each team member and a pace that fostered quality over quantity were essential to our team's success. Additionally, if the project is not a part of your daily work, be sure to set aside an appropriate amount of time to devote to the project each week to keep the project moving forward.

Transparency and accountability among team members: Establish transparency and accountability as team values and expectations. With team members working from different locations and with funding provided to different organizations within the team, maintaining open communication to establish and maintain trust among the group is vital.

6.5 Collaboration/creative partnerships

One of our greatest successes was the development of relationships with key stakeholders. Our relationship with the youth in foster care was most pivotal. By spending quality time engaging in conversation both formally in the classroom and informally through fun activities, we learned from the experts how best to make an impact in their lives. By consistently demonstrating our values of transparency and accountability along with hard work and dedication to this project, underdog DREAMS developed a reputation as trustworthy, knowledgeable team-players, thus allowing for these partnerships to form and grow.

7. Toolkit

7.1 underdog DREAMS Websites

- https://www.underdogdreams.org/
- Forms, additional charts and data can be accessed at the underdog DREAMS website.
    - http://clinicalscholarsnli.org/projects/underdog-dreams-improving-long-term-quality-of-life-outcomes-for-floridas-foster-youth-and-families/

7.2 Relevant websites

- U.S. Department of Health and Human Services Children's Bureau
    - https://www.acf.hhs.gov/cb
- U.S. Department of Health and Human Services Child Welfare Information Gateway
    - https://www.childwelfare.gov/topics/systemwide/statistics/
- Florida Department of Children and Families

  - https://www.myflfamilies.com
- Florida's Child Welfare Statistics
  - http://www.dcf.state.fl.us/programs/childwelfare/dashboard/
- Casey Family Programs
  - https://www.casey.org
- Center for Youth Wellness
  - https://centerforyouthwellness.org/
- American Academy of Pediatrics Health Foster Care America
  - https://www.aap.org/en-us/advocacy-and-policy/aap-health-initiatives/healthy-foster-care-america
- National Youth in Transition Database (NYTD)
  - https://www.acf.hhs.gov/cb/research-data-technology/reporting-systems/nytd
- Tracking the United States Congress
  - https://www.govtrack.us

7.3 Partnership websites

- Community-based Care Central Florida
  - http://www.cbccfl.org
- Move Live Learn
  - http://movelivelearn.com
- University of Central Florida Foundation
  - https://www.ucffoundation.org
- First Start Central Florida Academy
  - https://www.firststar.org/our-academies/university-of-central-florida/
- UCF College of Community Innovation and Education
  - https://ccie.ucf.edu
- Orange County Parks and Recreation
  - http://www.ocfl.net/CultureParks/Parks.aspx?m=dtlvw&d=65#.Xesk5C2ZNN0

- Friends of Puerto Rico
    - https://www.friendsofpuertorico.org
- Lo Cal Guest
    - https://localguest.com
- Cavarocchi Ruscio Dennis Associates
    - https://www.dc-crd.com

A more comprehensive toolkit can be found at *https://clinicalscholarsnli.org/community-impact.*

Author details

Annette Bell[1], Slyving Bourdeau[1], Asha Davis[1], Amanda Stanec[2] and Derrick Stephens[1*]

1 First Step Care, Florida, United States

2 Move Live Learn, Missouri, United States

*Address all correspondence to: dstephens@underdogdreams.org

References

[1] Felitti VJ, Anda RF, Nordenberg D, Williamson DF, Spitz AM, Edwards V et al. Relationship of childhood abuse and household dysfunction to many of the leading causes of death in adults. American Journal of Preventive Medicine. 1998; 14(4):245-258. DOI:10.1016/s0749-3797(98)00017-8.

[2] Pecora PJ, Jensen PS, Romanelli LH, Jackson LJ, Ortiz A. Mental health services for children placed in foster care: an overview of current challenges. Child Welfare. 2009;88(1):5-26.

[3] Dunnigan A, Thompson T, Jonson-Reid M, Drake FM. Chronic health conditions and children in foster care: Determining demographic and placement-related correlates. Journal of Public Child Welfare. 2017;11:4-5, 586-598.

[4] Jackson Y, Cushing CC, Gabrielli J, Fleming K, O'Connor BM., Huffhines L. Child maltreatment, trauma, and physical health outcomes: The role of abuse type and placement moves on health conditions and service use for youth in foster care. Journal of Pediatric Psychology. 2016;41(1):28-36.

[5] Turney K., Wildeman C. Mental and physical health of children in foster care. Pediatrics. 2016;138(5).

[6] Szilagyi MA, Rosen DS, Rubin D, Zlotnik S. Health care issues for children and adolescents in foster care and kinship care. Pediatrics. 2015;136(4):e1142-66.

[7] U.S. Department of Health and Human Services. The AFCARS Report. 2018. Available from: https://www.acf.hhs.gov/sites/default/files/cb/afcarsreport25.pdf.

[8] Florida Institute for Child Welfare. 2015. FY 2014-2015 Annual Report. Available from: http://centerforchildwelfare.org/kb/LegislativeMandatedRpts/FICWAnnualReportFY14-15.pdf.

[9] Florida Department of Children and Families. Florida's Child Welfare Statistics [Internet]. 2019. Available from: https://www.myflfamilies.com/programs/childwelfare/dashboard/. [Accessed 2019-11-30].

[10] U.S. Department of Health and Human Services. Child and Family Services Reviews: Florida Final Report [Internet]. 2016. 38 p. Available from: http://centerforchildwelfare.org/qa/CFSRTools/2016%20CFSR%20Final%20Report.pdf. [Accessed 2019-11-30].

[11] Armstrong MI, Greeson MT. The Florida child welfare services gap analysis report [Internet]. Tampa, FL: University of South Florida, College of Behavioral and Community Sciences; 2014 . 561 p. Report No. 288. Available from: http://centerforchildwelfare.org/kb/flres/GAP_Report040814.pdf. [Accessed 2019-11-30].

[12] Florida Department of Children and Families. 2017 Annual Performance Report [Internet]. 2017. 85 p. Available from: https://www.myflfamilies.com/service-programs/child-welfare/docs/2017LMRs/2017%20Annual%20Performance%20Report_ROA.pdf. [Accessed 2019-11-30].

[13] Metzler M, Merrick MT, Klevens J, Ports KA, Ford DC. Adverse childhood experiences and life opportunities: Shifting the narrative. Children and Youth Services Review. 2017;72:141-149. DOI:10.1016/j.childyouth.2016.10.021.

[14] Radcliff E, Crouch E, Strompolis M. Srivastav A. Homelessness in childhood and adverse childhood experiences

(ACEs). Maternal and Child Health Journal. 2019;23:811-820. DOI:10.1007/s10995-018-02698-w

[15] Harris NB. The Deepest Well: Healing the Long-Term Effects of Childhood Adversity. Boston, MA: Houghton Mifflin; 2018. p. 272.

[16] Hansen DM, Larson R. The youth experience survey 2.0: Instrument revisions and validity testing. Urbana-Champaign, IL: University of Illinois. 2005.

[17] Kennedy F, Pearson D, Brett-Taylor L, Talreja V. The life skills assessment scale: measuring life skills of disadvantaged children in the developing world. Social Behavior and Personality: an international journal. 2014;42(2):197-209.

[18] Quarmby T, Pickering K. Physical activity and children in care: A scoping review of barriers, facilitators, and policy for disadvantaged youth. Journal of Physical Activity and Health. 2016;13(7):780-787.

[19] Gilligan R. Enhancing the resilience of children and young people in public are by mentoring their talents and interests. Child Family Social Work. 1999;4:187-196.

[20] National Physical Activity Plan Alliance. The 2018 United States Report Card on Physical Activity for Children and Youth. Washington, DC: National Physical Activity Plan Alliance; 2018.

[21] Ward J. Effects of choice on student motivation and physical activity behavior in physical education. Journal of Teaching in Physical Education. 2008;27(3):385-398.

[22] Quarmby T, Sandford R, Pickering K. Care -experienced youth and positive development: An exploratory study into the value and use of leisure-time activities. Leisure Studies. 2019;38(1):28-42.

[23] Braveman P, Arkin E, Orleans T, Proctor D, Plough A. What is Health Equity [Internet]. 2017. Available from: https://www.rwjf.org/en/library/research/2017/05/what-is-health-equity-.html [Accessed 2019-11-30].

[24] Centers for Disease Control and Prevention. Social Determinants of Health: Know What Affects Health [Internet]. 2018. Available from: https://www.thegrowthfaculty.com/blog/BrenBrowntoptipassumeothersaredoingthebesttheycan. [Accessed 2019-11-30].

[25] Kininmonth C. Brené Brown Top Tip: Assume Others are Doing the Best They Can [Internet]. 2019. Available from: https://www.thegrowthfaculty.com/blog/BrenBrowntoptipassumeothersaredoingthebesttheycan. [Accessed 2019-11-30].

Chapter 9

Creating a Culture of Mental Health in Filipino Immigrant Communities through Community Partnerships

Aviril Sepulveda, Dean M. Coffey, Jed David, Horacio Lopez, Kamil Bantol and Joyce R. Javier

Abstract

One out of five children in the United States has a mental, emotional, or behavioral health diagnosis. Behavioral health issues cost America $247 billion per year and those with mental health disorders have poorer health and shorter lives. Evidence-based parenting interventions provided in childhood have proven to be effective in helping parents to prevent disruptive, oppositional and defiant behaviors, anxiety and depressive symptoms, tobacco, alcohol, and drug misuse, aggression, delinquency, and violence. Yet, few parents participate in such programs, especially hard-to-reach, underserved minority and immigrant populations. The Robert Wood Johnson Foundation has identified a culture of health action framework that mobilizes individuals, communities, and organizations in order to examine ways to improve systems of prevention, invest in building the evidence base for such systems, and provide evidence-based information to decision makers. The overarching goal of this effort was to create a *culture of mental health* among Filipinos, a large, yet understudied immigrant community that is affected by alarming mental health disparities, including high rates of adolescent suicide ideation and attempts. Our impact project focused on increasing the reach of the Incredible Years® because maximizing the participation of high-risk, hard-to-engage populations may be one of the most important ways to increase the population-level impact of evidence-based parenting programs. If the approach succeeded with Filipinos, comparable strategies could be used to effectively reach other underserved populations in the U.S., many of whom are reluctant to seek behavioral health services. In this chapter we discuss 1) the state of the literature on the topic of Filipino adolescent mental health disparities; 2) our wicked problem and the impact project aimed at ameliorating this issue; 3) how our team formed and implemented our impact project; 4) outcomes and results of our efforts; 5) challenges we faced and how they were overcome; 6) the leadership and health equity skills that were most helpful in addressing our problem; and 7) a toolkit that could assist other communities addressing youth mental health and prevention of suicide and depression.

Keywords: Filipino, suicide prevention, mental health stigma, community-based participator research

1. Introduction

1.1 Filipinos are a large yet invisible minority affected by significant youth behavioral health disparities

According to the 2010 US Census, Asians surpassed Hispanics as the largest group of new immigrants to the United States [1]. With a population of over 3.4 million, the Filipino population is the second-largest Asian subgroup in the United States and the largest Asian population in California. Despite their size, Filipinos are among the least studied groups when it comes to health, due to a lack of research that disaggregates Asian ethnic groups. In contrast to the "model minority myth" ascribed to Asians in general, the few studies on Filipino youth reveal higher rates of behavioral problems such as depressive symptoms, anxiety, and substance use compared to other Asian subgroups and ethnic groups [2–14]. For example, data from the US Youth Risk Behavioral Surveillance System found that Filipino youth have higher rates of adolescent female suicidal ideation (45.6%) compared with non-Hispanic white (26.2%), Hispanic (33.4%), and African-American (25.3%) females [13]. Filipino parents are exposed to multiple adversities, including intimate partner violence, loss of social status, discrimination, and high rates of major and postpartum depression, placing their children at risk for future behavioral health problems [15–24].

Despite these disparities, Filipino adults and children have low rates of mental health care utilization, including low engagement in parenting interventions, particularly in Los Angeles County [4, 16, 19, 25–30]. Due to stigma associated with mental health problems, many Filipinos access mental health services at lower rates and often as a last resort [7, 14, 15]. They are encouraged to keep problems within the family to avoid bringing shame (*hiya*) to the family [7, 11]. Given these unique aspects of the U.S. Filipino immigrant population, one of the authors (JJ) used a community-partnered participatory approach over the past 16 years to optimize the well-being of Filipino families [4, 5, 7, 8, 10–12, 28, 29, 31–33]. She learned that trusted community-based organizations such as churches can serve as gatekeepers to behavioral preventive services, such as parenting programs [8, 11].

1.2 Harsh discipline may be associated with Filipino youth's increased risk for mental health and behavioral health problems

The prevalence of physical punishment in the Philippines is 75% [34]. In a population-based study in the Philippines, the number of abused children from 1998 to 2002 increased five-fold; 90% of adolescent respondents endorsed having been physically maltreated while 60% reported being psychologically abused at least once in their lifetimes [35]. An international study of harsh discipline found that compared to five other countries, Filipino mothers reported the highest rates of harsh verbal discipline (71%) and harsh physical discipline with an object (56%) [34]. In our pilot work, 82% of Filipino immigrant parents of children ages 6–12 years old reported using physical punishment. Growing evidence also suggests that harsh discipline may be associated with Filipino youth's increased risk for subsequent unhealthy coping, low self-esteem, depression, anxiety, and physical abuse [23, 36–40].

1.3 Parenting plays a critical role in the development of childhood behavior problems

Parenting practices strongly affect child behavior problems, perhaps even playing a causal role [41]. Child behavior affects parenting in a transactional manner [42–45]. Children's challenging behaviors (e.g., high activity level and poor emotional regulation) can elicit coercive and detached parenting, with low nurturance/affection [46]. This parenting style may exacerbate the child's behavior problems [41, 47–49]. In contrast, parental affection, supervision and firm behavioral control predict long-term positive outcomes [50–54]. Parent training programs alter parents' behavior and, presumably in response, children's behavior [55, 56]. They also prevent punitive parenting and challenging child behaviors early, and interrupt this dysfunctional coercive cycle before the child's behaviors become more serious, requiring more intensive treatment.

1.4 Parenting interventions during middle childhood may have the potential to decrease harsh discipline in Filipino immigrant families

Middle childhood is a distinct developmental period with respect to understanding children's perceptions of their parents' behavior and how these perceptions relate to children's behavioral and psychological adjustment. Dramatic changes in cognitive development take place between the ages of 5 and 7 years [57, 58]. For example, children's beliefs become better predictors of their subsequent behavior [59, 60]. About the age of 8 years, the meaning that children attach to their parents' behavior becomes more salient. They notice differences among the discipline practices of their own parents and parents of peers [61]. This is relevant to Filipino immigrant families in the United States because of differences in child rearing practices between mainstream U.S. culture and Filipino culture [62, 63]. For example, Filipino parents are more likely to show their love indirectly through actions, while there is more emphasis on verbal communication of love and praise in mainstream U.S. culture [64].

The *Incredible Years® Parent Training Program* (IY) developed by Dr. Carolyn Webster-Stratton is one of the best-studied evidence-based parent training programs [55, 65]. The Incredible Years® programs are published in a series by developmental level for babies, toddlers, preschool and school age children. There is also the Advanced IY Program that is focused on promotion of positive communication within the family and between adults. Current evidence suggests that parent behavior-management programs like IY are promising treatments for reducing internalizing symptoms in clinically-referred preschool children and high-risk Chinese immigrant school-age children who have been referred to child protective services [66–69].

Filipino children growing up in the United States acculturate at a faster rate than their foreign-born parents, leading to conflict in the home [67–71]. These weakened family bonds have been linked with negative psychological outcomes such as depression among children of immigrants [72, 73]. For Filipinos, family conflict is significantly associated with depression, suicide-related behaviors, and substance use [74, 75]. Social cognitive theory suggests that childhood internalizing symptoms may have roots in dysfunctional parenting behaviors and family environments [76]. For instance, depressive behaviors may be both modeled and selectively reinforced by parents [77]. IY addresses problems associated with differential rates of acculturation between immigrant children and parents and targets many of the proposed mechanisms and risk factors for internalizing distress, such as harsh and unpredictable or critical parenting behaviors. Parents also learn cognitive strategies for themselves that they are encouraged to model and teach their children, such as self-praise; how to challenge negative thoughts; how to give positive attention through academic, social and emotional coaching; and how to get support.

2. Wicked problem impact project (WPIP) description

Our work together as a team in the Robert Wood Johnson Foundation (RWJF) Clinical Scholars Program was built on the foundation created by our Team Leader

(JJ). This included a needs assessment of the Filipino community that generated the consensus that the greatest community needs were the behavioral problems among Filipino adolescents that were exacerbated by the low utilization rates of services to address these problems. A suggested solution was also offered by the community to use an evidence-based parenting intervention during middle childhood before the children in this age group became adolescents [8, 11]. The importance of this first step cannot be stated too strongly. This project began as a community-defined problem with a community-defined solution.

The feasibility of such a project was tested with a pilot study that showed the intervention was acceptable by the parents participating in the first four IY pilot groups. Parents in the group reported lower parenting stress, increased use of positive verbal discipline and decreased use of physical punishment [10]. Focus groups conducted at the end of the pilot study identified a significant barrier to recruitment of immigrant Filipino parents as the cultural stigma associated with seeking help outside the extended family system [30]. These same groups proposed the novel solution to this problem of producing video recordings of testimonials by Filipino parents who participated in the groups about how the groups improved their parent–child relationship and how parents could incorporate their Filipino family values when using these parenting techniques [29].

The culturally-tailored video of parent testimonials was produced in partnership with a Community Advisory Board (CAB) using constructs from the Health Belief Model and Theory of Planned Behavior [78, 79]. We evaluated the video, entitled "*Para Sa Kinabukasan Ng Ating Mga Anak*: For Our Children's Future" (https://www.youtube.com/watch?feature=player_embedded&v=Md3jOFiXhtc) in a randomized controlled trial that involved screening nearly 600 Filipinos over a 16-month period in 23 community sites. A total of 215 parents and grandparents enrolled in the study. Compared to a control video, caregivers who watched the culturally-tailored video had significantly greater odds of enrolling in IY parent groups [4].

The RWJF Clinical Scholars Program to create a culture of health in the United States through the support and leadership training of teams to address a *wicked* health problem was a good fit for the next steps to bring about change in the community. Dr. Javier recruited an interdisciplinary team consisting of a well-respected Filipino community pediatrician (HL), a senior psychologist who was an expert in IY training and implementation (DC), an occupational therapist who was a cultural arts leader in the Filipino community (JD), and another occupational therapist who was promoting community action to address the problem of post-partum depression in new mothers (AS). Together, we formed Team Kapwa, named for a word which signifies a Filipino cultural value of shared identity. Participation in the Clinical Scholars Program caused us to narrow our focus to one wicked problem – the high rates of suicidality among Filipino adolescents, while expanding our influence and impact through high quality leadership training.

During the laying of the foundation and initial pilot research, the wicked problem grew more implacable. Suicide became the leading cause of death among Asian American and Pacific Islander youth ages 12–19 years; and among 10 to 14-year-old Asian or Pacific Islander females in the United States, suicide was tied with unintentional injuries as the leading cause of death [80, 81]. Our challenge was to use the positive parenting interventions from Incredible Years School Age Parent Program with the communication interventions from the IY Advanced Program with Filipino parents of children ages 8 to 12 years. Together, we believed that these two programs, focused on enhancing the parent–child relationship and developing effective family communication, would increase two protective factors against suicide: family connectedness and other adult caring to reduce these high rates of adolescent suicidality in the Filipino community.

3. Methods

3.1 Project

Evidence-based parenting programs do a wonderful job assisting parents who enroll in them. However, our biggest challenge was getting parents to participate, especially parents living in low-income, under-resourced communities. We could not address the wicked problem of mental health disorders among Filipino youth in our healthcare system alone. Our project used a community based participatory research model to connect our interdisciplinary team with service providers, community and faith leaders, consumers, and researchers to address the barriers to participation in behavioral health programs and prevent the wicked problem of adolescent suicidality in the Filipino community. The project addressed systemic gaps in our community that continue to contribute to the lack of utilization of mental health services and parenting programs in our community.

Exacerbating these systemic gaps to participating in effective parenting programs was the barrier of stigma associated with discussing mental health issues like suicide (i.e., suicide ideation and attempts may be under-reported because of its non-acceptance by the Catholic church and the associated shame to the family. We addressed this challenge by continuing to engage faith-based leaders in our planning and implementation activities. We offered IY as a prevention program rather than restricting it to children with behavior problems in order to overcome the stigma associated with accessing parenting programs, and the shame related to having a child with mental health problems.

3.2 Conceptual framework

Based on Bronfenbrenner's social ecological model, our strategy to implementing parenting interventions addresses multiple levels of influence [82]. Bronfenbrenner's social ecological model describes the levels of relationship among the family and the social systems and institutions that impact the functioning of the family (**Figure 1**). For example, we addressed the personal level by promoting the social and emotional competence of the child and teaching effective coping strategies to parents. On the interpersonal level we promoted healthy caregiver-child interaction, family functioning, school functioning, the home environment, while enhancing positive family/peer norms and the development of social networks. At the community level we offered IY as a community resource and promoted positive community norms (ie, decreasing the stigma associated with participation in parenting programs) (**Figure 2**).

3.3 Approach

Our project was designed to reflect the first two phases of a three-phase community-based participatory research initiative [83]. Phase 1 was the partnered planning of the initiative. Phase 2 was the implementation of the initiative, which from a community perspective is a pilot to determine what works in the community. Phase 3 was the initiation of community dissemination beyond agencies in the implementation phase based on a partnered analysis of Phase 2. Each phase has a cycle of activities that we refer to as the plan-do-evaluate cycle.

Phase 1 involved a series of meetings to address barriers and needs in the community in order to develop a shared understanding of mental health, by which we could facilitate implementation of a culturally-congruent educational campaign that can improve mental health awareness in our community. We formed a Steering

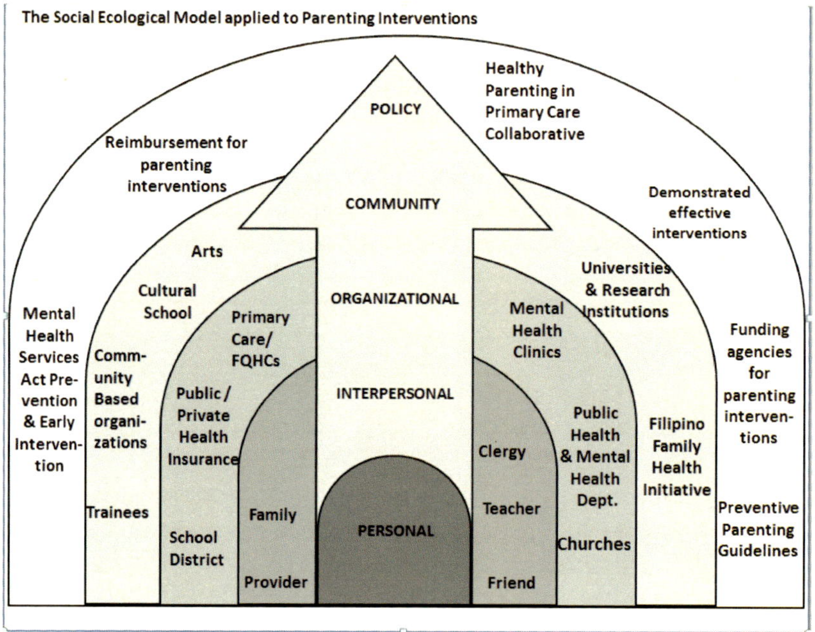

Figure 1.
Social ecological model applied to parenting interventions.

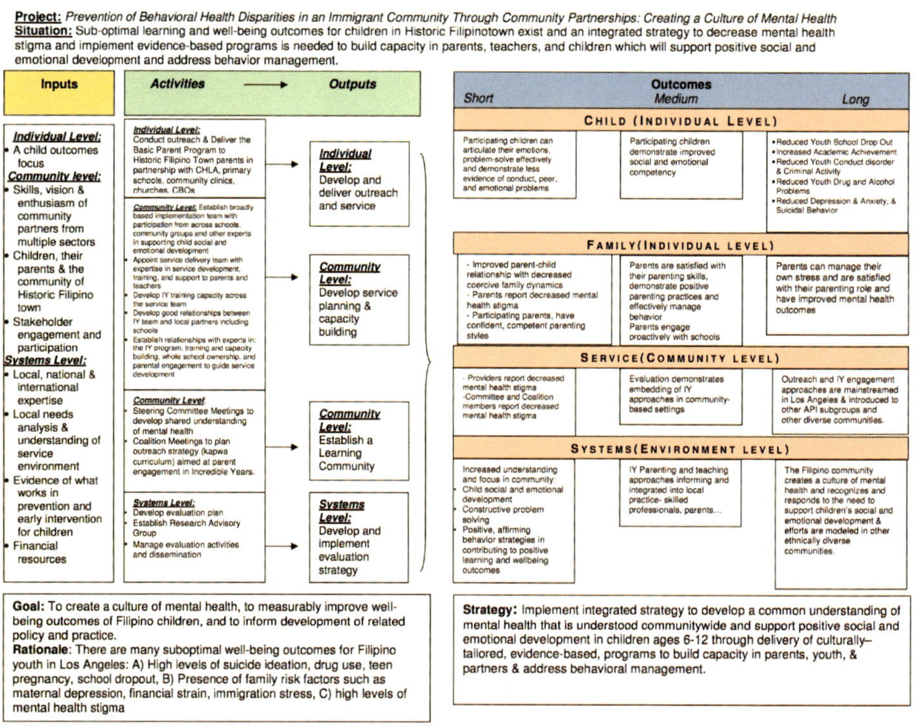

Figure 2.
Logic model for creating a culture of mental health in Filipino immigrant communities through community partnerships.

committee of seven members who would meet monthly to plan activities and conduct focus groups with Filipino community members and create a shared definition of mental health for Filipino youth. Based on prior studies, we developed an educational campaign strategy and planned a conference that combined science, art, and faith to engage the community in a dialog about mental health. This conference included activities such as presentations about mental health issues in the Filipino community by consumers, researchers, and community leaders; trainings in discussion of mental health issues; and screening of digital stories and dance performances about mental health stigma in the Filipino community. Our primary community partners included: Asian Pacific Counseling and Treatment Center; local churches; schools (both parochial and public); *Kayamang ng Lahi*, a Philippine cultural music and dance troupe; Search to Involve Pilipino Americans; and the Filipino Cultural School.

Phase 2 included training providers and community members to be group leaders in the Incredible Years® Parent Training Program and implementing the program. We continued to meet with our CAB, which was comprised mostly of Filipino parents who have helped us determine best practices/strategies for engaging parents to participate in the Incredible Years®. From our CAB we learned to incorporate *kapwa*, a core Filipino value defined as community, togetherness, or a sense of shared identity, and adopted the name Team Kapwa for our impact team. In order to contribute to the lack of research on Filipino youth prevention efforts and lack of preventive programs for depression and suicide in this community, we conducted a pilot study evaluating the Incredible Years® School Age Basic and Advance Program to Filipino parents of children ages 8–12 years old.

4. Outcomes

4.1 Creating a shared definition of mental health in the Filipino community

With the goal of creating a shared definition of childhood mental health in the Filipino community, we conducted focus groups in community organizations serving a large number of Filipino Americans. A total of thirty-seven (37) adults participated, many of whom were parents/grandparents, primary care or mental health providers, Incredible Years graduates, college students, and community advocates. Ages ranged from 18 to 79 years old which allowed the groups to have a depth in perspectives from multiple generations. A majority of participants also had previous experience working with Filipino youth, namely as caregivers or health providers.

We first asked participants to share words--both positive and negative--that came to mind when hearing "Filipino" and "mental health". The results highlighted the prevalence of mental health stigma. Participants commonly used the words judgmental, shame, crazy, and defect, indicating that mental illness continues to be negatively viewed in the community. Participants also described mental health as "hereditary" which coincides with the belief among Filipinos that mental health issues are solely genetic and passed down from generations. We used a word cloud to visualize these results (**Figure 3**). Remarkably, the most frequently shared word was "family" to describe mental health. Participants noted that an individual's mental health status is often dependent on family dynamics and communication. This reinforced the importance of our work with the Incredible Years® parenting workshops, given that fostering strong family relationships was seen as having the most influence in improving mental health status of Filipino youth.

Next, we provided focus group participants with several definitions of mental health. These included definitions by the World Health Organization, Centers for Disease Control and Prevention, and Philippine Mental Health Association. Using the choices that were reviewed and identified by our steering committee, we then asked participants to highlight words and phrases regarding mental health that they felt most resonated with Filipino parents. Word cloud results showed that

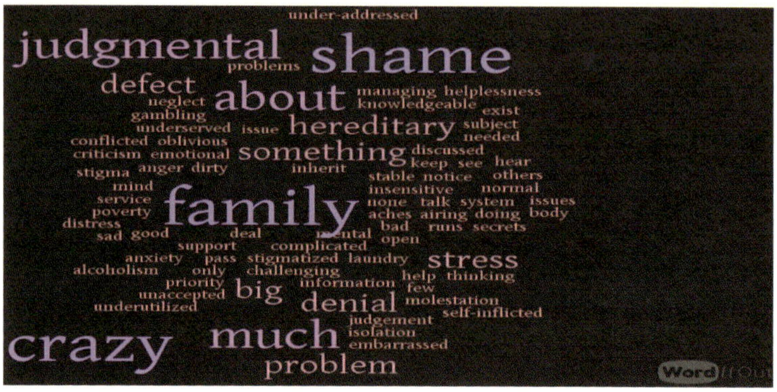

Figure 3.
Initial impressions of focus group participants to the terms, Filipino and Mental Health.

there was great variability in what the community sees as optimal mental health (**Figure 4**). For instance, participants chose the words and phrases, "well-being, peace of mind, productive, sense of identity, contribute to community, coping with normal stressors, and self-worth." These words are interconnected, yet they also describe different ways to achieve mental health and well-being. This served as a lesson for Team Kapwa: When approaching people about our project, we must appeal to the various mental health goals that the community values. We highlighted not just the potential for academic and social skill development, but also lessons on coping skills and dealing with everyday stressors.

4.2 Filipino family wellness - community conversations

Team Kapwa conducted a community-wide conference that sought to decrease mental health stigma and create a culture of mental health in the Filipino community. Flyers were sent to all previous study participants and disseminated in our team's social

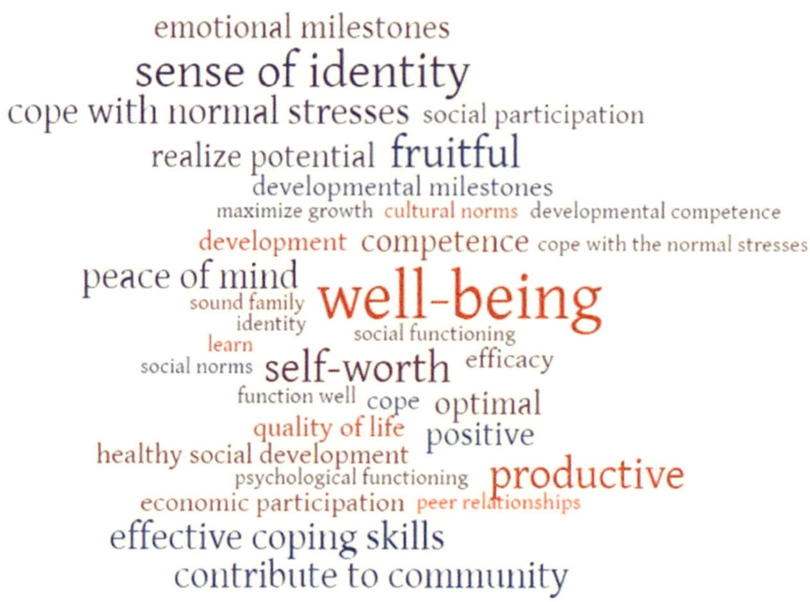

Figure 4.
Community preferred definitions of mental health synthesized from four standard definitions of mental health.

media site (facebook.com/filipinofamilyhealthLA). Our partners also distributed flyers throughout their organizations. In total, 130 people attended the event, many of whom were community members, students, parents, children, and IY graduates.

The conference successfully combined science and the arts to engage the community in a dialog about mental health. Dr. Javier presented compelling mental health statistics about suicide and health disparities among Filipino youth and also included a screening of the culturally tailored video, *Para Sa Kinabukasan Ng Ating Mga Anak* (For Our Children's Future). This was followed by a screening of Silent Sacrifices: Voices of the Filipino American Family, which was presented by Dr. Judy Patacsil. Silent Sacrifices was a documentary that tackled issues such as family conflict, generational gaps and depression among Filipino youth. Several community members shared their mental health experiences through a segment called "*Kwentuhan*" (Storytelling). The purpose of these stories was to highlight the prevalence of mental health disorders and the importance of seeking help. For example, one speaker shared how, despite being a nurse in a hospital Neonatal Intensive Care Unit (NICU), she was unsuccessful in helping her daughter cope with postpartum depression.

The conference also featured programs by Filipino organizations, including a folk dance by the group, *Kayamanan Ng Lahi*, and a play by the drama group, StanD, that addressed the stigma of mental illness among family members. Lastly, we offered breakout sessions to introduce participants to mental health resources in the community. These sessions introduced resources such as One Degree--a nonprofit that works with low-income families, the Los Angeles Department of Mental Health, and demonstration of the Incredible Years®. A copy of the program can be found in **Figure 5**.

After the conference, we asked participants to give us feedback on why they attended the event. Their answers highlighted the growing change in attitudes regarding mental health in the Filipino community. We learned that the community was ready to start conversations about mental health. According to one participant, "I think it's important to create discussion and dialogue as a form of normalizing [mental health] and education."

Other comments showed that the community was starting to see the importance of mental health care. One participant noted, "[I attended the event] to learn more about mental health and wellness specifically within the Pilipino community." Most importantly, we learned that the Filipino community was ready to take action and combat mental health stigma. One participant stated simply but powerfully, "We can no longer afford to be a silent minority. Too many of our youth are dying."

4.3 Sustainability

Sustainability required building upon the strength of our community organizations. To accomplish this, Team Kapwa developed partnerships with 12 new organizations that included public and private schools, school districts, a Filipino cultural school, community-based organizations and churches. Additionally, 15 Incredible Years® parent graduates became members of our Community Advisory Board, allowing us to hear directly from parents and learn ways to tackle mental health stigma in the Filipino community. We trained 45 health care professionals, parent champions, and community members to be Incredible Years® group leaders. We also started a social media group to reach the community digitally and have accumulated over 200 followers in the first 8 months. Finally, we have several pre-health and pre-mental health undergraduate and graduate level students, including our fifth author, who have dedicated their time to participate in and volunteer for this initiative. Team Kapwa believes it is critical to train the next generation of providers to conduct community-based participator research in the Filipino community.

FILIPINO FAMILY WELLNESS - COMMUNITY CONVERSATIONS

9:30 - 10:00	**Registration and Light Refreshments**
10:00 - 10:50	**Welcoming Remarks** **Filipino Family Wellness & Best Practices for Raising Kids in the U.S.: Our Story** Joyce Javier, MD, MPH, MS Team Kapwa Lilian Fabros Bando, JD, MSW
10:50 - 11:50	**Feature Film and Presentation** **Silent Sacrifices: Voices of the Filipino American Family** Judy Patacsil, PsyD, MFT
11:50 - 12:35	**Kwentuhan - Community Features** Mellissa Veluz-Abraham, MPA Riann De Los Reyes, RN, BSN Millie Pagett, RN
12:35 - 1:35	**Lunch and Cultural Arts Presentations** Philippine Classics - Piano and Violin Angela Reyes and Erica Abrina Family, Wellness and Healing in Philippine Folk Arts Kayamanan Ng Lahi Philippine Folk Arts
1:35 - 2:25	**StanD** A play to help break the stigma of mental illness
2:25 - 2:30	**Mindfulness Break** Rachel Gonzalez, RYT 200 Registered Yoga Instructor
2:30 - 3:20	**Break-Out Sessions** How to Easily Find the Right Community Resource: An Intro to One Degree Irving Pineda Everything You Want to Know About Mental Health Adrienne Cedro-Hament, LCSW When the Talking Stops: Promoting Family Communication Ana Jayme and Joyce Javier, MD, MPH, MS Thirty Years Too Late: Making Relationships Stronger Dean Coffey, PsyD and Horacio Lopez, M
3:20 - 3:35	**Closing Remarks**

Figure 5.
Filipino family wellness community conversations conference program.

Beyond this project, Team Kapwa's ultimate goal was to offer the Incredible Years® program to all families beginning from infancy to adolescence. We took several steps to achieve this. Drs. Javier and Sepulveda received funding to conduct IY Baby pilot groups, offering the groups in primary care and for mothers with postpartum depression who have babies in a NICU. We also successfully advocated for the Los Angeles County Department of Mental Health to add the briefer Incredible Years® Attentive Parenting Program as a billable prevention intervention. The goal to create sustainability accomplished its first steps with families in the Filipino community. To date, 100 Filipino parents have completed IY School Age groups, 70 new parents have enrolled, and at the end of the impact project funding period, Team Kapwa continued to work toward sustainability by expanding the research base with Filipino families and youth by conducting a program evaluation using a randomized pilot study to offer the Incredible Years® Advance Program for parents of children ages 8–12 years old. A notable difference in the recruitment for this new study were several parents who joined the study to address early indications of depression and self-harm in their pre-adolescent children.

This chapter describes the seminal work to address the wicked problem of suicide among Filipino adolescents by the Robert Wood Johnson Foundation

Clinical Scholars Program. Team Kapwa promoted the protective factors of family connectedness and other adult caring by offering Incredible Years® parenting workshops suggested by the Filipino immigrant community. The approach used by Team Kapwa may best be discussed in terms of the three guiding principles of the American Psychological Association's Task Force on Immigration [84]. The first principle is that "immigrants are resilient and resourceful" (p. 132). This impact project could not have been done without the involvement of community partners who defined the problem and offered their community defined solution, to provide parent training to parents of Filipino pre-adolescents to enhance the parent–child relationship before the children became adolescents. One of the strengths of this work with immigrant families was the partnership of the team with the community agencies and leaders as well as with parents participating in the workshops.

The second guiding principle is that "immigrants, like all human beings, are influenced by social contexts" (p. 134). Trust between the research team and the community, together with a sense of *kapwa,* the Filipino cultural value of shared identity with one another, produced a relationship that grew over years of interaction between the team and community members. This is especially true of cultures that are collectivistic. The use of the Incredible Years,® which was suggested during the community needs assessment, was very adaptable to the cultural values of the parents. Out of this relationship came a cohesive Community Advisory Board and willingness to participate in the production of a culturally tailored video for recruitment of parents to participate in groups with other Filipino parents. Melissa Veluz-Abraham, a mother who participated in a parent group described her experience this way:

"We strongly believe the cultural sensitivity that these classes provide is important to the Filipino parents and grandparents participating in the program. There is a sense of kapwa, a Filipino term that refers to connection with another person. That connection can be through shared experiences as Filipinos; ... experiences of how we were raised and the challenges those experiences may bring in our own child-rearing realities today. Kapwa also refers to consideration for the other; a sense of empathy for another human being. This was strong in our parent group that met every Saturday. There was a sense of support in that we all wanted to become better parents and caregivers, and we provided each other encouragement and compassion as we tried out and practiced the useful concepts and exercises that the program shared with us. The honesty that participants had in this space allowed us to learn from one another and helped us become the best caregivers that we can be for our children."

The use of Bronfenbrenner's social ecological model was effective in identifying avenues of influence and opportunities to promote change through considering the multiple levels of social context within the Filipino community and greater. It provided a conceptual foundation for the work of Team Kapwa.

Perhaps, the third guiding principle will be the most important for teams working with other cultural groups; to "use the lens of culture with the increasingly diverse immigrant-origin population." Team Kapwa completed focus groups with diverse generations within the Filipino community to create a shared definition of mental health (manuscript in preparation). In this activity, Team Kapwa again engaged the community to obtain their wisdom and expertise around the very culturally loaded and often stigmatized topic of mental health. The information obtained informed a values-based approach to engaging the community to increase engagement and participation in community activities to promote mental health. This was demonstrated in their use of the culturally-tailored video produced by members to the team prior to involvement in the RWJF Clinical Scholars Program that enhanced engagement of the Filipino community. The low-cost video production and digital storytelling by Team Kapwa and families from the Filipino community increased the impact and acceptance of their work in the Filipino community and beyond.

5. Key challenges for the future

There is still much to be done in the areas of engagement and sustainability. A reliable plan for sustainability is essential now with Filipino parents using the Incredible Years® parent workshops as less stigmatized avenues to seek mental health treatment services for their children in their own communities. To that end, Team Kapwa has applied for $250,000 in outreach funds from the Los Angeles County Department of Mental Health as part of the California Department of Public Health's California Reducing Public Disparities Project (CRDP) to fund these ongoing outreach parent groups in the Filipino community.

While this impact project had a focus on a specific problem in the Filipino community, there are lessons that were learned by Team Kapwa that may be helpful to other interprofessional teams and community activists interested in addressing wicked problems in their own communities. Without a doubt, the most effective part of such a project is beginning with a thorough community needs assessment that engages community leaders to identify and define the problem as well as to offer their ideas for solutions. The ongoing development of a Community Advisory Board is desirable to engage ongoing community support for the project. In terms of having an impact with a low budget, the use of culturally tailored engagement video and digital storytelling (available at filipinofamilyhealth.com) can amplify the voices of the community and enhance the willingness of the community to listen to important public health messages and respond. It is one way to use the lens of culture to engage diverse and hard-to-reach immigrant communities. The Leader Learning section that follows has suggestions for leadership skills that Team Kapwa found helpful in promoting a culture of health within the Filipino community and beyond.

6. Leader learning

Addressing complex problems calls for a variety of leadership skills that are necessary to understand and tackle abstract issues around the problem, engage the community, and produce systems to promote change. Awareness is one lesson that resonated with all the leaders in the group. Awareness of self, others, the culture, the community and the systems are catalysts to understanding the problem. Joyce Javier considered self-awareness as an important skill in her understanding what motivates her and others. Apple Sepulveda's recognition of the commonality of her own experiences and that of the community and how sharing her story was not only healing to her but also helped heal and empower other members of the community. Jed David's self-awareness has led him to take a deeper dive to knowing himself. The self-assessments that were an integral part of the Clinical Scholars Program led him to understand himself as a leader, identify areas for individual growth and increase impact. Dean Coffey grew in his conscious awareness of the inequities in the healthcare system; inequities created and sustained by poverty with wide gaps in economic resources that resulted in significant differences in the opportunity to live healthy lives. Horacio Lopez expressed appreciation for the development of his own leadership skills and growing awareness needed to acquire more skills to become an even more effective leader.

Communication, the exchange of ideas through language, gesture, and written information, was an essential leadership tool. Learning to communicate with each other as a team and with members helped Team Kapwa exchange clear ideas with one another. This communication fostered collaboration and partnership that helped us expand our networks and partners. The art of conversation that comes with effective communication skills helped us make adaptations to our messages to fit the varied types of audiences.

Negotiation, the art and method for reaching agreements, was not only important in accomplishing tasks but also in achieving outcomes. In solving complex problems, the solutions are often ambiguous. Critical solutions require negotiation skills to engage the interests of two opposing ideas. Negotiation in engaging stakeholders, community members, and even the team members was very useful in not just accomplishing the objectives of the project but also in persuading others to increase motivation and buy-in of key community leaders and organizations.

Experiential learning in the Clinical Scholars Program was transformational through a variety of learning experiences that met the needs of different learners where they were and helped us to move forward through a deeper understanding of ourselves and others. The training was transformative for us in further developing our educational philosophy that learners learn best when they are actively engaged and interested in the subject matter being taught. It is a process of collaboration that works best when the learner is relaxed, engaged and enjoying the process, even when it is more challenging for her/him/them.

Conflict management, the process of mitigating the negative impacts of the conflict and increasing its positive aspects, was also a very useful skill. As leaders, it is important to be able to manage conflict necessary to promote the performance and learning of the team. We acknowledged that conflict is a part of life and a learning opportunity. The different leaders on this team had different styles, and by knowing the different patterns of approaching conflicts and the different alternatives we can embrace, improves relationships among one another and with our community partners.

Collaboration was essential. Leadership is not working alone. As one of our trainers stated, "Power shared is power multiplied." One of the important transformations experienced is the realization that leadership is not an individual skill but a shared skill. Each person on a leadership team brings a unique skill set and influential personality qualities that empower the team in different ways. Being a lone leader is not as effective, but together, much more can be achieved. Fostering collaboration entails partnering with the community. Listening to the community and asking them for ways to help with solving the complex problems they are facing. The phrase, "Nothing about us, without us," is a tenet we hold dear and follow. By listening to and partnering with stakeholders to identify community-defined solutions to health disparities in the Filipino community, this is how we can most effectively address these issues.

7. Tool kit

This toolkit is to provide communities with a collection of related information, resources, and tools that they can use to guide and adapt as they address similar issues:

https://clinicalscholarsnli.org/wp-content/uploads/2020/07/Toolkit-for-Prevention-of-Behavioral-Health-Disparities-in-an-Immigrant-Community.pdf

7.1 Building a culture of mental health in immigrant Filipino families

This project aims to create a culture of mental health among Filipinos, a large, yet understudied immigrant community that is affected by alarming mental health disparities, including high adolescent suicide ideation and attempts. The project also entails to implement the Incredible Years in community settings and measure mental health stigma, parenting practices, parenting parental stress, and child problem behaviors.

Over the past 10 years, a series of studies that first identified Incredible Years as a community-defined solution to preventing Filipino adolescent behavioral health problems, then pilot tested Incredible Years to assess the feasibility and acceptability of this program, and finally developed a theory-based motivational video to increase enrollment rates in Incredible Years. The success of these pilots underscores our ability to build trust with community organizations serving large Filipino populations and to overcome logistical challenges involved in implementing the intervention.

7.2 Preliminary research

1. Pilot/Feasibility Study Conducted with Filipino Families

2. Development and Evaluation of Theory-based Recruitment Video to Promote Enrollment:

3. Creating a multidisciplinary team of clinicians and a steering committee to address barriers and needs in the community

4. Creating a Shared Definition of Mental Health through focus groups

5. Organized a conference that combined science, art, and faith to engage the community in discussing mental health issues, and screening of digital stories and dance performances about mental health stigma in the Filipino community.

6. Developing community partnerships

7. Implementation of Incredible Years Program to families

7.3 The team

The team members were recruited by the Principal Investigator, Joyce Javier, based on experience needed for the project. The team was comprised of these professionals who contributed in the following ways:

1. Joyce Javier, MD, MPH, MS, a General Pediatrician in an academic setting and project lead, oversaw project activities and evaluation, led the steering committee and coalition, identified systemic gaps and developed and implemented recommendations for change.

2. Dean Coffey, PsyD, a Clinical Psychologist, served as the agency mentor for Incredible Years® at Children's Hospital Los Angeles. He provided expertise, training and supervision in the Incredible Years® implementation.

3. Jed David, an Occupational Therapist at CHLA, had been on the Community Advisory Board for prior projects of Dr. Javier. He is a Tagalog and

Visayan-speaking Occupational Therapist with public policy background, a Tagalog-speaking Incredible Years® workshop leader, and a Philippine cultural arts liaison who provided input regarding use of the arts to engage Filipinos in mental health services.

4. Horacio Lopez, MD is a Tagalog-speaking Community Pediatrician who serves the Historic Filipinotown in Los Angeles and worked with Dr. Javier in her past projects. He also served as a liaison to Filipino community physicians and health care organizations.

5. Aviril Sepulveda, MS, OTD, OTR/L is a Tagalog-speaking Occupational Therapist and Incredible Years® workshop leader. She provided expertise in maternal depression and addressing barriers to mental health care.

6. Ana Jayme, AMFTis a Tagalog-speaking Marriage & Family Therapist, Steering Committee Member, and Incredible Years® Parent Groups Leader.

7. Shelina Miranda, MSW, MPH is Tagalog-speaking Associate Clinical Social Worker and Incredible Years® Parent Group Leader.

Primary funding for this initiative came from the Robert Wood Johnson Clinical Scholars Program.

7.4 Recommended articles and scientific literature

A. Filipino Health and Mental Health Disparities, Use of Community-Based of Participatory Research

1. Jocano, Landa, F. Filipino Value System: A Cultural Definition. Punlnad Research House. Metro Manila. 1997

2. Javier JR, Huffman LC, Mendoza FS. Filipino Child Health in the United States: Do Health and Health Care Disparities Exist? Preventing Chronic Disease. April 2007;4(2):A36. PMID:17362627.

3. de Leon, Mendoza, F. Celebrating the Creative Living Presence: A Culture of Healing: Guideposts for Education, Governance, and Wellness in Philippine Society. Asian Societal Institute. 2017

4. Javier JR, Supan J*, Lansang A*, Beyer W, Kubicek K, & Palinkas LA. Preventing Filipino mental health disparities: Perspectives from adolescents, caregivers, providers, and advocates. *Asian American Journal of Psychology*. 5(4) 316–324. 2014 Dec. PMID: 25667725

5. Coffey DM, Javier JR, Schrager SM. Preliminary Validity of the Eyberg Child Behavior Inventory with Filipino Immigrant Parents. *Child & Family Behavior Therapy.* 37:1–15. 2015. PMID: 27087739

6. Flores N*, Supan J*, Kreutzer C, Coffey DM, Javier JR. Prevention of Filipino Youth Behavioral Health Disparities: Identifying Barriers and Facilitators of Participation in an Evidence-Based Parenting Intervention among Filipino Parents. *Prev Chronic Dis.* 12:E178. 2015 Oct 22. PMID: 26491813

7. Javier JR, Coffey DM, Schrager SM, Palinkas LA, Miranda J. Parenting Intervention for Prevention of Behavioral Problems in Elementary School-Age Filipino-American Children: A Pilot Study in Churches. *J Dev Behav Pediatr*. 37(9):737–745. 2016 Nov/Dec.PMID: 27626390

8. Javier JR, Galura K*, Aliganga FAP*, Supan J*, Palinkas LA. Voices of the Filipino Community Describing the Importance of Family in Understanding Adolescent Behavioral Health Needs. Fam Community Health. 2018 Jan/Mar;41(1):64–71. PMID:29135796

9. Javier JR, Reyes A*, Coffey DM, Schrager SM, Samson A*, Palinkas L, Kipke MD, Miranda J. Recruiting Filipino Immigrants in a Randomized Controlled Trial Promoting Enrollment in an Evidence-Based Parenting Intervention. J Immigr Minor Health. 2018 May 17. PMID:29774510

10. Javier JR. The use of an educational video to increase suicide awareness and enrollment in parenting interventions among Filipinos. *Asian American Journal of Psychology*. Vol.9, No 4, 327–333. 2018 December. DOI: 10.1037/aap0000144. PMID: pending

11. Javier JR, Coffey, DM, Palinkas LA, Kipke MD, Miranda J, Schrager SM. Promoting Enrollment in Parenting Programs Among a Filipino Population: A Randomized Trial. *Pediatrics*. pii: e20180553. 2019 Jan 24. doi: 10.1542/peds.2018-0553. [Epub ahead of print]. PMID: 30679379

12. Maramba DC, ed. Family and Educational Environments: Contexts and Counterstories of Filipino Americans. Charlotte, NC: Information Age Publishing, Inc.; 2013. Endo R. & Rong X, ed. Educating Asian Americans: Achievement, Schooling, and Identities.

13. Nadal KL, Monzones J. Filipino Americans and Neuropsychology. In: Fujii D, ed. The Neuropsychology of Asian Americans. Boca Raton, FL: Taylor and Francis; 2010:47–70.

14. David EJ. Cultural mistrust and mental health help-seeking attitudes among Filipino Americans. *Asian American Journal of Psychology.* 2010;1(1):57–66.

15. David EJ. A colonial mentality model of depression for Filipino Americans. *Cultur Divers Ethnic Minor Psychol.* 2008;14(2):118–127.

16. Wolf D. Family secrets: transnational struggles among children of Filipino immigrants. *Sociol Perspect.* 1997;40(3):457–482.

17. Javier JR, Chamberlain LJ, Rivera KK, Gonzalez SE, Mendoza FS, Huffman LC. Lessons learned from a community-academic partnership addressing adolescent pregnancy prevention in Filipino American families. *Progress in Community Health Partnerships.* 2010;4(4):305–313. PMID:21169708.

18. Pesigan IJ, Luyckx K, Alampay LP. Brief report: identity processes in Filipino late adolescents and young adults: parental influences and mental health outcomes. *J Adolesc.* 2014;37(5):599–604.

19. Hayes DK, Ta VM, Hurwitz EL, Mitchell-Box KM, Fuddy LJ. Disparities in self-reported postpartum depression among Asian, Hawaiian, and Pacific

Islander Women in Hawaii: Pregnancy Risk Assessment Monitoring System (PRAMS), 2004–2007. *Maternal and child health journal.* 2010;14(5):765–773.

B. Recommended Literature on Mental Health Stigma (the *Wicked Problem* identified in this project)

1. Developing a Research Agenda for Understanding the Stigma of Addictions Part I: Lessons From the Mental Health Stigma Literature

2. Developing a Research Agenda for Reducing the Stigma of Addictions, Part II: Lessons From the Mental Health Stigma Literature

3. Mental Health: Culture, Race, and Ethnicity: A Supplement to Mental Health: A Report of the Surgeon General. (Chapter 4 Mental Health Care for American Indians and Alaska Natives)

4. Combating Stigma Within the Michigan Mental Health System: A Toolkit for Change

5. Anti-Stigma: A Guide to Reducing Addiction-Related Stigma

6. Gee GC, Spencer MS, Chen J, Takeuchi D. A nationwide study of discrimination and chronic health conditions among Asian Americans. Am J Public Health. Jul 2007;97(7):1275–1282. PMID:17538055.

7. B4Stage4: Changing the Way We Think About Mental Health

8. Children's Mental Health Ontario's Youth Action Committee Mental Health Awareness Toolkit

C. Recommended Literature: Community-Based Participatory Research CBPR Principles and application:

1. Wells K, Miranda J, Bruce ML, Alegria MA, Wallerstein N. Bridging Community Intervention and Mental Health Services Research. American Journal ofPsychiatry. 2004;161(6):955–963.

2. Applying Community-Based Participatory Research Principles to the Development of a Smoking-Cessation Program for American Indian Teens: "Telling Our Story

3. Community Engagement Principles for Community-Campus Partnerships for Health

4. Understanding the Community and its Culture

D. Recommended Literature Learning from Others, Having Conversations about Health and Mental Health in Diverse Populations

1. Chung B, Jones L, Jones A, et al. Community Arts Events to Enhance Collective Efficacy and Community Engagement as a Means of Addressing Depression in an African American Community. American Journal of Public Health. 2009;99(2):237–244.

2. Corbie-Smith G, Goldmon M, Isler MR, et al. Partnerships in Health Disparities Research and the Roles of Pastors of Black Churches: Potential Conflict, Synergy, and Expectations. Journal of the National Medical Association.102(9):823–831.

3. Baezconde-Garbanati L, Murphy ST, Moran MB, Cortessis VK. Reducing theExcess Burden of Cervical Cancer Among Latinas: Translating Science into Health Promotion Initiatives. Californian journal of health promotion.11(1):45–57.

4. Native American Mental Health Model: West, A. E., Williams, E., Suzukovich, E., Strangeman, K., & Novins, D. (2012). A Mental Health Needs Assessment of Urban American Indian Youth and Families. American Journal of Community Psychology, 49(3–4), 441–453. https://doi.org/10.1007/s10464-011-9474-6

E. Recommended Literature: Promoting Mental Health Awareness in the Community

1. Promoting Mental Health Awareness With Public Service Announcements Public service announcements (PSAs)

2. Developing A Stigma Reduction Initiative Summary

3. Public Service Announcements: Placing Drop-In Articles: Flyers of our initiatives workshops have been included in church newsletters.

F. Recommended Literature: Promoting Parent–Child Relationships Using an Evidenced-Based Model:

1. The Incredible Years: A training series for the prevention and treatment of conduct problems in young children. 2nd ed. Washington, DC: American Psychological Association; 2005.

2. https://filipinofamilyhealth.com

3. Perceptions of Parenting: Mapping the Gaps between Expert and Public Understandings of Effective Parenting in Australia

4. Lau AS, Fung JJ, Ho LY, Liu LL, Gudiño OG. Parent Training With High-Risk Immigrant Chinese Families: A Pilot Group Randomized Trial Yielding Practice-Based Evidence. *Behavior therapy.* 2011;42(3):PMID: 21658524.

G. Recommended Tools: Action Planning Documents:

1. Creating a Vision: FastTrack Leadership Communication Compass

2. Team Charter: WPIP Team Charter

3. Team Values: FastTrack Leadership Values Checklist

4. Team member Individual Development Plan:

5. Models and Framework for Understanding Social Determinants of Health

6. Evaluation Planning: W.K. Kellogg Foundation Evaluation Handbook W.K. Kellogg Foundation Logic Model Development

7. University of Kansas Community Toolbox

8. Change Management Communication Strategies

9. Periodic Table for High Concern Communication

10. High Stress Risk Communications

11. Advanced Risk Communication/Message Mapping Template

12. Leading Systems Change

13. 5 R Framework

14. Creating Mental Model Using Causal Loop Diagramming.

15. Understanding Political Systems and Stakeholder Analysis

16. Decision Analyses Matrices

A more comprehensive toolkit can be found at https://clinicalscholarsnli.org/community-impact

8. Challenges, successes, and lessons learned

8.1 Challenges

The team was challenged by conflicting demands of clinical work, research, life events, and community outreach. We have tackled these challenges by keeping the lines of communication open, being flexible, and staying resilient, leveraging the team's strengths, and prioritizing projects and opportunities. Another challenge for us is community engagement as it takes time and effort, and some degree of patience. We have developed the tenacity and continue to build new relationships and nurture existing ones. We also use social networks and share our stories.

8.2 Shifts in thinking

While working on the project, we have developed new mindsets toward the value of authenticity, shared experiences, interconnectedness of the people experiencing the Wicked Problem, including the team members.

8.3 Successes

Through community presentations, we have increased the awareness about Filipino mental health and suicide. The Community Wellness Conference raised the visibility of the problem of suicide among adolescents and has ignited the interest of the Los Angeles County Department of Mental Health to continue the work. Through parenting workshops, we are contributing to strengthening parent–child relationships. Parents are also able to build a community and share experiences with other parents.

8.4 Community leadership

Community leadership starts with community. There is strength in numbers, the power of the team of 5, along with our partners, parents, and grandparents is so much more impactful than the power of one. Working with many sectors, disciplines, institutions, academia, sectors such as academia, school districts, governmental agencies, hospitals, schools, and community-based organizations have their own culture and ways of getting things done. Navigating the systems requires flexibility and adaptability to handle different styles.

8.5 Overall lessons learned

As a team, we learned that working with the community on wicked problems such as mental health is a marathon not a sprint. Community partnership takes time. Kapwa, the spirit of interconnectedness, is critical to this work. We are all connected, what happens to me, happens to you, what happens to him or her, happens to us. It takes some vulnerability to share our stories and transformation come with being able to share our personal stories with others, and theirs with us.

If you are going to tackle this issue in your community, the FIRST thing you should do is ... involve the community. Ask the community their needs, their strengths, their proposed solutions. Listen to them and include them in all aspects of the project.

If you are going to tackle this issue in your community, we would NOT recommend ... developing your own plan or recommendations without community buy-in or input.

Wisdom we wished we had at the start but learned along the way:

Dr. Joyce Javier: The importance of sharing our own stories. Focusing on what you are most passionate about gets things done.

Dr. Dean Coffey: How powerful the cultural concept of Kapwa (shared identity) is in working together as a team on a shared objective. His one piece of advice for doing projects like this is: work for a cause you believe in and the rest will fall in place.

Dr. Aviril Sepulveda: The power of vulnerability and sharing stories can make one more effective in getting crucial messages across; tapping into one's strength and empowering volunteers and community members is a strong way to achieve success.

Jed David: The importance of self-care for the team; leading with kapwa (shared identity) means leading with empathy.

Dr. Horacio Lopez: The Incredible Years is a powerful tool; when it comes to parenting skills, there is always more to learn and that makes each of us a better parent.

Author details

Aviril Sepulveda[1], Dean M. Coffey[2], Jed David[1], Horacio Lopez[3], Kamil Bantol[1] and Joyce R. Javier[1,2]*

1 Children's Hospital Los Angeles, California, United States

2 Keck School of Medicine, University of Southern California, California, United States

3 Hollywood Presbyterian Medical Center, California, United States

*Address all correspondence to: jojavier@chla.usc.edu

References

[1] Hoeffel EM, Rastogi S, Kim MO, Shahid H. The Asian Population: 2010. http://www.census.gov/prod/cen2010/briefs/c2010br-11.pdf. Accessed August 5, 2019.: US Census Bureau;2012.

[2] Choi Y, Lahey BB. Testing the model minority stereotype: Youth behaviors across racial and ethnic groups. Social Services Review. 2006;80(3):419-452.

[3] Javier JR, Huffman LC, Mendoza FS. Filipino Child Health in the United States: Do Health and Health Care Disparities Exist? Preventing Chronic Disease. 2007;4(2):A36. PMID:17362627.

[4] Javier JR, Coffey DM, Palinkas LA, Kipke MD, Miranda J, Schrager SM. Promoting Enrollment in Parenting Programs Among a Filipino Population: A Randomized Trial. Pediatrics. 2019;143(2):pii: e20180553. PMID: 30679379.

[5] Javier JR, Chamberlain LJ, Rivera KK, Gonzalez SE, Mendoza FS, Huffman LC. Lessons learned from a community-academic partnership addressing adolescent pregnancy prevention in Filipino American families. Progress in Community Health Partnerships. 2010;4(4):305-313. PMID:21169708.

[6] Javier JR, Lahiff M, Ferrer RR, Huffman LC. Examining Depressive Symptoms and Use of Counseling in the Past Year Among Filipino and Non-Hispanic White Adolescents in California. Journal of Developmental & Behavioral Pediatrics. 2010;31(4):295-303. PMID:20431400.

[7] Javier JR, Supan J, Lansang A, Beyer W, Kubicek K, Palinkas LA. Preventing Filipino Mental Health Disparities: Perspectives from adolescents, caregivers, providers, and advocates. Asian American Journal of Psychology. 2014;5(4):316-324.PMID: 25667725

[8] Javier JR, Supan J, Lansang A, Beyer W, Kubicek K, Palinkas LA. Preventing Filipino Mental Health Disparities: Perspectives from Adolescents, Caregivers, Providers, and Advocates. Asian Am J Psychol. 2014;5(4):316-324. PMID: 25667725.

[9] Javier JR, Festa N, Florendo E, Mendoza FS. Children in Immigrant Families: The Foundation for America's Future. Adv Pediatr. 2015;62(1):105-136.

[10] Javier JR, Coffey DM, Schrager SM, Palinkas LA, Miranda J. Parenting Intervention for Prevention of Behavioral Problems in Elementary School-Age Filipino-American Children: A Pilot Study in Churches. J Dev Behav Pediatr. 2016;37(9):737-745.PMID: 27626390.

[11] Javier JR, Galura K, Aliganga FAP, Supan J, Palinkas LA. Voices of the Filipino Community Describing the Importance of Family in Understanding Adolescent Behavioral Health Needs. Fam Community Health. 2018;41(1):64-71. PMID: 29135796. .

[12] Javier JR, Reyes A, Coffey DM, et al. Recruiting Filipino Immigrants in a Randomized Controlled Trial Promoting Enrollment in an Evidence-Based Parenting Intervention. Journal of immigrant and minority health. 2018;21(2):324-331. PMID: 29774510.

[13] Kann L, Warren C, Harris W, et al. Youth Risk Behavior Surveillance UnitedStates 1993,. Morbidity and Mortality Weekly Report. 1995(44):1-56.

[14] Wolf D. Family secrets: trans-national struggles among children of Filipino immigrants. Sociol Perspect. 1997;40(3):457-482.

[15] David EJ. A colonial mentality model of depression for Filipino Americans. Cultur Divers Ethnic Minor Psychol. 2008;14(2):118-127.

[16] HM G, Tarraf W, West BT, Chan D, Miranda PY, Leong FT. Antidepressant use among Asians in the United States. Depression Anxiety. 2010;27(1):46-55.

[17] Aczon-Armstrong M, Inouye J, Reyes-Salvail F. Depression and chronic illness: Asian/Pacific Islander adults in Hawaii. Issues Ment Health Nurs. 2013;34(3):169-179.

[18] Sentell T, Unick GJ, Ahn HJ, Braun KL, Miyamura J, Shumway M. Illness severity and psychiatric hospitalization rates among Asian Americans and Pacific Islanders. Psychiatric services (Washington, D.C.). 2013;64(11):1095-1102.

[19] Kim HJ, Park E, Storr CL, Tran K, Juon HS. Depression among Asian-American Adults in the Community: Systematic Review and Meta-Analysis. PLoS One. 2015;10(6):e0127760.

[20] Okamura KH, Ebesutani C, Bloom R, Higa-McMillan CK, Nakamura BJ, Chorpita BF. Differences in internalizing symptoms across specific ethnic minority groups: An analysis across Chinese American, Filipino American, Japanese American, Native Hawaiian, and White youth. Journal of Child and Family Studies. 2016;25(11):3353-3366.

[21] Small R, Lumley J, Yelland J. Cross-cultural experiences of maternal depression: associations and contributing factors for Vietnamese, Turkish and Filipino immigrant women in Victoria, Australia. Ethn Health. 2003;8(3):189-206.

[22] Hayes DK, Ta VM, Hurwitz EL, Mitchell-Box KM, Fuddy LJ. Disparities in self-reported postpartum depression among Asian, Hawaiian, and Pacific Islander Women in Hawaii: Pregnancy Risk Assessment Monitoring System (PRAMS), 2004-2007. Maternal and child health journal. 2010;14(5):765-773.

[23] Esteban EJ. Parental verbal abuse: culture-specific coping behavior of college students in the Philippines. Child Psychiatry Hum Dev. 2006;36(3):243-259.

[24] Sanapo MS, Nakamura Y. Gender and physical punishment: the filipino children's experience. Child Abuse Review. 2011;20(1):39-56.

[25] Appel HB, Huang B, Ai AL, Lin CJ. Physical, Behavioral, and Mental Health Issues in Asian American Women: Results from the National Latino Asian American Study. Journal of Women's Health.20(11):1703-1711.

[26] Gong F., Gage S.J.L., Tacata L.A. Help Seeking Behavior Among Filipino Americans: A Cultural Analysis of Face and Language. Journal of Community Psychology. 2003;31(5):469-488.

[27] Sanchez F, Gaw A. Mental health care of Filipino Americans. Psychiatric services (Washington, D.C.). 2007; 58(6):810-815. PMID:17535941.

[28] Javier JR, Lahiff M, Ferrer RR, Huffman LC. Examining depressive symptoms and use of counseling in the past year among Filipino and non-Hispanic white adolescents in California. J Dev Behav Pediatr. 2010;31(4):295-303.

[29] Javier JR. The use of an educational video to increase suicide awareness and enrollment in parenting interventions among Filipinos. Asian American Journal of Psychology. 2018;9(4):327-333. PMID:31565181

[30] Flores N, Supan J, Kreutzer CB, Samson A, Coffey DM, Javier JR. Prevention of Filipino Youth Behavioral Health Disparities: Identifying Barriers and Facilitators to Participating in "Incredible Years," an Evidence-Based Parenting Intervention, Los Angeles, California, 2012. Prev Chronic Dis. 2015;12:E178. PMID: 26491813.

[31] Javier JR, Chamberlain LJ, Rivera KK, Gonzalez SE, Mendoza FS,

Huffman LC. Lessons learned from a community-academic partnership addressing adolescent pregnancy prevention in Filipino American families. Prog Community Health Partnersh. 2010;4(4):305-313.

[32] Coffey DM, Javier JR, Schrager SM. Preliminary Validity of the Eyberg Child Behavior Inventory With Filipino Immigrant Parents. Child Fam Behav Ther. 2015;37(3):208-223. PMID: 27087739

[33] Javier JR, Coffey DM, Filipino Family Health Intitative Community Advisory Board. Para Sa Kinabukasan Ng Ating Mga Anak: For Our Children's Future (Available at https://youtu.be/AkOrzHIdEN8) 2014.

[34] Runyan DK, Shankar V, Hassan F, et al. International Variations in Harsh Child Discipline. Pediatrics. 2010;126(3):e701-e711. PMID: 20679301.

[35] Ramiro L, Madrid B, Amarillo M. The Philippines WorldSAFE Study (Final report). International Clinical Epidemiology Network, Manila;2000.

[36] Hindin MJ, Gultiano S. Associations between witnessing parental domestic violence and experiencing depressive symptoms in Filipino adolescents. Am J Public Health. 2006;96(4):660-663.

[37] Ansara DL, Hindin MJ. Perpetration of intimate partner aggression by men and women in the Philippines: prevalence and associated factors. Journal of interpersonal violence. 2009;24(9):1579-1590.

[38] Fehringer JA, Hindin MJ. Like Parent, Like Child: Intergenerational Transmission of Partner Violence in Cebu, the Philippines. Journal of Adolescent Health. 2009;44(4):363-371. PMID: 19306795.

[39] Mandal M, Hindin MJ. Keeping it in the family: intergenerational transmission of violence in Cebu, Philippines. Maternal and child health journal. 2015;19(3):598-605.

[40] Pesigan IJ, Luyckx K, Alampay LP. Brief report: identity processes in Filipino late adolescents and young adults: parental influences and mental health outcomes. J Adolesc. 2014;37(5):599-604.

[41] GR Patterson. Continuities-A search for causal mechanisms: Comment on the special section. Developmental Psychology. 1998;34:1263-1268.

[42] Bates JE, Pettit GS, Dodge KA, Ridge B. Interaction of Temperamental Resistance to Control and Restrictive Parenting in the Development of Externalizing Behavior. Dev Psychol. 1998;34(5):982-995 PMC2791965.

[43] Belsky J, Hsieh K, Crnic K. Mothering, fathering, and infant negativity as antecedents of boys' externalizing problems and inhibition at age 3: Differential susceptibility to rearing influence? Development and Psychopathology. 1998;10:301-319 PMID: 9635226.

[44] Kochanska G. Children's Temperament, Mothers' Discipline, and Security of Attachment: Multiple Pathways to Emerging Internalization. Child Development. 1995;66(3):597-615.

[45] Kochanska G. Multiple pathways to conscience for children with different temperaments: From toddlerhood to age 5. Developmental Psychology. 1997;33(2):228-240 PMID: 9147832.

[46] O'Connor TG , Deater-Deckard K, Fulker D, Rutter M, Plomin R. Genotype-environment correlations in late childhood and early adolescence: Antisocial behavioral problems and coercive parenting. Developmental Psychology. 1998;34:970-981.

[47] Stormshak EA, Bierman KL, McMahon RJ, Lengua LJ. Parenting

Practices and Child Disruptive Behavior Problems in Early Elementary School. Journal of clinical child psychology. 2000;29(1):17-29. PMID: 10693029

[48] Loeber R. Disruptive and antisocial behavior in childhood and adolescence: Development and risk factors. In: In: Hurrelmann K LF, eds. Health hazards in adolescence, ed. Prevention and intervention in childhood and adolescence. Vol 8. Oxford, England: Walter De Gruyter; 1990:233-257.

[49] Brennan PA, Le Brocque R, Hammen C. Maternal Depression, Parent–Child Relationships, and Resilient Outcomes in Adolescence. Journal of the American Academy of Child & Adolescent Psychiatry. 2003;42(12):1469-1477 PMID: 14627882.

[50] Galambos NL, Barker ET, Almeida DM. Parents Do Matter: Trajectories of Change in Externalizing and Internalizing Problems in Early Adolescence. Child Development. 2003;74(2):578-594 PMID: 12705574.

[51] Patterson GR, Chamberlain P. A Functional Analysis of Resistance During Parent Training Therapy. Clinical Psychology: Science and Practice. 1994;1(1):53-70.

[52] Patterson GR, Forgatch MS, DeGarmo DS. Cascading effects following intervention. Development and Psychopathology. 2010;22(4):949-970 PMID: 20883592.

[53] Reid MJ, Webster-Stratton C, Beauchaine TP. Parent training in head start: a comparison of program response among African American, Asian American, Caucasian, and Hispanic mothers. Prev Sci. 2001;2(4):209-227.

[54] Tolan PH, Gorman-Smith D, Henry DB. The developmental ecology of urban males' youth violence. Developmental Psychology. 2003;39(2):274-291 PMID: 12661886.

[55] Brestan EV, Eyber SM. Effective psychosocial treatments of conduct-disordered children and adolescents: 29 years, 82 studies, 5,272 kids. Journal of clinical child psychology. 1998;27:180-189.

[56] Serketich WJ, Dumas JE. The effectiveness of behavioral parent training to modify antisocial behavior in children: A meta-analysis. Behavior Therapy. 1996;27:171-186.

[57] Sameroff AJ, Haith MM. The five to seven year shift. Chicago: University of Chicago Press; 1986.

[58] Siegler RS, Alibali MW. Children's thinking. 4th edition. Upper Saddle River, NJ: Prentice Hall; 2004.

[59] Davis-Kean PE, Huesmann LR, Jager J, Collins WA, Bates JE, Lansford JE. Changes in the relation of self-efficacy beliefs and behaviors across development. Child Dev. 2008;79(5):1257-1269.

[60] Huesmann LR, Guerra NG. Children's normative beliefs about aggression and aggressive behavior. Journal of personality and social psychology. 1997;72(2):408-419.

[61] Lansford JE, Chang L, Dodge KA, et al. Physical discipline and children's adjustment: cultural normativeness as a moderator. Child Dev. 2005;76(6): 1234-1246.

[62] Nadal KL. Pilipino American Identity Development Model. Journal of Multicultural Counseling and Development. 2004;32:44-61.

[63] Tompar-Tiu A, Sustento-Seneriches J. Depression and other mental health issues: The Filipino American experience. San Francisco: Jossey-Bass Publishers; 1995.

[64] Maramba DC, ed Family and Educational Environments: Contexts and Counterstories of Filipino

Americans. Charlotte, NC: Information Age Publishing, Inc; 2013. Endo R. & Rong X, ed. Educating Asian Americans: Achievement, Schooling, and Identities.

[65] Chambless DL, Hollon SD. Defining empirically supported therapies. Journal of Consulting and Clinical Psychology. 1998;66(1):7-18 PMID: 9489259.

[66] Herman KC, Borden LA, Reinke WM, Webster-Stratton C. The Impact of the Incredible Years Parent, Child, and Teacher Training Programs on Children's Co-Occurring Internalizing Symptoms. School psychology quarterly : the official journal of the Division of School Psychology, American Psychological Association. 2011;26(3):189-201.

[67] Webster-Stratton C, Herman KC. The impact of parent behavior-management training on child depressive symptoms. J Couns Psychol. 2008;55(4):473-484.

[68] Lau A, Fung J, Yung V. Group parent training with immigrant chinese families: enhancing engagement and augmenting skills training. Journal of Clinical Psychology. 2010;66(8):880-894. PMID:20564684.

[69] Lau AS, Fung JJ, Ho LY, Liu LL, Gudino OG. Parent training with high-risk immigrant chinese families: a pilot group randomized trial yielding practice-based evidence. Behav Ther. 2011;42(3):413-426.

[70] Chung P.J., Borneo H., Kilpatrick S.D., et al. Parent-adolescent communication about sex in Filipino American families: a demonstration of community-based participatory research. Ambul Pediatr. 2005;5(1):50-55.

[71] Heras P, Revilla LA. Acculturation, generational status, and family environment of Pilipino Ameircans: A Study in Cultural Adaptation. Family Therapy. 1994;21(2):129.

[72] Hwang W-C, Wood JJ. Acculturative family distancing: links with self-reported symptomatology among Asian Americans and Latinos. Child psychiatry and human development. 2009;40(1): 123-138.

[73] Rumbaut R. The Crucible Within: Ethnic Identity, Self-Esteem, and Segmented Assimilation among Children of Immigrants. International Migration Review. 1994;28(108):748-794.

[74] Lim NE. Family closeness, parental role fulfillment and immigration stress: A study on Filipino American young adults' satisfaction with parental upbringing 2012.

[75] Guerrero AP, Hishinuma ES, Andrade NN, Nishimura ST, Cunanan VL. Correlations among socioeconomic and family factors and academic, behavioral, and emotional difficulties in Filipino adolescents in Hawai'i. Int J Soc Psychiatry. 2006 ;52(4):343-359.

[76] Bandura A. Social foundations of thought and action: A social cognitive theory. Englewood Cliffs, NJ, US: Prentice-Hall, Inc; 1986.

[77] Hawkins WE, Clarke GN, Seeley JR. Application of social learning theory to the primary prevention of depression in adolescents. Health Values: The Journal of Health Behavior, Education, and Promotion. 1993;17:31-39.

[78] Rosenstock I. The health belief model: Explaining health behavior through expectancies. In: Glanz K et al, ed. Health behavior and health education: Theory, research, and practice. San Francisco: Jossey-Bass; 1990:39-62.

[79] Ajzen I. The theory of planned behavior. Organ Behav Hum Decis Process. 1991;50.

[80] Centers for Disease Control and Prevention DoHaHS. WISQARS

Leading Causes of Death Reports, 1981-2016. Retrieved from https://webappa.cdc.gov/sasweb/ncipc/leadcause.html. 2018.

[81] Centers for Disease Control. Leading Cause of Death in Males and Females, United States. 2015. Available at https://www.cdc.gov/healthequity/lcod/index.htm. Accessed August 8, 2019.

[82] Bronfenbrenner U, Ceci SJ. Nature-nurture reconceptualized in developmental perspective: a bio-ecological model. Psychological review. 1994;101(4):568-586.

[83] Chung B, Jones L, Dixon EL, Miranda J, Wells K, Community Partners in Care Steering C. Using a Community Partnered Participatory Research Approach to Implement a Randomized Controlled Trial: Planning the Design of Community Partners in Care. Journal of health care for the poor and underserved.21(3):780-795.

[84] American Psychological Association. Crossroads: The psychology of immigration in the new century. Report of the APA Presidential Task Force on Immigration. Washington, DC; 2012.

Chapter 10

Addressing the Under-Representation of African American Public Health Researchers: The Flint Youth Public Health Academy

Kent Key

Abstract

In order to meet the health needs of a culturally diverse population, the United States public health workforce must become ethnically diversified to provide culturally competent care. The underrepresentation of minority, specifically African American public health professionals may be a contributing factor to the high rates of preventable health disparities in the African American community. Studies have shown that racial/ethnic communities bear the highest disparities across multiple health outcomes. African Americans, when compared with European Americans, suffer the greatest rates of health disparities, thus providing the justification to increase minority public health professionals. In addition, studies suggest that minorities are more likely to seek medical and health services from individuals of the same ethnicity. This will assist in decreasing language and comprehension barriers and increase the cultural competence of the health providers who serve populations from their ethnic/cultural origin. This chapter will highlight a 2014 study designed to explore and identify motivators for African Americans to choose public health as a career. African American public health professionals and graduate students were engaged to discuss their career and educational trajectories and motivators for career choice. Using qualitative research methods, this study was guided by the following research question: what are the motivating factors to engage African Americans into careers in public health? The study was approved by the Walden University Institutional Review Board and was conducted in 2014. The results of this study have served as the blueprint for the creation of the Flint Public Health Youth Academy (FPHYA). Coincidently the 2014 study was wrapping up at the genesis of the Flint Water Crisis (FWC). The FWC impacted residents of all ages in Flint. Specifically, the youth of Flint were exposed to lead (a neuro-toxin) and other contaminants through the water system which impacted them physically and cognitively. National media outlets disseminated headlines across the world that Flint youth would have behavioral (aggression) issues and struggle academically as a result of their exposure to lead. The FPHYA was designed to provide positive messages to and about Flint youth. It is an introduction to careers in public health, medicine, and research for Flint Youth. It creates a space for Flint youth to work through their lived experience of the FWC while learning the important role public health and research plays in recovering from an environmental public health

IntechOpen

crisis. More importantly, it is a pathway to public health careers providing didactic sessions, local mentors and internships.

Keywords: Youth Engagement, Public Health Careers, Health Disparities, Career Pipeline, Public Health Workforce, African American

1. Introduction

In the United States (US) and in other parts of the world, people have been classified and identified by various factors. These factors include race, socio-economics, gender, sexual orientation, and religious belief to name a few. Once categorized, these groups of people are often compared with one another, and in many instances are treated differently causing disparities. In the US, these disparities have historically been supported by systems, structures and laws. Thus, racism, sexism and many other "isms" have manifested both overtly and covertly and have impacted generations of people. These systems, structures and laws have made it easier for some groups to excel, while at the same time, making it difficult for others. For example, even in 2019, men generally make more money than women who are doing the exact same job. African Americans and other people of color are accepted and graduate from college at lower rates than European Americans. African Americans make up some of the lowest percentages of medical doctors, public health professionals, researchers, dentists and nurses when compared to European Americans. Ironically, the health disparities rates of the African American community are the highest when compared to those of European Americans. The motivators for this project are racial and ethnic health disparities and the under-presentation of African American and other minority health professionals. In this chapter we will explore key challenges (barriers) for African Americans to pursue careers in public health, and motivators and strategies used to offset those challenges [1–10].

1.1 The problem

This chapter will focus on the Wicked Problem: the underrepresentation of African Americans and other minority public health professionals which contributes to health disparities in communities of color; and the negative impact the FWC has had on Flint youth.

African Americans are grossly underrepresented in public health, medicine and research disciplines [1–5]. A national panel of experts commissioned by the federal government posits that the underrepresentation of African Americans and other minority public health professionals contributes to health disparities in communities of color [2, 3]. Understanding the impact of cultural nuances, beliefs and norms, trust, historical experiences and communication methods play important roles in engaging marginalized minority communities, particularly in engaging them in seeking health care [2, 3, 5–10]. In addition, early exposure to careers is critical for career trajectory. Youth of color, specifically, African American youth typically are not exposed to these careers [11]. Furthermore, Flint youth were exposed to lead and other bacteria through their drinking water. Scientists have shared that Flint youth will have issues with cognitive and behavioral development due to exposure to poisoned water. News headlines stated that Flint youth would have behavioral and cognitive issues which could result in poor academic performance due to the exposure to lead and the effect that the neurotoxin has on the body. This could negatively impact pursuing post-secondary education [12].

The hypothesis and rationale for this study which served as the precursor to the FPHYA is lifted from the Sullivan Commission Report. This report entitled, Missing Persons: Minorities in the Health Professions provided an overview of diversity in the nation's healthcare workforce (https://campaignforaction.org/wp-content/uploads/2016/04/SullivanReport-Diversity-in-Healthcare-Workforce1.pdf). This commission was named after the former US Secretary of Health and Human Services, Dr. Louis Sullivan, and was composed of a cross-sector team of professionals who at the conclusion of their study proposed new approaches and a new model for making the health professions workforce more diverse to improve the overall health of our nation. One crucial recommendation from this report's conclusion is: in order to decrease health disparities in communities of color we must increase public health, medical and researchers from communities of color [2, 3].

1.2 Addressing the problem

In order to address racial and ethnic disparities a multifaceted approach must be enacted. Cross-sector collaboratives and policy changes must occur to institutionalize this effort. The 2014 study in Flint is one small contribution towards working to address health disparities. It was designed to identify motivators to engage African Americans in careers in public health. This is one step towards addressing the racial and ethnic health disparities plaguing the African American community. Furthermore, the results of this study (found in the next sections of this chapter) served as a guidance and precursor to inform the creation of a Flint youth empowerment program designed to engage Flint's (a majority African American city) youth into careers in public health. The FPHYA, will empower Flint youth to pursue careers in public health, medicine and research; serve as a catalyst for early career exposure, mentoring and role modeling for African American youth; and create a pathway to careers while addressing the underrepresentation of African American and other people of color in public health, medicine and research. The FPHYA utilizes the Flint Water Crisis as a real-life scenario to create an interest in public health and research. Finally, the FPHYA will engage African American and other minority youth in interactive didactic educational sessions, science-based exploratory projects, and research-based inquiry.

2. Methods

The methods used in this study included two critical phases: first those used to conduct the 2014 study, and second, those used to create the FPHYA. The 2014 study was conducted as part of Dr. Key's dissertation research prior to his participation in the Culture of Health Leadership Program. Out of this research arose recommendations, motivators and barriers for minorities, particularly African Americans, pursuing careers in public health and medicine. Data from this research was used to develop the curriculum for FPHYA, which was launched in the third year of the Culture of Health program.

2.1 Phase one: the 2014 study

The study was designed to explore and identify motivators and barriers for African Americans to choose public health as a career. African American public health professionals and graduate students, who had attained or were pursuing a Bachelors, Masters, DrPH or PhD degree in public health, were engaged to discuss their career and educational trajectories and motivators for career choice.

Qualitative methods were chosen for this study to gain a critical in-depth understanding of experiences shared by participants through extensive exploration [13, 14]. Grounded theory was used to complement the qualitative process. Grounded theory is derived from observational interviewing in which themes and codes are captured through dialog via interviews, focus groups and community dialogs. This method allowed for questions to be used that focus on how individuals experienced the process of career choice, while identifying motivators, barriers and other critical steps to the process. Focus groups were used to engage participants in dialog and to collect data for this study. The motivators discussed during the focus groups answered two key grounded theory questions: what was central to the process; and what influenced or caused the phenomenon to occur [15].

A sample size of 20 participants was used for this study. Creswell posits that a sample between 20 and 30 participants is appropriate to reach a point of saturation when developing a theory [14]. Three focus groups were conducted consisting of faculty, staff, and students from a local university in the state of Michigan; also faculty, staff, and interns of a local county health department also in Michigan. After receiving permission to recruit from the Dean and the County Health Officer, recruitment invitations were emailed electronically via listservs. The recruitment invitation clearly listed eligibility criteria and explained the purpose of the study. A follow-up email provided logistics for focus groups to all who replied to the recruitment invitation.

The research instrument (interview guide) was developed by the researcher for this study. Prior to use during focus groups, the research instrument was reviewed by two researchers, one an expert specializing in health disparity research, and the other an expert in qualitative research. The research instrument was used to conduct the focus group dialogs and was guided by the literature concerning career motivators. The questions in the interview guide covered a range of topic areas to identify motivators for career choice. The questions provided a platform for participants to answer freely and honestly without any leading prompts from the researcher. The interview guide covered four main domains: 1) participants' initial engagement into public health; 2) career trajectory experiences; 3) motivators to maintain trajectory; and 4) barriers encountered and methods used to overcome set barriers. The focus groups began with introductions, explaining focus group ground rules, reminding participants of their right to withdraw from the study at any time, and sharing that the focus groups would be digitally recorded, and all records would be kept confidential. A general demographic questionnaire was then distributed to ascertain the demographics of the sample (i.e. gender, age, employment status, educational status).

To ensure trustworthiness (credibility, transferability, and dependability) in this study, triangulation was used [14, 16–18]. Two digital audio recorders were used to record each focus group (Device A and Device B). Device A was used to generate transcripts. Once the transcripts were generated, Device B was used to verify the accuracy of the transcripts to ensure reliability/dependability and validity/credibility. The researcher also took notes during each focus group, recording words as well as any emphasis or change in tone as conveyed by participants. Once transcription was complete and themes were identified, they were shared with study participants to ensure that the message was captured and interpreted accurately and to identify any discrepant responses. The researcher also kept a journal to aid in self-reflection to address any possible past experiences, prejudices, and orientations of potential issues of bias and prejudice. This journaling process ensures credibility, reliability and objectivity [14, 16, 18]. Utilizing a purposeful sampling strategy along with a thick description of the phenomena in this study ensured transferability [16, 18, 19].

The interview data is presented using verbatim statements from study participants in the following five discussion topics: (a) introduction to public health, (b) public health as a career choice, (c) career motivators, (d) barriers to career obtainment, and (e) African American students' exposure to public health careers. Discussion frequencies were tabulated by dividing the total number of responses per identified theme by the total number of responses per that discussion topic yielding the percentile reflected in the interview data.

2.2 Phase two: the FPHYA

As a Culture of Health Leader from the Robert Wood Johnson Foundation, health equity, interdisciplinary and cross-sector collaboration, and policy are critical components of the methodology used to establish the FPHYA. Beginning in 2017, two years were spent creating an interactive curriculum which includes didactic sessions, experiential learning, mentoring and role modeling experiences, community assessment activities, and youth ambassador policy training. This was completed with the guidance of a team of professionals which included: Community Based Organization (CBO) leaders, Faith-Based leaders, Academicians/Researchers, local Public Health Professionals, Public School Officials, local Water Crisis Activists, Policy Makers, Flint ReCast leaders, parents and most importantly youth. In 2019 we expanded our stakeholder collaborative to include two new partners, the City of Flint- Office of the Mayor and the YouthQuest program. The curriculum was tested and piloted at a local high school in the spring of 2019. The stakeholder team met and discussed process evaluation recommendations, implemented those recommended changes and two subsequent summer camps were conducted in the summer/early fall of 2019.

Moving forward, the youth from the FPHYA will connect to other national youth groups focused on community health and well-being. The FPHYA conducted community assessments and will submit for presentation at the 2020 American Public Health Association's (APHA) Community Based Public Health Caucus (CBPHC). The CBPHC has a youth department comprised of youth from across the country doing public health work in their city. The FPHYA youth participants will be encouraged to join this youth caucus to continue their journey of engagement into careers in public health.

3. Outcomes

The outcomes in this section will be discussed in two-phases: first the outcomes of the 2014 study which guided the development of the FPHYA; and second the outcomes of the first year of FPHYA programming.

3.1 Phase 1: the 2014 study

Across 3 focus groups, participants identified both motivators and barriers for African Americans pursuing a degree in public health. The demographic information was based on self-reported data (see **Table 1**). There were 20 participants total, 16 females and 4 males. The majority of participants were females affiliated with the university either as faculty, staff, or graduate students. For both women and men, degree levels were equally distributed among Master's and Doctoral degrees.

3.2 Discussion topic 1: introduction to public health

Two main questions were asked in this discussion topic: When were you introduced to public health? How did you become involved in public health? Seventy five

Participants Demographic Profile (N = 20)				
	Female		Male	
	N	%	N	%
	16	80	4	20
Organization type:				
Academia	14	70	2	10
Government	2	10	2	10
Other	0	0	0	0
Education level:				
Bachelor	2	10	0	0
Master	7	35	2	10
Doctoral	7	35	2	10

Table 1.
Demographic profile of participants.

percent of study participants reported they were introduced to public health during their undergraduate studies. Fifteen of the participants shared they were introduced to public health while in high school, while ten percent of participants were introduced to public health while in their graduate program.

Participants identified key events and activities that initiated their involvement into public health. Over half of the participants were introduced to public health through community projects. Others (15%) were introduced to public health via job/internship; yet another fifteen percent were introduced by taking a public health related course. Ten percent of the participants were introduced to public health through interaction with a public health professional. Finally, five percent of participants were introduced via career fair, and likewise, and the remaining five percent through a family member or parent.

3.3 Discussion topic 2: career choice

Discussion Topic 2, career choice was centered on the question: at what point did participants choose public health as their career choice? An overwhelming majority of participants (15 out of 20) chose a career in public health as a career choice during the end of their undergraduate school years.

3.4 Discussion topic 3: career motivators

Career motivators were the focus of discussion topic three. Participants shared their experiences along their educational and career trajectories while identifying key motivators that aided them in reaching their career choice and obtaining a degree in public health. The Facilitator began the discussion by asking participants if they experienced any educational or career motivators, what those motivators were and if any motivators were more significant than others. Noteworthy, many participants shared they experienced several motivators throughout their trajectory so motivators were not always experienced singularly.

The following motivators were identified by participants during the focus group discussions: helping others/helping the community, race/racial identity, mentor(s), social support, family/parental support, social justice/health disparities, lived sickness/injury and job/finances. Discussion frequencies were calculated by taking the

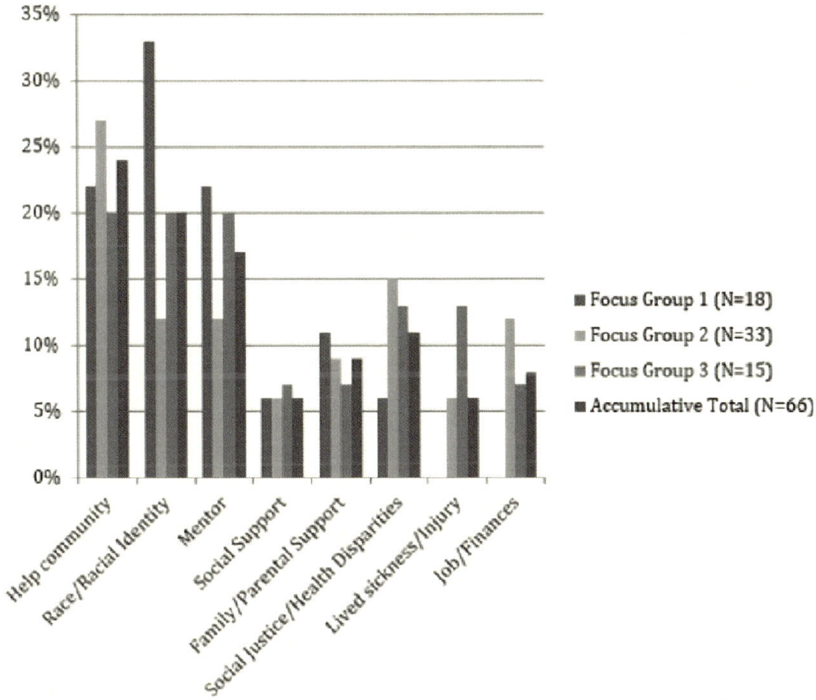

Figure 1.
Motivator frequency discussed.

number of responses per motivator/theme and dividing that number by the total number of responses for all motivators (See **Figure 1**). Representative quotes of participant motivations for their career choice are presented in **Table 2**.

3.5 Discussion topic 4: barriers

The focus of discussion topic four was the career barriers experienced by participants. Barriers that discouraged or negatively impacted success in achieving their career choice and obtaining a degree in public health were identified. This discussion began by asking participants if they experienced any barriers, what those barriers were and what helped them to overcome those barriers? Similarly to motivators, the participants shared that barriers were not always experienced singularly but at times may have been coupled with other barriers as they continued on their career trajectory.

The following barriers were identified by participants during the focus group discussions: first generational college ignorance, race/racism/stereotyping, lack of social support, lack of mentor(s), lack of networking, self-esteem/confidence, lack of family support, and job/finances. Discussion frequencies were calculated by taking the number of responses per identified barrier and dividing that number by the total number of responses for all barriers (See **Figure 2**).

3.6 Discussion topic 5: African American students exposure to public health careers

Discussion Topic 5 focused on African American students' exposure to public health. This discussion explored how early should African American students be introduced to careers in public health and how should that introduction to public

Motivator Quotes	Barrier Quotes	Feedforward Model
Race	***Funding and Faculty Support***	***Forethought***
"Well, my motivation for public health was because I did not see anybody who looked like me. I was doing work in a field where primarily the people who were most impacted were African-American, but the people who were doing all the services and providing all the help were not African-American. So I did not think that they were – it was my opinion that some of the services or some of the things that were offered were not the most appropriate resources or means for folks of color."	"So I went to speak with my first year advisor and we were talking about classes. "Oh that's great. That's good. I'm glad you are succeeding. You're doing great." And then as soon as the word funding came out of my mouth he said, "Well you know, grad school funding – you just have to go and find what you can." Not once – And he was the head of the department – of my department. I'm like, "You are the top. Like at the top it's just us. You're supposed to be helping me out. I'm your – You were assigned to me.""	"In order for African American youth to consider public health as a profession, they must be exposed to it. We know this does not happen often in our community. We need afterschool programming, summer internships, and youth engaged research activities to create this interest so they will think about public health as they choose their college trajectories."
Social Justice	***Racism/Prejudice***	***Planning***
"So that was kind of my area as a undergrad in history, was looking at social movements. And many of the social movements that I looked at actually had health components. You know, so you can look at this later on and realize that. But at the time, I did not realize that. And when I was community organizing, the community organizing I saw as part of the social movements, but it was also the place and space in which people are. So the history of a place has an impact and implication for the health of that place. And so for me, it all kind of tied, and I probably did not know of tied, and I probably did not know it at the time, that that's kind of where I was headed. So really talking a lot about place when I was community organizing, and empowerment, how communities organize, so community organization, and a lot of it was always tied to health issues."	"And – well, I went to a private school in Georgia, so – and there were about six of us in my particular public health program. So we had to be a unit if we wanted – we had to support each other. So I – and we – to this day, we talk about how there would be group assignments, and of course, we would gravitate towards each other, and do presentations in front of the class And there were a few times when we had to have meetings with our professor and the dean because it was clear that we were scored more harshly, or we – things were not fair. So there were – there were plenty of barriers, and I think that's why we are so close to this day, because we all had to go through the same thing."	"Because I was exposed early to public health, I knew the type of classes in high school that I would need to pursue public health. I went to youth public health retreat, this happened one time in my city. It changed my life. From that time, I had a plan, volunteered at the health department while in high school and war on my way. I was one of the lucky ones."

Motivator Quotes	Barrier Quotes	Feedforward Model
Parent/Family Support	***First Generation College Ignorance***	***State of being proactive***
"My dad's always been a motivator for me. He's an environmental health scientist and I've always grown up knowing that that was his field but it never occurred to me that that was public health until maybe a year ago. Just seeing the effect that he has – He's always been – how can I put this? He's never been like, "have to go into public health." But I think he saw in me that I was interested so he constantly would put public health in front of me."	"I did not know about public health, so I, you know, let us say I stumbled upon it. But just navigating things, you do not know what you do not know. And if you did not have someone, whether you are first generation, who kind of helped pave the path before you, it's – it makes it difficult, or it takes you longer to get there, because you do not have that support or knowledge to help you get there.	"Once I understood while in undergrad that I wanted to be an epidemiologist, I applied for a scholarship to attend the American Public Health Association. My experience at APHA was a game changer. I met others across the country and networked with other students and presenters to prepare for my graduate application to the School of Public Health. Many of those contacts I met at APHA wrote me letters of support for my application for SPH."

Table 2.
Quotes: Motivators, barriers, feedforward model.

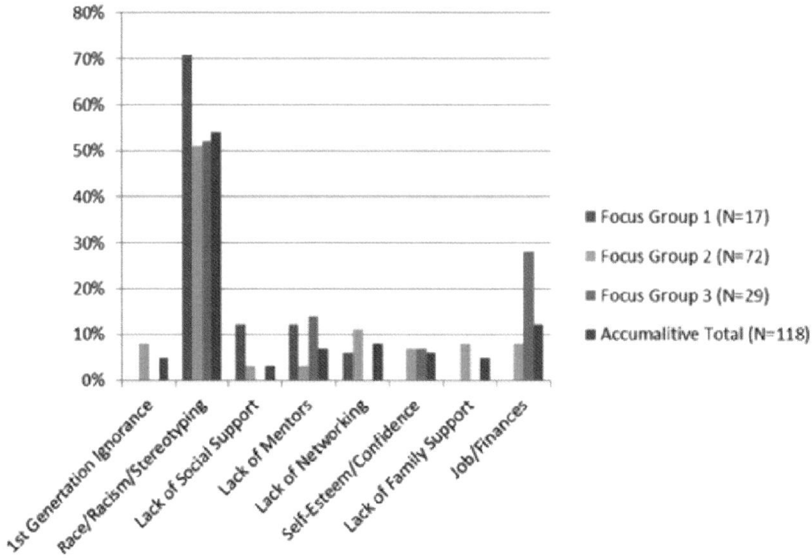

Figure 2.
Barrier frequency discussed.

health be packaged and presented to them. Over half of the participants (55%) felt that African American students should be introduced to public health careers while in elementary school. A strong thirty percent (30%) of participants felt African American students should learn about it in middle school. The remaining participants (15%) felt like high school years were the critical years when African American students should be exposed to public health careers.

As participants discussed critical issues regarding exposure and visibility, six recommendations were identified as effective ways to package and present public health to African American students. Those six recommendations were:

1. *Visibility through branding and marketing:* Develop marketing and branding campaigns to promote careers in public health to youth of color; promote representation of people of color in public health by highlighting individuals working in the field and the types of positions available.

2. *Caped warrior/celebrity approach*: Engage celebrities (music artists, actors, athletes, etc.) who are people of color to be public health ambassadors and use their platforms to bring national awareness to specific public health causes.

3. *Framing as social justice*: Recognize the intersectionality of public health issues and apply existing frameworks (social determinants of health, socio-ecological model) to address issues like racism systemically and advance health equity. The Community-Based Participatory Research approach, for example, seeks to improve the health of communities through a social justice lens.

4. *Role models/mentors:* Identify local public health professionals working in academia, government, or with local CBOs and connect them with youth through organized events like talks, webinars and workshops. Young people need to first know and see local mentors working in this space; these connections can then lead to opportunities for professional development and pathways to employment in public health.

5. *Packaging public health with behaviors:* Understand that public health is a science, but also involves observing and understanding people's behaviors. Mental health issues like trauma, depression and stress contribute to overall health and should be embedded in public health interventions.

6. *Summer employment with a public health focus:* Connect students with internships at public health organizations where they have the opportunities to make substantive contributions to public health research and projects in their communities.

3.7 Phase 2: the FPHYA

Two important outcomes have risen from the first two years of FPHYA programming. Approximately 70 youth participants were engaged in 2019. As a result, the YouthQuest program (who provides afterschool programming to the Flint Community Schools) has invited the FPHYA to partner with summer camp programming and to partner to provide afterschool programming during the 2019–2020 calendar school year to Flint Schools and some local area charter schools. In addition, the City of Flint and the ReCast program partnered with the FPHYA for an additional summer cohort. This cohort resulted in the creation of the new youth initiative, Youth Unlimited Productions (YUP) a program of the FPHYA, Flint ReCast and the Mayor's office and have submitted a grant application for $120,000.00 to fund 2020 activities for YUP. Currently program assessments from program participants are being analyzed and data will be shared through future dissemination efforts.

4. Discussion

The 2014 study participants had a sophisticated understanding of the motivators to engage African American students into careers in public health. They identified motivators and recommendations that, if used in a feedforward model (explained below), would be promising for increasing the number of African American students in public health. Their comments related to motivators such as race/racial identity, role models/mentors, family support and social support were consistent with the literature regarding African Americans and career choice. Concerns around the common barriers that participants experience, such as: racism/prejudice, lack of social support, lack of family support, and the lack of mentors were also consistent with the literature regarding African Americans and career choice. **Table 2** shares quotes that speak to the motivators, barriers and Feedforward model lifted from the transcripts of the 2014 study.

The following section discusses the Feedforward model in Ref. to the 2014 study and finally in the context of the FPHYA.

4.1 Feedforward model and the 2014 study

The feedforward model served as the conceptual framework for the 2014 study. This model is a decision-making framework that is based on the feedforward concept. The feedforward concept utilizes knowledge and planning which produces action based on the knowledge acquired [20–22]. The premise of the feedforward model consists of three stages: (a) forethought, (b) planning, and (c) state of being proactive; in layman's terms, motivation leads to behaviors, and those behaviors lead to actions [11, 21]. The findings of this study can offer support for the three stages of this model. The eight motivators identified by participants in this study were fluid and could be found in one or all of the stages of the feedforward model.

The findings in this study suggest that forethought for career choice begins with the participants' introduction to public health and careers in public health. In this study, 75% of participants were introduced to public health while in undergraduate school; 15% were introduced to public health while in high school; and 10% were introduced to public health while in graduate school. Furthermore, study participants suggested that African American students should be introduced to public health and careers in public health in elementary school.

In the planning stages of the feedforward model, participants identified many planning activities that were initiated as a result of the forethought stage. The planning activities identified by participants in this discussion varied. Participants identified applying for graduate school as a result of their plans to pursue a degree in public health. Participants who were introduced to public health and public health careers while in high school were motivated to apply for undergraduate school and enroll in courses that would either result in a bachelor's degree in public health or to enroll in classes that would prepare them to pursue a master's degree in public health. In addition, participants attributed their ability to maintain their educational trajectory of obtaining a degree to many of the motivators identified in this study. Other participants attributed pursuing and applying for public health positions, jobs and promotions based on the motivators that they received in the forethought stage. Participants also attributed preparing for and taking the GRE test to get into graduate school based on the motivators and information they received in the forethought stage. Study participants shared their actions that resulted from the planning and the forethought stages as it related to choosing a career in public health. Participants took several courses of action in their experiences in the proactive stage. Study participants identified maintaining class enrollment and overcoming barriers to their educational attainment as proactive steps to secure their career. Taking classes to fulfill the course requirements, maintaining passing grades, securing employment in public health job positions, working in internship and fellowship programs, connecting with other African American students to form networks and group accountability were all cited as proactive steps taken by participants. Finally, accountability to their mentors and role models and following through on their advice and guidance proved to be key proactive steps as identified by several of the study participants.

4.2 The feedforward model and the FPHYA

As a result of the 2014 study. The FPHYA administration and stakeholder team wanted to ensure that all three phases of the feedforward model were incorporated in FPHYA programming. In the forethought stage: FPHYA participants (many of them for the first time) were introduced to the field of public health. Through active engagement activities, online games, real life case studies and the lived experience of the Flint Water Crisis, students were provoked to consider public health as a career and the impact that this career could have on them, their community and the nation. FPHYA participants were also exposed to local minority public health professionals who will serve as role models and mentors to guide them towards subjects to take in high school that will prepare them for a career in public health.

In the planning phase, FPHYA participants shared how they would like to be engaged. The FPHYA participants developed the Youth Unlimited Productions to merge and marry public health and health communication (messaging) with music, arts, and pop culture. In addition, participants are exploring what college courses and prerequisites are needed to complete a public health degree. Others are exploring how to connect other degree disciplines like social work, communications and history and how to utilize those in a public health capacity to impact population health.

In the state of being proactive, FPHYA participants are actively seeking funding to support future programming and projects. FPHYA participants have created a set of policy recommendations based on their youth photo voice project to keep parks and other recreational spaces safe for youth. Their current focus is youth diabetes and obesity. They are engaged in creating a campaign to keep Flint City parks clean, efforts to provide summer jobs for Flint youth to monitor and clean the parks and an inventory of youth serving organizations in Flint who could benefit from the FPHYA's YUP.

5. Recommendations

Participants offered six recommendations to increase the number of African American students engaged in public health careers. Although study participants identified and shared the motivations that began their career trajectory in public health, what remains still is the lack of knowledge of public health among African Americans, little to no visibility of minority professionals in the field and relatively low enrollment of African American and other minority groups in Schools of Public Health across the country. Based on the data collected from focus group participants in this study, it is recommended that future researchers focus on the following: (a) visibility through branding and marketing, (b) utilizing a caped warrior/celebrity model, (c) framing public health with social justice, (d) the effectiveness of role models/mentors, (e) packaging public health with behaviors, and (f) creating summer employment centered around public health.

These six recommendations for future research may prove to be successful in recruiting African American and other minorities into public health. They can also inform workforce planners how to curtail effective strategies, create effective marketing strategies, and engage the interest of African American and other minority students at a young age in careers in public health. Furthermore, these recommendations could be implemented into current pipeline and recruitment programs for researchers and modified to be public health specific.

For *public health research*, these recommendations may inform future research initiatives. Implications for future research based on these recommendations could include measuring the effectiveness of public health marketing and branding initiatives. Using an ecological model to access the effectiveness on personal, family, and community levels is most strongly recommended. As an example research project to test marketing and branding effectiveness: Implement a city-wide billboard campaign while concentrating on specific zip code areas to implement the socioecological tailored intervention and compare the results of the zip codes (with similar demographic and SES factors) between those with and those without the intervention.

More specifically for *public health practice*, creating opportunities for current African American public health professionals to be paired with students can create both role/modeling and mentoring relationships. Visibly exposing African American students to African American public health professionals may generate interest in the field, become the genesis of network development, and possibly provide the opportunity for internships and other employment opportunities. Another example of an intervention in public health practice includes designing and implementing programs that package public health with behaviors. Research projects, programs and interventions centered on connecting behaviors to health outcomes could be implemented and testing this approach could be used to assess if the intervention was successful in reducing unhealthy behaviors and increasing health outcomes, while simultaneously introducing African Americans to public health and exposing them to the field.

5.1 Implementing the 2014 study recommendations

As a result of the 2014 study, the six recommendations were used to guide the development of the Flint Public Health Youth Academy (FPHYA) in Flint Michigan. The FPHYA will continue to draw from the recommendations of the study in the following three main domains: 1) Community Assessment, 2) Learning Academy, and 3) Advocacy and Policy. Flint youth will be equipped to share their perspective regarding the water crisis, exposed to careers and mentors in public health and medicine and empowered to advocate for policy change to prevent future possible public health and environmental health disasters in Flint.

In conclusion, there are many implications of the 2014 study highlighted in this chapter and the development of the FPHYA. Most importantly are the social changes as shared below.

5.1.1. Implications for social change

The results of this study identified key motivators that have proven to aid African Americans in securing a career in public health. The results also identified key barriers that negatively impact the progression of African Americans pursuing a career in public health. Participants generated a list of recommendations for presenting public health to African American youth to engage them early on and possibly pique their interest to pursue public health as a career. The anticipated social change as a result of this study is the awareness of the motivators that may effectively engage African American students into careers in public health, and the identified barriers to obtaining those careers. This study was designed to provide insight for addressing the underrepresentation of African American public health professionals, with broader implications for serving as a blueprint for designing pathways to careers for other ethnic minority groups, keeping in mind that each minority group may have variance in cultural norms and cultural values, yet, this study could serve as a blueprint for tailoring and adapting similar research, interventions and programs specific to that minority population. Secondly, this study may be used to address a larger effort to reduce/eliminate the negative impact of racial and ethnic health disparities and the preventable deaths and illnesses that these disparities cause yearly. Implications for social change will result from a greater understanding of the motivators to increase the number of African American public health professionals. The results of this study may lead to (a) establishing best practices in diversifying the public health workforce, (b) creating educational pipelines or pathways for African Americans and other minority students, and (c) the increase of African American public health professionals may play a critical role in the reduction of health disparities the negatively affect the social, economic, and physical health of the African American community.

Findings from this study can be incorporated into existing programs by adding the identified motivators as components into those programs to increase the chances for effectively recruiting African Americans into careers in public health positively impacting the current social trend of underrepresented African Americans in public health, thus creating social change. A broader social change implication, as supported by the Sullivan Report and other national reports, may also be experienced by increasing the number of African American students introduced to public health and thus increasing the number of African American public health professionals. It is predicted that there will be a decrease in health disparities in African American communities after achieving a change in the make-up of the workforce to reflect the composition of those communities. This may also result in a decrease in the number of African Americans who die from preventable diseases as a result of health disparities.

6. Tool kit

- Additional resources:

   a. Community Engagement Studio Flint: Flint Public Health Youth Academy Website

Author details

Kent Key
Division of Public Health, College of Human Medicine, Michigan State University, Michigan, United States

*Address all correspondence to: kent.key@hc.msu.edu

References

[1] U.S. Census Bureau. U.S. Census News: Nation's population one third minority. 2012. Retrieved from: http://www.census.gov/PressRelease/www/2012

[2] Sullivan LW, Mittman IS. The state of diversity in the health professions a century after Flexner. Academic Medicine. 2010;85(2):246-252.

[3] Sullivan Commission. Missing person: Minorities in the health professions: A report of the Sullivan Commission on diversity in the healthcare workforce. 2004. Retrieved from: http://www.aacn.nche.edu/media/pdf/sullivanreport.pdf.

[4] Mitchell DA, Lassiter SL. Addressing health care disparities and increasing workforce diversity: The next step for the dental, medical, and public health professions. American Journal of Public Health. 2006; 96(12):2093-2097.

[5] Annang L, Richter DL, Fletcher FE, Weis MA, Fernandes PR, Clary LA. Diversifying the academic public health workforce: strategies to extend the discourse about limited racial and ethnic diversity in the public health academy. Association of Black Nursing Faculty Journal. 2010; 21(2):39-43.

[6] Calender A. Recruiting underrepresented minorities to chiropractic colleges. Journal of Chiropractic Education. 2006;20(2): 123-127.

[7] Gabard, DL. Increasing minority representation in the health professions. Journal of Allied Health. 2007;36(3):165-175.

[8] U.S. Department of Health and Human Services (USDHHS), Bureau of Health Professions. (2009, April). Evaluating Programs to Recruit Minorities into Health Professions. Retrieved from http://www.bhpr.hrsa.gov/healthworkforce/.../EvalHealth CareerCollege EnrichmentProgApril 2009.pdf .

[9] Grumbach K, Mendoza R. Disparities in human resources: Addressing the lack of diversity in the health professions. Health Affairs. 2008;27(2):413-422.

[10] Smith SG, Nsiah-Kumi PA, Jones PR, Pamies RJ. Pipeline programs in the health professions, Part 1: Preserving diversity and reducing health disparities. Journal of the National Medical Association. 2009;101(9):836-847.

[11] Gibbons MM, Shoffner MF. Prospective first-generation college students: meeting their needs through social cognitive career theory. Professional school counseling. 2004;8(1):91-97.

[12] Hanna-Attisha M, LaChance J, Sadler RC, Champney Schnepp A. Elevated blood lead levels in children associated with the Flint drinking water crisis: a spatial analysis of risk and public health response. American Journal of Public Health. 2016;106:283-290.

[13] Polkinghorne, D. Language and meaning: Data collection and qualitative research. Journal of Counseling Psychology. 2005;52(2):137-145. DOI:10.1037/0022-0617.52.2.137

[14] Creswell JW. eds. Qualitative inquiry & research design: Choosing among five approaches. 2nd ed. Thousand Oaks, CA: Sage; 2007.

[15] Creswell JW. eds. Research design: Qualitative, quantitative, and mixed methods approaches. 3rd ed. Thousand Oaks, CA: Sage; 2009.

[16] Lincoln YS, Guba EG. Naturalistic Inquiry. London, England: Sage; 1985

[17] Guba EG, Lincoln YS. Fourth Generation Evaluation. London, England: Sage; 1989

[18] Shenton AK. Strategies for ensuring trustworthiness in qualitative research projects. Education for Information. 2004;22:63-75.

[19] Tuckett AG. Part II. Rigour in qualitative research: complexities and solutions. Nurse Researcher. 2005;13(1): 29-42.

[20] Agarwal R, Umphress D. A flexible model for simulation of software development process. Proceedings of the 48th Annual Southeast Regional Conference. 2010;40:204-218.

[21] Basso D, Belardinelli MO. The role of the feedforward paradigm in cognitive psychology. Cognitive Process. 2006;7:73-88.

[22] Capelo C, Dias JF. A feedback learning and mental models perspective on strategic decision making. Education Technology Research Development. 2009;57(5), 629-644.

Chapter 11

Violence: A Prescription of Hope for a Vulnerable Population

Tonita Smith, Edith Amponsah and Lia Garman

Abstract

Violence is a preventable disease that has long term effects on health. In the United States, violence has become an epidemic that disproportionately affects the African American community. Risk factors that contribute to the perpetration of youth violence include a combination of individual, relationship, community, and societal factors. Individual risk factors include a personal history of victimization of violence, high emotional stress, and exposure to violence and conflict. Family risk factors include low parental education, low income, poor family functioning and low parental involvement. Community risk factors include diminished economic opportunities, high concentration of poor residents, and socially disorganized neighborhoods – all of which are prevalent in communities with high rates of violence. Preventive strategies aimed at reducing violence need to be collaborative and community based. This multi-city project, A Prescription of Hope, aims to educate community members from Illinois and Missouri on the long- term effects of exposure to violence. The target population for Missouri is Ferguson, a small community with an approximate population of 21,035 (2017); however, it is recognized nationally for the demonstrations and unrest that erupted after the August 9, 2014 shooting death of 18-year-old Michael Brown. Worldwide, an estimated 200,000 homicides occur each year among youth aged 10–29 years, accounting for 43% of all homicide annually.

Keywords: Violence prevention, youth violence, health disparities, faith-based community intervention, youth mentorship

1. Introduction

Exposure to violence has long-term implications for mental, physical, and emotional health and wellbeing. In the U.S., individuals that experience high levels of violence face increased risk of mental health and behavioral disorders such as depression, posttraumatic stress disorder (PTSD), personality and conduct disorders, anxiety, sleep and eating disorders, substance abuse, and suicide and suicide attempts [1]. Injuries and violence are the leading causes of death among children, adolescents, and young adults in the U.S., and disproportionately affect young people of color [2]. The epidemic of gun violence in the United States claims thousands of lives every year [3]. During 2015–2016, the U.S. Centers for Disease Control and Prevention (CDC) reported a total of 27,394 firearm homicides, including 3,224 (12%) among persons aged 10–19 years [3].

Across the U.S., systemic inequities make some communities more vulnerable to violence than others. Studies show males, ethnic minorities, and urban residents are at increased risk for witnessing violence [4]. At the societal level, high levels of income inequality, structural disadvantage and racism contribute to the perpetration of multiple forms of violence [1]. African Americans and Hispanics are more likely to be victims of violent crimes than are Caucasians, and African Americans are disproportionately victims of homicide compared with Caucasians or Hispanics [5]. Those from low-income households are also much more likely than others to experience violent crime [5].

Addressing violence at the community level is often complicated by a lack of trust between at-risk members of the community and the criminal justice system. The U.S. has a much higher rate of police homicide compared to other high-income countries, with an estimated 1,000 civilians killed annually [6]. Studies have shown police officers are likely to use more force with African American civilians than Caucasians, and African Americans are three times as likely to have their cars searched by a police officer during a stop [7]. Biased policing harms historically disadvantaged groups, and disproportionately subjects racial and ethnic minorities to suspicion, surveillance, and intrusion that can have deadly consequences [7].

In recent years, several high-profile police killings of unarmed Black men have put a media spotlight on police brutality and racialized policing. The killing of 18-year-old Michael Brown in Ferguson, Missouri on August 9, 2014 set off a wave of national protests and demonstrations against police brutality. The militaristic police response included the dispatch of rooftop snipers, police dogs and military vehicles, and tear gas that was widely used on protestors. Ineffective communication and coordination across the 50 law enforcement agencies involved in the protest response exacerbated the already weak relations between the Ferguson and St. Louis communities and the local police.

The violence during the Ferguson protest occurred in a "sociopolitical context of long-standing racial, economic, and societal disparities" [7]. Historically, these disparities have contributed to the high violence and crime rates in Ferguson and beyond. Missouri is among the states with the highest firearm mortality rates [8]. Data gathered by the Mayor's Office in 2012 showed that the city's firearm death for youth was more than three times the national rate, and the St. Louis metro area was ninth in the nation for the number of youth murdered by guns [9]. Almost half (46%) of all victims are under age 25 while over half (51%) of all suspects are believed to be under age 25 [9].

The citizens and police officers involved in the protests had an extensive history of prior trauma exposure, increasing the risk for negative mental health outcomes [10]. Exposure to violence has a unique impact on youth, who are in critical stages of physical, emotional and mental development. Youth exposed to community violence exhibit increased rates of aggression and high-risk behavior, with the neighborhood having a significant influence on violent behaviors [11]. Neighborhood disorganization in conjunction with individual level exposure to violence has a measurable effect on trauma symptoms among youth [12]. Exposure to trauma is also linked to increased risk of PTSD, which manifests differently in youth and adults [13]. Research on PTSD among youth indicates that there can be long-term biological alterations produced by exposure to trauma, including increased heart rate, elevated or lower cortisol levels, and chronic sleep disturbance [4].

2. Wicked problem impact project (WPIP) description

Violence and trauma are separate yet connected complex problems with complicated risk factors. The interconnectedness of the two presents even greater challenges and is confounded by several variables. Many treatment programs and interventions targeting youth offer effective interventions, but often fail to consider the community context [11]. Initial formative research and interactions with the community illustrated a lack of role models and indicated a population of youth with no fear of death and dying. Our team wondered why this was occurring. What caused the disconnect? We wanted to look at ways to tackle bridging the gap between the community and law enforcement. From this early formative discovery, we agreed that a faith-based program with an emphasis on mentorship would be beneficial to this particular population. Engaging with the community in the planning and implementation of this project ensures that the project will appropriately address the needs of the community and be impactful long after conclusion of the project.

This project, A Prescription of Hope, was developed with the intent to promote awareness by educating community members on the effects of violence on health and was initially led by a two-person team consisting of a public health nurse (TS) and a pharmacist. It was also informed by the understanding that social support is a protective factor for youth exposed to trauma and violence. Studies show social resources, including relational support, neighborhood cohesion, and neighborhood satisfaction contribute to mental health resistance and resilience following trauma exposure [14]. Youth mentoring, after-school programs, and the involvement of community faith-based organizations have been proven to be valuable sources of support for youth in communities impacted by violence. This project intended to capitalize on those findings and implement similar strategies in local at-risk communities in Ferguson, Missouri.

3. Methods

3.1 Motivation

Initial inspiration for this project stemmed from the tragic death of Michael Brown, an 18-year old African American male who died in a police shooting at the hands of a 28-year old white officer in Ferguson, Missouri. As a nurse (author TS), a native of St. Louis, and a mother of three African American boys, the incident impacted me on a personal level. I had the unfortunate experience of viewing this young man's body lie in a street very familiar to me for up to four hours. I felt helpless and could not erase the memories of what I had witnessed. As with many who live in the city of Ferguson, this situation began to negatively impact my daily work, my communication with other people, my sleep, my eating habits, and more. Reflecting on my own response to the event, I began to think of the young adults reliving the trauma daily, and the residual effects that this incident would have on the community.

The idea for this project emerged through connecting with my colleague, Dr. Lachell Wardell. We had a shared vision for community-based models of healing the trauma being suffered by the local population--wounds that were magnified by the daily re-traumatizing exposures portrayed in the media. Our vision for our Clinical Scholars Wicked Problem Impact Project encompassed solutions to assist the youth in coping with the aftermath of the riots and violence and implement ways to prevent future generations from becoming victims or perpetrators of violence.

Knowing that no single approach could solve the myriad problems facing the community, we narrowed our focus and set our sights to target our priority objectives. Our priority objectives were faith-based (Faith, Love, Hope, and Resilience), meaning showing love to one another, promoting hope, and fostering examples of resiliency. The education component of the project was designed to include peer-to-peer engagement, scenario-based skits that promote healthy life skills, and addressing anger management, conflict resolution and coping skills. We named this project A Prescription of Hope.

3.2 Planning

Planning process for our project encompassed four primary components: formative research, the development of an advisory board, engagement of community stakeholders, and networking and building partnerships. At the end of the first year of implementation, the project leads decided to diversify our focus through a project phase we called "A Tale of Two Cities", with one arm active in the Ferguson community and the other active in the Chicago, Illinois area. This chapter focuses solely on the Ferguson branch of A Prescription of Hope.

3.2.1 Formative research

Parents and youth were recruited through local schools and Believers Temple Word Fellowship Church (BTWF) in St. Louis. We made announcements to the BTWF congregation about the program, and got permission to distribute flyers to members and leave them in the lobby. Believers Temple has a building separate from the main sanctuary for youth, where we were able to speak to youth directly about the program. We were also granted permission from elementary, middle and high schools in the Ferguson school district to send flyers about the program home with students.

We targeted youth between the ages of 10–18, initially focusing just on youth who lived in Ferguson, but later expanding to include neighboring communities. We requested that participants commit to a minimum of 75% of sessions over the 12-week project period.

Once we had recruited participants, we gathered formative data through interviewing parents (n = 108) who volunteered to share concerns regarding their child's behavior, friends, and issues at school or in the community. These interviews helped to gage parents' beliefs and immediate needs, guided what resources were needed, and built trust between parents and program directors. After receiving parental consent for all youth participants, we further surveyed each child that attended the educational and mentoring sessions at the start of the program (n = 478). The Developmental Assets Profile (DAP) served as our survey tool. This assessment consists of 58 questions that aim to measure the internal strengths and external supports that influence a youth's success in school and in life [15]. Data collected through the DAP assessment showed us which children were being affected directly or indirectly by violence and allowed us to tailor direct support to those in need.

The program was implemented through monthly sessions, with multiple "cohorts" participating in the program over a year. In the summer, we held two sessions per month which yielded increased participation (**Figure 1**). Small groups were 10 participants with one mentor/facilitator. Participants were divided based on the number of youths that were present at any given session.

The program included the implementation of a 12-week curriculum, which was developed to be interactive and engaging. A total of eight adult volunteer facilitators led group activities with the youth, which included scenario-based games, role plays, speaker presentations, field trips, and other activities.

The curriculum centered on the four core values of faith, love, hope and resilience, with each module involving unique peer-to-peer activities in group settings. For the faith module, we explored belief systems, moral systems, perceptions of right and wrong, and making good, conscious choices. In the love module, we

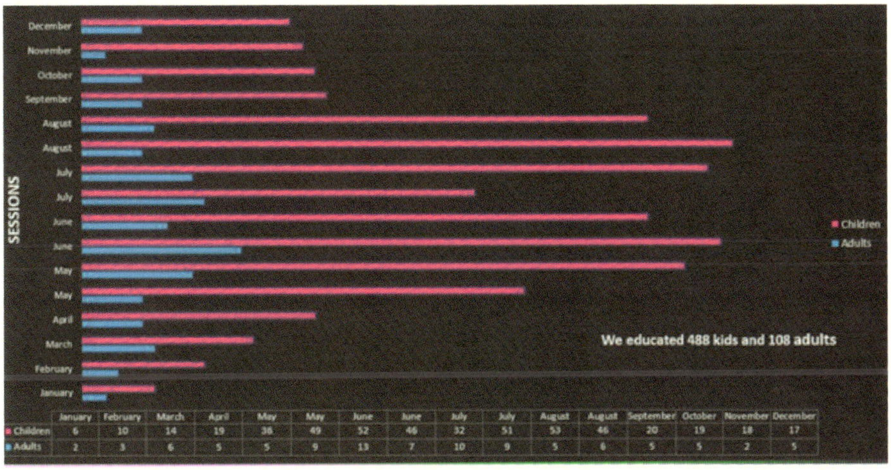

Figure 1.
Youth mental health screenings.

facilitated activities and conversations that centered on compassion, giving back to the community and working together. This module included a field trip to a homeless shelter where the youth participants volunteered. In the hope module, we created vision boards, did affirmations and positive self-talk work, and conducted self-esteem and confidence building exercises. In the final module, resilience, we focused on conflict management, coping, building strengths, and strategies for putting the components into the curriculum into action. We surveyed participants in the beginning, halfway through, and at the conclusion of the curriculum to assess what they learned and how their perspectives changed. The content of the curriculum stayed the same throughout; the only change made over the course of implementation was moving some participants into different groups based on their needs and availability.

Of the 478 youth that were assessed and participated in the educational and mentoring sessions, 307 received referrals for clinical mental health care and 98 of those referred (32%) attended 3 or more appointments with their providers.

3.2.2 Advisory board

A wide array of community-based organizations and local experts collaborated with our efforts to put the A Prescription of Hope project plans into action. These organizations were the BTWF, a youth program called Young People's Leadership Academy (YPLA), a local social worker, a professor from Creighton University, and a psychologist. After the project diversified, the St. Louis branch of the project continued the same partnerships with BTWF Church (Bishop Calvin Scott) and the local social worker. The Advisory Board expanded to include a community member who had lost their son to gun violence and a community-based health center. In addition, the St. Louis Prayer Project Inc., a non-profit founded by author TS joined the advisory board as a youth-focused organization that uses the "Developmental Relationships Framework" to serve as the emphasis of the youth-mentorship program [16].

3.2.3 Community engagement

In addition to implementing the curriculum, A Prescription of Hope collaborated on several projects with local middle and high schools in the community. The social worker we engaged with as one of our advisory board members performs

PTSD assessments on at-risk children that are referred to her by teachers and office staff from school; and refers at-risk children to our program. She has been instrumental in getting children referred for counseling services on an in-patient or outpatient basis. She also works directly with the children's families to connect them to resources, including job skills training and life coaching, and obtain counseling referrals for them.

An important element of our program's success has been our ability to leverage the resources available in our community. The local community-based health center serves as a resource for mental health services and counseling for children referred by our staff and by the social worker. We meet quarterly for updates, and as needed in-between, to discuss the focus of care and plans of action identified to assist the children moving forward. The pastor of the church also supports our program by providing an avenue for our team to share information, post flyers, and participate in church-community based activities that further inform the community about our services.

3.2.4 Networking and building partnerships

Social media has been an important tool for A Prescription of Hope to spread awareness of the impact of violence as related to PTSD among youth through an anti-violence PSA. The video PSA (St. Louis Youth A Prescription for Hope, Violence Prevention) features several of the youth that participated in the program. It was shown at schools, the local community partner health center, and shared on other social media platforms. The video showcases an interview with a high school student sharing a personal story. While his story is dramatic, it represents a role-model success story in that he was later referred for counseling services and is currently doing well and attending college on a fully supported scholarship.

3.3 Project goals

The goals of the first year of A Prescription for Hope were to empower parents, teens, and key stakeholder residents, reduce health disparities by providing sustainable interventions through screening at-risk youth, and advocating for policies that provide after-school care to at-risk children. For year two, we expanded the goals to include developing a curriculum which incorporated mental health, resiliency training, and the effects of violence on health. Our second goal for the year was to launch a campaign of speaking engagements that promote awareness.

Despite the conclusion of the formal Clinical Scholars 3-year experience, A Prescription for Hope continues to work towards educating youth on anti-violence and the impact of PTSD through the curriculum-based program that can be implemented in schools for youth, parents, and school staff. We continue to foster relationships with local organizations, including one that collaborates with police officers. We are also working towards having a scholarship funded after-school community-based facility.

In the long term, A Prescription for Hope would like to have our own facility that can house youth in a structured after-school program. This would provide a safe space for them to come to receive mentorship, love, and participate in recreational activities that would build skills to promote healthy living and successful futures.

4. Outcomes

To date, youth ages 10–18 years of age in the city of St. Louis have benefitted the most from the A Prescription for Hope project. We've been able to show

how faith-based after-school programs that have an emphasis on mentorship with classes focused on conflict resolution, anger management, coping skills, resiliency training, and communication can make a positive difference in at-risk young adults. Furthermore, we directly connected hundreds of youth to mental health services through providing referrals so they could obtain the clinical care they needed.

We recognized youth who were nominated by peers, family members, teachers, church members, etc. monthly who were making positive decisions in their homes, schools, churches, and communities. We included them on our website's blog, on social media platforms, and sent them an award basket filled with a Prayer Project t-shirt, a certificate of achievement, a prayer journal, and a $100 Foot Locker gift certificate.

While the three years of project visioning, planning and implementation resulted in several newly developed collaborations, the development of educational curricula, the launching of faith-based resiliency intervention programs, and clinical referrals for professional care for at-risk youth in need, the most important outcomes are the stories of youth who were impacted. Some anonymized exemplar youth success stories are presented below:

- A high school male who was suffering from severe PTSD and depression as a result of trauma exposure and violence participated in our program. Before participating in the program, he was contemplating quitting school and the football team. As part of A Prescription for Hope services, he and his mother were counseled on trauma and its effects. One year later, he is still attending counseling services, and is now attending a university on a football and academic scholarship.

- A middle school young girl was having behavioral issues in school including fighting, getting suspended, and receiving failing grades. She was also suffering from PTSD due to trauma she suffered from the violent death of her father being killed by his neighbor. She and her brother started receiving counseling services and mentorship through our program and she became an honor roll student. She is now an eighth-grade graduate looking forward to starting high school next school year.

- A twelve-year-old boy was suffering from severe depression due to his father being incarcerated and being left home alone to care for himself every day after school while his mother worked. He was receiving failing grades and was suffering from a mild case of failure to thrive due to low weight. He started receiving mentoring and counseling services and is now participating in after-school sports programs and gets to visit with his dad on a regular basis. They share a healthy relationship and he's looking forward to his father's release from prison soon.

5. Discussion

Community partnered interventions are important tools to helping heal communities traumatized by violence. When these community partnerships are broad and inclusive of many sectors, the outcome is stronger. A Prescription for Hope included faith-based organizations, clinicians, non-profits, academicians, parent voices and youth voices. The diversity of that chorus strengthens and informs approaches, making them richer and extending their impact.

The voices of the youth are essential to creating youth-centered programs that are effective; not only does it empower them to share and engage with others; it also promotes trust among the group. We were able to get to know each other and build meaningful partnerships that allowed us to educate them using non-traditional methods. As a facilitator and mentor many times, the lead author (TS) had the opportunity of observing peer-to-peer interactions which by far were the most rewarding. Listening to them share real-life, transparent stories of traumatic experiences, hopes, and aspirations with others in small group sessions allowed them to let their defenses down. These interactions resulted in their peers showing genuine concern, empathy, and self-expression. It was in these moments that real breakthroughs took place. The youth were able to be vulnerable and it was apparent that the safe space that we were hoping to create had been achieved. The presence of the social worker brought reassurance and offered strategies to prevent the communication from turning to an undesired direction.

The impacts of community-based interventions on youth are positive and dramatic, as indicated by the exemplar stories above. While millions of dollars in federal investment to rebuild schools and communities would be wonderful, it is striking the degree of difference that love, attention, counseling, support, role-modeling and mentoring can make in a child's life, even a child who is dealing with the complexities that result from violence. Surely, these kinds of approaches can be augmented to benefit many children who are at-risk across many communities. Particularly in times of economic contraction or recession, the resources for extensive revitalization might not exist. Yet, this project demonstrates the potential impacts of smaller-scale interventions that are doable at the community level.

Making a difference in communities is more than just having passionate advocates--it is about giving those advocates voice, enhancing their skills, giving them the tools and support to launch impactful programs. While the financial support was not large in comparison to many grant-based programs ($35,000/year), the combination of financial resources and sophisticated skills training augments the ability of passionate advocates to make real differences in communities that need it the most.

6. Leader learning (TS)

My personal experience with the RWJF, Clinical Scholars program over the 3-year period has been nothing short of "Excellence." My learning experience has included a greater respect for diversity among other professionals and peers, personal enrichment in improving my personal life and the life of others, improved self-awareness, and increased self-confidence as a leader in the field of Public Health.

Working with community partners provided me with the opportunity to participate in community projects which enhanced my networking skills with local stakeholders, improved my communication skills, leadership skills, and problem-solving skills. I was able to build long lasting trusting relationships as well as plan for future projects and opportunities.

My experience with the youth has humbled me in ways that are unimaginable. My goals were to educate them and leave a lasting impression, but they were the ones who educated me. I am forever grateful and forever changed. I can only hope that I've done the same for them. I told myself going into this project that if I could help to positively change one child's outcomes then I've done my job. Lastly, I learned that in order to reach youth you have to be willing to give a lot of yourself while expecting nothing in return. Your motives have to be genuine or they will see through you and you will never gain their trust. Patience and love have to be your strength or you will never reach them. I am stronger and better as a result of every young person I've encountered.

7. Toolkit and other resources

- St. Louis Prayer Project Website
- St. Louis Prayer Project Facebook Page
- St. Louis Prayer Project Instagram

A more comprehensive toolkit can be found at https://clinicalscholarsnli.org/community-impact

Author details

Tonita Smith[1*], Edith Amponsah[2] and Lia Garman[3]

1 St. Louis Prayer Project Inc., Missouri, United States

2 Tulane University School of Medicine, Louisiana, United States

3 University of North Carolina Chapel Hill Gillings School of Global Public Health, North Carolina, United States

*Address all correspondence to: tonitasmith3@gmail.com

References

[1] Sumner SA, Mercy JA, Dahlberg LL, Hillis SD, Klevens J, Houry D. Violence in the United States: Status, challenges, and opportunities. Journal of the American Medical Association. 2015;314(5):478-488. DOI: 10.1001/jama.2015.8371.

[2] Cohen L. Communities are not all created equal: Strategies to prevent violence affecting youth in the United States. Journal of Public Health Policy. 2016;37(1):81-94. DOI: 10.1057/s41271-016-0005-4.

[3] Kegler SR, Dahlberg LL, Mercy JA. Firearm Homicides and Suicides in Major Metropolitan Areas — United States, 2012-2013 and 2015-2016. CDC Morbidity and Mortality Weekly Report. 2018;67(44):1233-1237. DOI: http://dx.doi.org/10.15585/mmwr.mm6744a3.

[4] Buka SL, Stichick TL, Birdthistle I, Earls FJ. Youth exposure to violence: prevalence, risks, and consequences. American Journal of Orthopsychiatry. 2001;71(3):298-310. DOI: 10.1037/0002-9432.71.3.298.

[5] Sacket D. Neighborhoods and Violent Crime. Office of Policy Research and Development, U.S. Department of Housing and Urban Development [Internet]. 2016. Available from: https://www.huduser.gov/portal/periodicals/em/summer16/highlight2.html

[6] Hemenway D, Azrael D, Conner A, Miller M. Variation in rates of fatal police shootings across US states: The role of firearm availability. Journal of Urban Health. 2019;96(1):63-73. DOI: 10.1007/s11524-018-0313-z.

[7] Kahn KB, Martin KD. Policing and race: Disparate treatment, perceptions, and policy responses. Social Issues and Policy Review. 2016;10(1):82-121. DOI: 10.1111/sipr.12019.

[8] Centers for Disease Control and Prevention. Firearm Mortality by State [Internet]. 2020. Available from: https://www.cdc.gov/nchs/pressroom/sosmap/firearm_mortality/firearm.htm.

[9] Filler C. City of St. Louis Youth Violence Prevention Partnership. Washington University in St. Louis Institute of Public Health. 2016. Available from: https://publichealth.wustl.edu/city-of-st-louis-youth-violence-prevention-partnership/

[10] Galovski TE, Peterson ZD, Beagley MC, Strasshofer DR, Held P, Fletcher TD. Exposure to violence during Ferguson protests: Mental health effects for law enforcement and community members. Journal of Traumatic Stress, 2016;29:283-292. DOI: 10.1002/jts.22105.

[11] Harden T, Kenemore T, Mann K, Edwards M, List C. The truth n' trauma project: addressing community violence through a youth-led, trauma-informed and restorative framework. Child and Adolescent Social Work Journal. 2015;32(1):65-79. DOI: 10.1007/s10560-014-0366-0.

[12] Butcher F, Galanek J, Kretschmar JM, Flannery DJ. The impact of neighborhood disorganization on neighborhood exposure to violence, trauma symptoms, and social relationships among at-risk youth. Social Science & Medicine. 2015;146:300-306. DOI: 10.1016/j.socscimed.2015.10.013.

[13] McLaughlin K. Posttraumatic stress disorder in children and adolescents: Epidemiology, pathogenesis, clinical manifestations, course, assessment, and diagnosis. In: Brent D, Solomon D, editors. UpToDate. Waltham: MA. 2019. Available from: https://www.uptodate.com/contents/

posttraumatic-stress-disorder-in-children-and-adolescents-epidemiology-pathogenesis-clinical-manifestations-course-assessment-and-diagnosis.

[14] Galovski TE, Peterson ZD, Fox-Galalis A. Trajectories of Posttraumatic Stress and Depression in Police and Community Members Following the Violence during Civil Unrest in Ferguson, Missouri. American Journal of Community Psychology. 2018;62:433-448. DOI: 10.1002/ajcp.12273.

[15] Search Institute. The Developmental Assets Profile (DAP) [Internet]. 2019. Available from: https://www.search-institute.org/surveys/choosing-a-survey/dap/. [Accessed 2020-05-15].

[16] Search Institute. The Developmental Relationships framework [Internet]. 2018. Available from: https://www.search-institute.org/developmental-relationships/developmental-relationships-framework/.

Chapter 12

The MHISTREET: Barbershop Embedded Education Initiative

Nnemdi Kamanu Elias, Alfred Larbi, Kevin Washington and Erin Athey

Abstract

The United States (US) is in the midst of a mental health crisis. More than one in four (26.2%) adults experience a diagnosable mental health disorder each year, and 46% of the population will do so in their lifetime. Collectively, mental health disorders are a leading cause of disability and account for one-third of all years lived with disability and premature mortality. Black Americans constitute about 12% of the US population, but they make up more than 18% of the population affected by mental disorders. Black men are 30% more likely than non-Hispanic white men to report having a mental illness but are less likely to receive proper diagnosis and treatment. Black adults are 20% more likely to report serious psychological distress than white adults. Despite this, many Black people do not seek mental health care for various reasons. Causes of higher morbidity and non-care seeking behavior in Black people and Black men in particular include racism, discrimination, stigma, and distrust of the healthcare system. Across the District of Columbia (DC), Black Americans are twice as likely as other ethnicities to report a serious mental disorder, especially if they live in poverty and did not complete high school. In the project service area of Ward 8 in Southeast DC, 92% of the population is Black, 30.7% live in poverty, and only 85% of the population age 25+ completed high school. Evidence shows common mental health disorders are distributed according to a gradient of economic disadvantage across society; the poor and disadvantaged suffer disproportionately from common mental health disorders. In Southeast DC, this negative impact on mental health is compounded by the geographic concentration of underemployment, lack of economic opportunity, poverty, and underutilization of mental health services. Improving mental health literacy is a non-systemic intervention shown to increase mental health care-seeking behaviors. Mental health literacy is the knowledge of, attitude about, and behavior toward mental health issues and mental health services. The goal of the Mental Health Improvement through Study, Teaching, Rebranding, Embedded Education, and Technology or (MHISTREET) initiative is to improve mental health in Black men through embedded education in non-traditional spaces such as barbershops.

Keywords: black mental health, depression, black American, community-based interventions

1. Introduction

1.1 Mental Health in the United States

The United States (US) is in the midst of a mental health crisis [1–7]. More than one in four (26.2%) adults experience a diagnosable mental health disorder each year, and 46% of the population will do so in their lifetime [1, 2]. Collectively, mental disorders are a leading cause of disability, accounting for one-third of all years lived with disability and premature mortality [3].

Despite the heavy burden of disease, availability of mental health care services is inadequate. Available care services are often underutilized because mental health disorders impair one's ability to seek and adhere to care, delaying the receipt of effective treatment. Screening, early detection, and effective ongoing treatment of mental health disorders can have a positive impact on the quality and quantity of life. Unfortunately, this often does not occur; many people experience their introduction to mental health treatment in emergency settings at a late stage in the course of the disease. Elements influencing mental health treatment-seeking behaviors include systemic factors, knowledge, beliefs, attitudes, and stigma [4].

1.2 Mental Health in black Americans

More than 18% of people in the US who experience mental health morbidity are Black, but Black people account for only 12% of the population [4]. Black adults are more likely to have feelings of sadness, hopelessness, and worthlessness than are white adults [6]. Despite this higher morbidity, many Black Americans do not seek mental health care [4]. Multiple factors contribute to the higher burden of mental health morbidity in Black Americans and include, but are not limited to, racism and other forms of discrimination, stigma, distrust of the health care system, a perception of bias and lack of cultural sensitivity in the health care system in general, inadequate mental health literacy, and poverty.

1.2.1 Racial discrimination, stress, and trauma

Hankerson et al. cited individual and institutional racial discrimination as a risk factor for depression [8]. Institutional racism results from policies and practices within organizations that contribute to discrimination for a group of people [9]. Living with a plethora of discriminations that manifest as police brutality and other forms of racial harassment can result in racial stress and have a deleterious effect on the health and well-being of Black people. Racial stress often occurs as a result of repeated everyday discrimination known as micro-aggressions. Research shows that repeated acts of micro-aggression are a more consistent predictor of depressive symptoms than single instances of major discrimination [10, 11].

The persistent psychological assault of racial stressors culminates in the form of racial trauma. Racial trauma occurs when African Americans are surrounded by constant reminders of the dangers of being African American [12]. Washington called these reminders a form of Persistent Enslavement Systemic Trauma (PEST) [13]. PEST describes a specific dimension of the trans-generational trauma pervasive in all walks of Black American life. PEST is a systemic trauma that has residual effects on the daily activities of African/Black people and influences multiple aspects of their lives. Washington asserts PEST affects the entire psychological well-being of people of African descent, including their physical bodies, minds, perceptions of reality and themselves, relationships with themselves and others, and notions of what it means to be a person [13].

1.2.2 Stigma

Stigma is a collection of attitudes, beliefs, and behaviors that assign shame to an individual who exhibits actions or traits outside of a perceived norm [14]. Connor et al. posited that both public stigma (negative attitudes held by the public) and internal stigma (negative attitudes held by stigmatized individuals about themselves) are important barriers to successful mental health treatment [15]. Their study found Black American adults as a whole tended to internalize the stigma of mental illness and sought treatment at half the rate of non-Hispanic white Americans [15]. Upon seeking treatment, Black people were reported to skip sessions and terminate treatment at higher rates than their white counterparts [15].

1.2.3 Distrust of the health care system

The history of deliberate medical and scientific mistreatment of Black people in the US is well-chronicled [8]. One of the most significant events was the 1932 Tuskegee Syphilis Experiment, in which Black men with syphilis were followed by the US Public Health Service to observe the course of the disease [16]. Researchers withheld treatment allowing the disease to progress and, in some cases, to infect wives and children of the subjects. The Tuskegee Experiment was one in a series of events throughout history that instilled social norms of medical mistrust in the Black community.

Qualitative studies show that some Black Americans today have a fear of being used as "guinea pigs" [16]. This fear drives decreased healthcare utilization, treatment compliance, and decreased willingness to participate in research and clinical trials [8, 17].

Some Black Americans identified the mental health system specifically as a stressor [15]. Many perceived that Black Americans had a more difficult time accessing mental health services and expressed frustration with the process of seeking care.

1.2.4 Bias and lack of cultural sensitivity

Multiple studies of the US health care system have documented implicit bias—thoughts and attitudes that exist outside conscious awareness. In one such study, Hall et al. examined 15 articles and used the Implicit Association Test to assess implicit bias. They concluded that most health care providers appear to have an implicit bias in terms of positive attitudes toward whites and negative attitudes toward people of color [18].

Several studies have shown Black Americans strongly prefer mental health providers of their same ethnic background [8, 15, 17]. However, Black people make up only 3.9% of psychologists [5] and 5% of physicians [17], a visible reminder of why Black Americans perceive the mental health system as being culturally insensitive.

1.2.5 Inadequate mental health literacy

An important factor related to seeking mental health support is mental health literacy, which is the "knowledge and beliefs about mental disorders which aid their recognition, management, or prevention" [19, 20]. In a 2010 study of Black Americans, participants were able to recognize their symptoms (trouble sleeping, excessive drinking, sadness, and fatigue) but did not relate them to depression [21]. Upon learning the relationship, a majority of participants believed they needed to deal with them on their own and were averse to the idea of seeking treatment. Many believed that treatment would be ineffective or feared the idea of taking medication [21]. Many Black people do not perceive a need for mental health care as shown in a 2017 study using data from the National Survey of Drug Use and Health (NSDUH). Only 9.4% of Black Americans reported a perceived need for mental health care compared with 17.9% of their white counterparts [14].

1.2.6 Poverty

Economic challenges prevalent within the Black community also affect psychological well-being. Black adults living below poverty are two to three times more likely to report serious psychological distress than those living above poverty [6]. A 2013 review of depression in Black men found that higher-income served as a protective factor against depression, and job security correlated with a lower frequency of depressive episodes [22]. In a 2011 study of Black men, major depressive disorder (MDD) was associated with lower income, less education, and being unmarried [23].

1.3 Mental Health in Black American men

Black men, in particular, have increased morbidity due to mental illness. Data from the US Department of Health and Human Services show Black men are 30% more likely than non-Hispanic white men to report having a mental illness [5]. Suicide attempts among Black males are 1.6 times higher than white males [5]. A 2017 Health and Human Services study found the death rate from suicide for African American men was more than four times greater than for African American women [6].

Racial stress contributes to the total burden of stress on Black men and impacts mental health outcomes. In a 2006 longitudinal prospective study of over 700 Black men, racial discrimination was strongly associated with poor physical and mental health [24]. A 2011 study using data from the National Survey of American Life found that Black American men below the age of 30 had greater depressive symptoms, experienced greater perceived discrimination, and had a lower perception of mastery than their counterparts above the age of 54 [11]. Belgrave & Brevard state African American boys have many potential stressors, even relative to African American girls, that negatively impact their psychological well-being throughout their lives [9].

A 2012 review analyzing beliefs of masculinity among men of color found an association between "machismo" or traditional masculinity beliefs and the inability or unwillingness to describe emotions - "taking it like a man" [25, 26]. Masculinity is often associated with certain expectations and standards a man must uphold. In a 2019 qualitative study, Black men reported endorsing the role of caretaker, someone who needs to display strength for their family [26]. Displays of emotion or vulnerability were perceived as a weakness and negatively affected mental health treatment-seeking behaviors [27, 28].

Research by Holden et al. showed Black men are more likely to struggle with describing depression and their emotional state [5], making acknowledging the need for care increasingly difficult. Even if Black men recognize the symptoms of depression, they are less likely than Black women to believe mental health treatment would be effective. Younger Black men were the least open to the idea of seeking mental health treatment as compared with older African American men and women of all ages [4]. Cook et al. and others have shown Black American men have lower rates of use of psychotropic medication than their white counterparts [8, 29].

1.4 The Initiative's service area

The broad geographical area within the District of Columbia (DC) where the initiative operates is referred to as "Southeast DC" or "East of the Anacostia River". The unemployment rate across DC is four times the national average with twice the rate of alcohol abuse, twice the rate of alcohol-related driving deaths, and 20 times the violent crime rate [30]. Most of these figures are driven by data from Southeast DC, the service area for the **M**ental **H**ealth **I**mprovement through **S**tudy, **T**eaching, **R**ebranding, **E**mbedded **E**ducation, and **T**echnology or MHISTREET.

Life expectancy in Southeast DC can be up to 10 years less than other neighborhoods three miles away, with limitations due to physical or emotional health more common. More than 10 times as many families as those who live in other areas of DC reside in poverty, and child poverty rates are as high as 47.1% compared with 20.3% nationally [31]. Additionally, one in five (20.3%) Southeast DC residents is unemployed.

In MHISTREET's specific area of Ward 8 in Southeast DC, 92% of the population is Black, 30.7% of the population lives in poverty, and 85% completed high school [7]. Southeast DC is unfortunately emblematic of numerous disenfranchised communities in the US [32]. African Americans living here experience the highest rates of mental health disorders in DC [33]. Contributing factors include constant exposure to environmental factors such as discrimination, violence, limited health service access, and poverty [34, 35]. Each factor is a significant barrier to mental health service utilization and exists at multiple social-ecological levels including individual/interpersonal, provider/mental health system, community, and societal levels [33]. Devising effective systematic approaches for improving the mental health of Black men living in Southeast DC must reflect an understanding of the ecological and system perspective.

2. Wicked problem impact project (WPIP) description

Wicked problems are unique in that they have no definitive formulation. They are interdependent, codependent, and symptoms of other wicked problems. Wicked problems have no true endpoints and no template to follow. As laid out in the introduction, poor mental health and wellbeing in Black Americans, particularly Black men, fit this description. It is an elusive, complex, "*wicked problem*" with no clear solution [36].

The selection of poor mental health and well-being among African Americans in Southeast DC is based on the authors' experiences at a medical clinic treating people living with HIV/AIDS. The clinic is located within the United Medical Center hospital, the only hospital in Southeast DC. United Medical Center operates as a safety-net hospital in the only designated mental health professional shortage area of the city. The authors surmised that the impact of negative social determinants (racism, discrimination, and underemployment) on the physical health of their predominantly Black and low-income patients was compounded by unaddressed mental health issues. Their patients who had mental health disorders (depression, anxiety, post-traumatic stress disorder) also had difficulty adhering to their care and treatment goals and consequently had poorer health outcomes. These outcomes also informed the authors' view that improving access to and utilization of mental health services in Ward 8 of Southeast, DC should be a key priority, and the first step should be increasing mental health literacy in the community to reduce the barriers to treatment.

3. Methods

3.1 Approach

The project design changed dramatically over the first few months and continued to evolve over the course of the initiative. Project evolution was possible because the team drew from community-based participatory research (CBPR) principles [37, 38] and used an action research approach [39].

3.1.1 CBPR principles

- Use community settings and involve the community in the project design and implementation
- Build on strengths and resources within the community
- Focus on problems relevant to the community
- Use an ecological perspective that attends to multiple determinants of health and disease
- Openly address race, racism, ethnicity, and social class

3.1.2 Five-step action research approach

- Problem identification
- Organization of plan of action
- Data collection
- Organization and analysis of data
- Planning for future action

3.2 Original project design

The initial proposal was to design a community hospital-based clinical support program at the patient, provider, and population levels. At the patient level, the plan was to screen primary care patients for mental health disorders and social needs and link them to mental health care and social services. For the providers, the intent was to support mental health education of Southeast DC private Medicaid primary care providers and share community mental health resources. Lastly, at the population level, the goal was to train community members on *Mental Health First Aid* and implement a social marketing program. After extensive qualitative and quantitative data collection among patients, healthcare providers, and community members, this original design within a traditional health care setting was abandoned.

3.3 Current project design

The project became predominantly community-based and was implemented outside the traditional health care setting to have a wider reach and deeper resonance within the community. After many cycles of the action research process, the focus became African American men, and the core intervention became an educational program for barbers and community members to increase mental health using the culturally safe space of the barbershop to deliver "embedded education".

3.4 Project development and implementation

3.4.1 Formation of a mental health sub-committee of the Ward 8 Health council

The authors were regular attendees of Ward 8 Health Council meetings, created by a former DC mayor to convene diverse stakeholders committed to improving the health of Ward 8 residents. The Council consists of stakeholders from local managed-care associations, hospitals, universities, community-based organizations, and DC residents, who meet monthly and share information and ideas. The issue of poor mental health in Ward 8 was a topic of frequent discussion. The authors were invited by the chair of the council to create a mental health sub-committee charged with promoting and enhancing policies and practices that increase access to mental and behavioral health services, decreasing stigma associated with mental health disorders, promoting mental health wellness, and improving mental health literacy and outcomes for individuals living in Ward 8. Sub-committee members reflected the diversity of the council and were influential in the decision to change the original project design.

3.4.2 Pre-implementation data collection

Through the authors' rigorous review of the literature and consultation with the mental health sub-committee and other community members, the program evolved into a community-based intervention. The authors strongly believed the intervention needed to reach residents who were not engaged with the traditional health system.

Quantitative Data Collection: The authors developed an academic partnership with the public health school of a local university. MHISTREET team members served as site directors for eight master's level research projects designed to gain a better understanding of the mental landscape in Southeast DC. Projects included mental health literacy surveys of providers and patients, use of GIS mapping data to analyze drivers of emergency room visits, and systematic literature reviews.

Qualitative Data Collection: The authors conducted a listening tour and hosted several community-engaged sessions and informational interviews, to hear various perspectives on mental health from community stakeholders. Meeting participants included church leaders, health department officials, community residents, medical professionals, representatives from the National Association on Mental Illness (NAMI, DC Chapter), and local core service agencies (outpatient mental health clinics).

3.4.3 Selection of mental health literacy as core intervention

Myriad factors relate to and influence mental health treatment-seeking behaviors. One important factor is mental health literacy, the knowledge and beliefs about mental health disorders which aid their recognition, management, or prevention [19, 20]. Literacy is a significant determinant of mental health and has the potential to improve both individual and population health. Mental health literacy is conceptualized by Bjornsen et al. [40–43] as having four domains:

- understanding how to obtain and maintain good mental health
- understanding mental health disorders and their treatments

- decreasing stigma against mental illness and
- enhancing help-seeking efficacy

Domains are consistent with the qualitative input collected from community partners and stakeholders about their concerns with stigma, misinformation, and misperceptions about mental health. Their experiences echoed research findings on stigma, medical mistrust, and cultural norms within the African American population.

As a result of strong community input and data collection, increasing mental health literacy became the goal of the intervention. Closing the existing literacy gap was determined to be essential to improve community mental health.

3.4.4 Selection of anchor institution

The authors' understood that an anchor institution was critical to successful program implementation. The term "anchor institution" was coined by Michael Porter in 2002 [44] and is defined as a community-dependent resource which capitalizes on opportunities to create shared value and be a major economic force within the community by controlling important levers for community development [45]. In a review of outreach strategies directed at Black men, the highest yield was produced using personnel of the same ethnicity to conduct face-to-face outreach [17]. Results were amplified when the outreach came from within the Black community [21].

Emerging literature highlights the power and potential of universities, hospitals, and other institutions with long-term rooted investments in an area to transform neighborhoods, cities, and regions [46]. Originally, the authors thought the local hospital would serve as the anchor institution. However, that idea was abandoned based on community perceptions of the hospital and the team's desire to reach individuals not currently engaged with the health care system.

The authors then considered the Black church, given its historical importance and service to the Black community. The team connected with an out-of-state program called PEWS (Promoting Emotional Wellness and Spirituality) at the Mental Health Association of New Jersey. PEWS trains faith leaders in mental health to address the need within their congregations. The authors explored replicating the PEWS model in Southeast DC with the Faith-Based Director of the local DC Department of Behavioral Health. However, a nascent program was already in place, and the committee advised that large segments of the population would not be reached through religious organizations.

After much discussion, with Black men as the primary focal point of the intervention, barbershops were selected as the anchor institution to implement mental health literacy programming. Unlike healthcare sites and religious organizations, barbershops are regarded as a trusted and equalizing space and barbers as trusted members of the community. In addition, barbershops are non-medical and non-religious settings with no "negative psychological baggage" [47].

3.4.5 Use of the black barbershop for increasing mental health literacy

The team conducted a systematic review of barbershop interventions to evaluate their effectiveness and seek best practices from several existing programs in the US and abroad. They consulted with the Lion's Den in the United Kingdom, a barbershop mental health program recognized by former Prime Minister Theresa May and Prince William. In the US, the authors found several health-related programs in barbershops. The most robust and well known was The Confess Project led by

DOI: http://dx.doi.org/10.5772/intechopen.98461

Lorenzo Lewis. Mr. Lewis's grassroots efforts in Arkansas and surrounding states were inspirational and confirmed the notion that the Black barbershop has long served an important social and cultural purpose.

Barbershops have historically been a safe gathering place for Black men, a place where people have received the news, registered to vote, and shared personal struggles. The barber often not only cuts hair but also serves as a confidant. The barber/client connection in Black communities places the barber in a unique position to be a strong partner and leader in increasing mental health literacy among Black men. In addition, the authors' speculated the Black barbershops' place in the community would enable interaction with women and children, so this health intervention could potentially impact families and the broader community.

The use of barbershops for health interventions dates to the 1980s. This model has been used to address Black American health issues such as hypertension, prostate cancer, and HIV/AIDS, but the MIHSTREET team found no published reports in peer-reviewed literature regarding its use for mental health interventions [48–50]. All intervention studies reviewed by the team found greater health improvement among those interacting with the barber [51–55]. The literature, composed of non-experimental studies, suggested that several common factors were present in successful barbershop interventions, including the training of the barber in health knowledge, referring clients to a healthcare provider (physician and/or primary care provider), and the use of a theoretical model to guide the intervention. These findings influenced the authors' approach to project design and implementation, specifically the training of the barbers and the need for an immediate connection to services.

3.4.6 Use of embedded education for increasing mental health literacy

MHISTREET chose embedded education, a recognized public innovation in governance tool, to deliver mental health information [56]. Embedded education is the practice of educating people through everyday interpersonal encounters within organizations that exist for non-educational purposes [57]. Embedded education uses existing social relationships and trust between individuals and organizations or within social networks, to deliver content that learners can immediately use and share [58]. By using the existing trusting environment of the barbershop and minimal additional supplies, MHISTREET's barbershop approach provides the potential to reach a mental health service-neglected population. As a client waits for or receives services, he becomes a learner in a health-related educational encounter. The encounter occurs between the barbers and their clients and/or between community residents/peer educators and the clients. The educational content is mental health information transmitted via conversations between barber and client or between a community resident/peer educator and clients.

3.4.7 Barbershop embedded education (BEE) curriculum development

With guidance from multi-disciplinary community partners on the Ward 8 sub-committee, the authors created a culturally relevant mental health education curriculum for embedded education in barbershops. The curriculum was based on the previous work of a collaborating partner, Dr. Kevin Washington, a professor of psychology, who had developed a mental health curriculum specifically designed for African American men. The final product was a six-module curriculum that incorporated pop-culture, race, and social justice themes, and used interactive lessons, music, video, and audio presentations.

3.4.8 BEE training

The program structure for BEE involved training barbers on mental health and having them engage with and share resource information with interested clients. A pilot cohort of barbers received the initial training in 2018 and provided structured feedback. Specific feedback included comments such as, "This was great; I hear people's problems all the time and I didn't know how to help them!" and "I used to think peoples' issues were too big to overcome and now I know there is help out there" and "I did not realize there is help out there for my brothers." Participants also stated the training was beneficial but too long. It interfered with their work schedules, led to a loss of earnings, and financial incentives provided for attendance were not enough to counterbalance lost income.

3.4.9 Program redesign

Feedback from barbers and input from community advisors led to program modifications. The revamped MHISTREET program included not only barbers but also 40 community members. The inclusion of community members was modeled

INPUTS →	ACTIVITIES →	OUTPUTS →	OUTCOMES
1. Literature review 2. Expert opinions 3. Surveys of patients, providers, and community members 4. Inventory Of community resources 5. GIS Mapping	1. Community Engagement meetings 2. Curriculum development 3. Barber and community resident training (BEE Squad) 4. BEE Squad presentations in the barbershops 5. Social media development	1. Number of barbershops 2. Number of clients per shop 3. Number of barbers and community members trained	**Short-term outcomes (knowledge change)** 1. *Kirkpatrick Training Evaluation* 2. BEE Squad's increase in mental health literacy 3. Barbershop Clients increase in mental health literacy **Medium-term outcomes (attitude and behavioral change)** 1. Clients are more inclined to seek MH care 2. Clients seek mental health care 3. Clients actively engage in a mental health care plan arid follow through **Long-term outcomes (changes in well-being)** 1. Reduced rates of untreated mental health disorders 2. A decline in mental health disparities among black men 3. Black men become agents over their own mental health with effects on the greater community

Table 1.
The "MHI-STREET" *initiative project logic model.*

after an existing program, The Confess Project in Arkansas [58], led by community mental health advocate Lorenzo Lewis. Mr. Lewis shared his moving story of adversity and the benefit he received from mental health counseling. Through storytelling, he was increasing the mental health literacy of barbershop clients in Arkansas and surrounding states.

3.4.10 Use of storytelling for mental health literacy

Storytelling is an evidence-based education method that increases the likelihood of behavior change based on the activation of neurotransmitters in the brain responsible for concentration, empathy, and connection [59]. Storytelling, particularly stories that resonate individually, has the ability to change one's attitudes, beliefs, and behavior, and can be a powerful vehicle for change.

3.4.11 Program expansion - barbershop embedded education squad

The authors used their original barber training to develop a program similar to The Confess Project [58]. The MHISTREET team hosted a one-day training event for the new iteration of the project. The authors then met monthly over six months with the new team affectionately referred to as the "BEE Squad". The six BEE Squad members learned more about mental health, rehearsed their stories, and practiced facilitation of group discussions.

3.4.12 Logic model

The logic model that the authors used as a framework to develop the Barbershop Embedded Education program. Provides the inputs, activities, outputs and outcomes related to the project (**Table 1**).

3.5 Inputs

3.6 Data collection and analysis

3.6.1 Resident/patient survey

The authors developed, administered, and analyzed a 200-patient mental health knowledge, behavior, and attitude survey in the only safety-net hospital in Southeast DC. Data showed that over 80% of respondents had some degree of knowledge about mental health but over half indicated significant stigma around using mental health services for themselves or loved ones.

3.6.2 Provider survey

The authors developed and administered a survey to six local Medicaid primary care providers on their knowledge and practices in mental health care. All of the providers reported that they were caring for many patients with mental health disorders and five of the six providers were interested in learning more about mental health and available services.

3.6.3 GIS mapping

In partnership with George Washington University (GWU), the team collaborated on geographic "hotspot" mapping in Ward 8 to determine whether a correlation existed between emergency room use and mental health diagnoses. While informative about the overall prevalence of mental health disorders, the analysis did not show any particular "hotspots" for the high prevalence of mental health disorders within the Ward 8 boundaries.

3.6.4 Service inventory

The authors' supervised eight GWU public health student projects. One project resulted in an inventory of Ward 8 mental health and social service resources as requested by stakeholders. Information from the inventory was incorporated into the BEE training curriculum.

3.7 Activities

3.7.1 Community engagement

Over the first two years, the authors built an active and engaged network of professionals from the Ward 8 Health Council, including several community-based leaders from around Washington, DC. The authors regard this as one of the project's strengths and earliest successes.

The MHISTREET creation and leadership of the Mental Health Sub-Committee Advisory Group of the Ward 8 Health Council allowed access to the insight and knowledge of thought leaders. It generated active collaborations with local clinics, DC managed care organizations and mental health professionals in order to gain a deeper awareness of local strengths, resources, and needs.

The sub-committee members also convened three Southeast DC faith leaders and organizations from the local community and around the US for advice and guidance. Among the most prominent organizations was the Mental Health Association in New Jersey through their PEWS program (Promoting Emotional Wellness and Spirituality).

Other community engagement activities implemented included:

- Convened a core group of five barbers to serve as an advisory team for the embedded education approach and curriculum development

- Met with three local Core Service Agencies, which are the DC Department of Behavioral Health funded MH outpatient clinics, to introduce the program and gauge interest in partnerships

3.7.2 Barbershop embedded education training

In 2018, the team piloted their curriculum with a cohort of five barbers (**Table 2**). Weekly 2-hour sessions were held for six weeks. Lunch, refreshments and $50 Visa gift card incentives were provided.

The team developed a partnership consisting of the Confess Project, members of the original advisory committee, and the DC Commission for Fatherhood, Men, and Boys (DCFMB) to expand the project to include community members. The training was a one-day conference with 40 men from the community recruited with support of the DCFMB. Twelve men stated a willingness to share their stories in barbershops and connect people to resources. Two-hour, monthly training sessions for six months followed the conference.

The BEE Squad conducted the barbershop trainings, in pairs, over the course of three months. The attendance of customers at the barbershops was highly variable.

Element	Description
Existing relationships	
Host	Barbershops
Encounter	1. Barber engages client during service 2. Peer Educator engages room of clients during services or while waiting for services
Target Individuals	Black American Men (barbers, owners, clients)
Community	Family and friends of the target population, barbershop visitors
Embedded Education Practice	
Content	Personal stories of mental health service use; positive accurate messaging on mental health
Learning Objectives	1. To increase mental health literacy 2. To increase knowledge of the local mental health resources in the Southeast, DC community,
Anticipated Change	Knowledge, attitude, and behavior change around mental health; increased likelihood of seeking mental health services
Pedagogy	Listening to peer educators, participatory interactive dialog
Tools	Peer stories, barber discussions
Activities	Connection to services if desired
Educators	Non-medical community residents/peer educators trained by program staff

Adapted from Embedded Education Case Study Barbershop [60].

Table 2.
Curriculum design elements.

Some shops had upward of 30 guests, while others had only 4 to 5 customers in the shop. The presentations were also highly variable due to the variance in presentation skills of the participants, as well as the layout of the shops, the time of day and the day of the week. In some cases, the presentations got curtailed due to distractions in the shop. Also, some of the presentations served refreshments. All of these factors influenced the learning environment of the embedded education sessions.

3.7.3 Social media

The team's third area of activity was the development of a social media presence. The purpose was not only to promote the program but also to stimulate conversations around mental health. One of the authors attended a Social Entrepreneurship training with SeedSpot at Booz Allen Hamilton to develop an "elevator pitch" to market the program and also enrolled in a graduate-level social marketing course at a local university to gain a better understanding of social marketing. The team hired a consultant and developed a social media presence for MHISTREET and the Barbershop Embedded Education (BEE) program (Web site: http://www.mhistreet.com/; Twitter: @MHISTREET; Facebook: The MHI Street Initiative) The team continues their work as members collaborate with public health communications trainee to develop additional marketing materials with positive mental health messaging and resources targeted to barbers and their clients.

4. Outputs

Between sessions, the authors and their team visited all of the barbershops in Ward 8 (n = 13) and approximately half the barbershops in Ward 7 (n = 6) to share information about the project. All but one barbershop showed interest in the BEE session. The authors then arranged the dates and times for the BEE Squad to perform the intervention.

5. Outcomes

The Kirkpatrick Training Evaluation Model was used to evaluate the core intervention of this initiative, embedded education with storytelling in the barbershop [61]. The Kirkpatrick Model is a four-level evaluation method for assessing learning processes and considers any style of training, both informal and formal, to determine aptitude based on four criteria: reaction, learning, behavior, and result.

5.1 Reaction: what learners thought or felt about the training

The authors and their partners used reflection and facilitation summary at the end of each barber and community member training session. Presenters elicited feedback from the audience to learn how they were interpreting the information by having 'check-in' points and pausing the education sessions periodically to talk through any misunderstandings or emotionally difficult topics. The lead facilitator was a trained psychologist and was able to debrief and provide feedback in a professional and therapeutic manner.

5.2 Learning: to what degree learners acquired intended knowledge, behavior, and attitudes

Post-then-Pre evaluations were conducted after the training sessions with the barbers during the pilot (N = 5) and the BEE Squad (N = 40). All of the barbers completed the evaluation and approximately half of the BEE Squad did so. Without exception, all of the trained team members reported an increase in knowledge related to mental health in their community. Additionally, at the beginning of each session with the barbers, the previous session's content was reviewed, and any comments, confusion or participant feedback were clarified.

5.3 Behavior: to what degree did learners apply what they learned; what was the extent of behavior and capability improvement and implementation

After educational sessions were completed, participants practiced their storytelling and presentations with the larger group. The group and facilitators provided feedback. When visiting barbershops, each BEE Squad presenter was accompanied by a BEE Squad 'buddy' and a member of the MHISTREET team to ensure the accuracy and proper delivery of the messaging. Presentation styles varied greatly, but the accuracy of the content was reportedly consistent among the BEE Squad.

5.4 Result: effects resulting from learners' performance

The MHISTREET team received IRB approval to collect data in the barbershops by distributing surveys after BEE Squad presentations. However, the team quickly determined that conducting surveys with clients in barbershops would not work. Clients were willing to talk and contribute informally but were not comfortable answering surveys. Consequently, barbershop sessions became brief presentations of storytelling with subsequent question and answer periods. This format also provided a forum for clients to share opinions, thoughts, and fears comfortably. The less-structured format removed barriers to delivery. Feedback on the format provided evidence for the feasibility and acceptability of this intervention as barbers and customers were highly engaged in conversation around mental health. Some reported that this was their first opportunity to speak about this topic. Barbers and barbershop owners became comfortable accepting flyers with information about local resources and mental health information. The team was able to leave materials in 85% of barbershops in Ward 8 at the conclusion of the Clinical Scholars' funding.

6. Discussion

The initial success of the MHISTREET initiative demonstrates the positive outcomes achievable when an engaged multidisciplinary and influential community network functions cohesively to improve mental health literacy through embedded education. Access to relevant data, purposed to inform the initiative, has driven the creation and maintenance of alliances in the built environment of Washington DC. Alliances between barbers, healthcare providers, and community stakeholders in the local Southeast DC community has proven to be of great benefit toward achieving the aim of this initiative, which is to provide a non-traditional, non-healthcare platform for black men to share and hear stories of mental health resilience, encourage mental health-related conversations among barbershop clients, and serve as a bridge to mental health services.

The MHISTREET initiative encouraged both barbers and BEE Squad members to recognize improving mental health literacy is a likely precursor to undertaking health-preserving actions necessary for mental health wellness and maintenance. BEE Squad members also recognize embedded education is a viable means of improving mental health literacy. Recognition was likely facilitated by the "autonomy-compatible interactions" among Black men, barbershop clients and barbers, and networks of professionals, community-based leaders, and organizations. When people assume responsibility for their own mental health as a direct result of improved literacy, they are making an autonomous decision. Autonomous decisions are likely to result in acts of health-preservation such as seeking medical care or sharing stories of lived experiences of mental health issues to help address them.

A key challenge faced by all involved in delivering the MHISTREET initiative was navigating the process of helping Black men and barbershop clients undertake health-preserving actions, without overriding or undercutting their autonomy to do so. This is a common challenge faced by consortia delivering initiatives designed to help others help themselves. In the context of this initiative, overcoming this challenge required all involved to recognize and uphold two self-evident truths: 1) Help must start from the present situation of the men who share their stories of resilience in the face of mental health issues, and 2) MHISTREET cannot be delivered as a benevolent gift or "plug-in" program. Rather, the focus should be on devising ways to cost-effectively replicate the initiative in other cities to maximize local support available for improving the mental health literacy of Black American men.

The MHISTREET initiative uses the benefit of non-traditional, proactive, and behaviorally-focused self-management support. Results suggest BEE may be an effective form of structured education by which self-management strategies for mental health issues can be learned and applied by Black men. Embedded education has the potential to both alleviate the pressure on and work in concert with health and social care services. If Black men make early informed decisions that result in early care-seeking, issues with mental health could potentially be less chronic at the point of care and less difficult to manage. Such efficiency could translate into less severe mental health disorders and fewer health and social care dollars spent on treatment and recovery. The MHISTREET team encourages like-minded groups in cities across the US and beyond to replicate this initiative to determine its true health and economic value when widely disseminated.

7. Leader learning

7.1 Building trust

Perhaps the most critical aspect of this work was building trust within the community. Being a professional and healthcare provider does not automatically grant one trust. The trust required to work with barbers, community stakeholders, and other concerned citizens comes with time and following through on your word. Without trust, none of this work is possible.

7.2 Partnerships and networks across sectors

One of the project goals was to work across sectors with a variety of healthcare and non-healthcare professionals. Being part of the Ward 8 Health Council was a good entrée, and networking continued by engaging with anyone and everyone who expressed an interest in this work. Through building diverse networks, the authors learned that having more thought diversity and perspectives on the team led to a greater understanding of the problem and more thoughtful and "real-world" solutions.

7.3 Flexibility and patience

New grass-root programs do not happen immediately but take time to develop. Progress occurs in "fits and starts" and does not follow a particular curve. You must be flexible with your model and not make assumptions when the work begins. In addition, opportunities may arise unexpectedly and you must be ready to take advantage of them. Plans also backfire or do not work as envisioned, and you must have a plan B, C, and D!

7.4 Community engagement

The strength of this and similar projects is the voice of the community. This work cannot be accomplished by outsiders, (clinicians, academics, etc.) without the collaborative effort of people who live, work, and play in the community. Community voices are invaluable and often lead to new insights and ideas. People who know the community know what will work and what will not. To have sustainability and buy-in, community engagement at all levels of the project is requisite.

8. Toolkit

A comprehensive toolkit can be found at: https://clinicalscholarsnli.org/community-impact.

Author details

Nnemdi Kamanu Elias[1], Alfred Larbi[2], Kevin Washington[3] and Erin Athey[4*]

1 MindFlower Group, Washington, DC, United States

2 Cambridge Clinical Trials Unit, Cambridge University Hospitals NHS Foundation Trust, Cambridge, United Kingdom

3 Grambling State University, Grambling, Louisiana, United States

4 George Washington University, Washington, DC, United States

*Address all correspondence to: eyeagley@email.gwu.edu

References

[1] Reeves WC, Strine TW, Pratt LA, et al. Mental illness surveillance among adults in the United States. MMWR. 2011;60(3):1-32. Atlanta, GA: Centers for Disease Control and Prevention. Available from http://www.cdc.gov/mmwr/preview/mmwrhtml/su6003a1.htm?s_cid=su6003a1_w

[2] Johns Hopkins Medicine. Mental Health Disorder Statistics [Internet]. Available from: https://www.hopkinsmedicine.org/health/wellness-and-prevention/mental-health-disorder-statistics#:~:text=An%20estimated%2026%25%20of%20Americans,substance%20abuse%20and%20anxiety%20disorders.

[3] Roberts LW, Louie AK, Guerrero APS, Balon R, Beresin EV, Brenner A, Coverdale J. Premature Mortality Among People with Mental Illness: Advocacy in Academic Psychiatry. Academic Psychiatry. 2017;41:441-446.

[4] Ward E, Wiltshire JC, Detry MA, Brown RL. African American Men and Women's Attitude Toward Mental Illness, Perceptions of Stigma, and Preferred Coping Behaviors. Nursing Research. 2013;62(3):185-194. doi: 10.1097/NNR.0b013e31827bf533

[5] Holden KB, McGregor BS, Blanks SH, Mahaffey C. Psychosocial, socio-cultural, and environmental influences on mental health help-seeking among African-American men. Journal of Men's Health. 2012;9(2):63-69. doi:10.1016/j.jomh.2012.03.002.

[6] U.S. Department of Health and Human Services Office of Minority Health. Mental and Behavioral Health - African Americans [Internet]. 2019. Available from https://minorityhealth.hhs.gov/omh/browse.aspx?lvl=4&lvlid=24

[7] DC Health Matters. 2020 Demographics [Internet]. 2020. Available from: http://www.dchealthmatters.org/demographicdata?id=131495.

[8] Hankerson SH, Suite D, Bailey RK. Treatment Disparities among African American Men with Depression: Implications for Clinical Practice. Journal of Health Care for the Poor and Underserved. 2015;26(1): 21-34. doi:10.1353/hpu.2015.0012

[9] Belgrave FZ & Allison KW. African American Psychology: From Africa to America. Sage Publications: Thousand Oaks, CA. 2019.

[10] Wheaton FV, Thomas CS, Roman C, Abdou CM. Discrimination and Depressive Symptoms Among African American Men Across the Adult Lifecourse. Journal of Gerontology Series B: Psychological Sciences and Social Sciences. 2018;73(2):208-218. doi: 10.1093/geronb/gbx077.

[11] Watkins DC, Hudson DL, Caldwell CH, Siefert K, Jackson JS. Discrimination, mastery, and depressive symptoms among African American men. Research on Social Work Practice. 2011;21, 269-277. doi:10.1177/1049731510385470

[12] Williams MT. The link between racism and PTSD [Internet]. 2016. Available from https://www.psychologytoday.com/blog/culturally-speaking/201509/the-link-between-racism-and-ptsd

[13] Washington K. Persistent Enslavement Systemic Trauma (PEST) of Blacks Under Trump. In: Lee BX, editor. The Dangerous Case of Donald Trump 27 Psychiatrists and Mental Health Experts Assess a President. New York, NY: Thomas Dunne Books; 2019.

[14] Breslau J, Cefalu M, Wong EC, Audrey Burnam M, Hunter GP, Florez KR, Collins RL. Racial/ethnic differences in perception of need for mental health treatment in a US national sample. Social Psychiatry and Psychiatric Epidemiology. 2017;52(8): 929-937. doi: 10.1007/s00127-017-1400-2.

[15] Connor KO, Carr Copeland V, Grote NK, Koeske G, Rosen D, Reynolds CF, Brown C. Mental health treatment seeking among older adults with depression: the impact of stigma and race. American Journal of Geriatric Psychiatry. 2010;18(6):531-543. doi: 10.1097/JGP.0b013e3181cc0366.

[16] Jones JH. Bad Blood. Simon and Schuster; 1993. 297 p.

[17] Graham LF, Scott L, Lopeyok E, Douglas H, Gubrium A, Buchanan D. Outreach Strategies to Recruit Low-Income African American Men to Participate in Health Promotion Programs and Research: Lessons From the Men of Color Health Awareness (MOCHA) Project. American Journal of Men's Health. 2018;12(5):1307-1316. doi: 10.1177/1557988318768602

[18] Hall WJ, Chapman MV, Lee KM, Merino YM, Thomas TW, Payne BK, Eng E, Day SH, Coyne-Beasley T. Implicit Racial/Ethnic Bias Among Health Care Professionals and Its Influence on Health Care Outcomes: A Systematic Review. American Journal of Public Health. 2015;105(12):e60-e76. doi: 10.2105/AJPH.2015.302903.

[19] Jorm AF, Korten AE, Jacomb PA, Christensen H, Rodgers B, Pollitt P. Mental health literacy: a survey of the public's ability to recognise mental disorders and their beliefs about the effectiveness of treatment. Medical Journal of Australia. 1997;166(4):182-186.

[20] Jorm AF. Mental health literacy: empowering the community to take action for better mental health. American Psychologist. 2012;67(3):231-243. doi: 10.1037/a0025957.

[21] Connor KO, Lee B, Mayers V, Robinson D, Reynolds CF, Albert S, Brown C. Attitudes and beliefs about mental health among African American older adults suffering from depression. Journal of Aging Studies. 2010; 24(4):266-277. doi: 10.1016/j.jaging.2010.05.007

[22] Ward E & Mengesha M. Depression in African American men: A review of what we know and where we need to go from here. The American Journal of Orthopsychiatry. 2013;83:386-397. doi:10.1111/ajop.12015

[23] Lincoln KD, Taylor RJ, Watkins DC, Chatters LM. Correlates of Psychological Distress and Major Depressive Disorder Among African American Men. Research on Social Work Practice. 2011;21(3): 278-288. doi: 10.1177/1049731510386122

[24] Borrell LN, Kiefe CI, Williams DR, Diez-Roux AV, Gordon-Larsen P. Self-reported health, perceived racial discrimination, and skin color in African Americans in the CARDIA study. Social Science & Medicine. 2006;63(6):1415-1427. doi: 10.1016/j.socscimed.2006.04.008.

[25] Griffith DM, Gunter K, Watkins DC. Measuring Masculinity in Research on Men of Color: Findings and Future Directions. American Journal of Public Health. 2012;102(Suppl 2): S187–S194. doi: 10.2105/AJPH.2012.300715.

[26] Hammond WP & Mattis JS. Being a Man About It: Manhood Meaning Among African American Men. Psychology of Men & Masculinity. 2005;6(2), 114-126. doi: 10.1037/1524-9220.6.2.114

[27] Eley NT, Namey E, McKenna K, Johnson AC, Guest G. Beyond the Individual:Social and Cultural Influences on the Health-Seeking Behaviors of African American Men. American Journal of Men's Health. 2019;13(1):1557988319829953. doi:10.1177/1557988319829953.

[28] Thompson VLS, Bazile A, Akbar M. African Americans' Perceptions of Psychotherapy and Psychotherapists. Professional Psychology: Research and Practice. 2004;35(1), 19-26. doi: 10.1037/0735-7028.35.1.19

[29] Lê Cook B, Carson NJ, Nilay Kafali E, Valentine A, Rueda JD, Coe-Odess S, Busch S. Examining psychotropic medication use among youth in the U.S. by race/ethnicity and psychological impairment. General Hospital Psychiatry. 2017;45:32-39. doi: 10.1016/j.genhosppsych.2016.12.004.

[30] Government of the District of Columbia Department of Health. Health Equity Report: District of Columbia 2018 [Internet]. 2018. Available from: https://www.streetsensemedia.org/wp-content/uploads/2019/06/HER-Report-FINAL_with-letter-and-table_02_08_2019.pdf.

[31] District of Columbia Office of Planning. 2013-2017 ACS Key Demographic Indicators [Internet]. Available from: https://planning.dc.gov/sites/default/files/dc/sites/op/page_content/attachments/Key%20Indicators%202013%20-%202017_0.pdf.

[32] Stein P. DC's Poorer Residents are Increasingly Concentrated East of the Anacostia [Internet]. Available from: https://www.washingtonpost.com/news/local/wp/2015/04/14/d-c-s-poorest-neighborhoods-now-more-concentrated-east-of-the-anacostia-study-shows/.

[33] Ganz O, Curry LE, Jones P, Mead KH, Turner MM. Barriers to Mental Health Treatment Utilization in Wards 7 and 8 in Washington, DC: A Qualitative Pilot Study. Health Equity. 2018; 2(1): 216-222. DOI: 10.1089/heq.2017.0051.

[34] Naveed M. Income Inequality in DC Highest in the Country [Internet]. 2017. Available from: https://www.dcfpi.org/wp-content/uploads/2017/12/12.15.17-Income-Inequality-in-DC.pdf.

[35] Neighborhood Info DC. Ward 8—Profile of Health and Socio-Economic Indicators [Internet]. 2015. Available from: http://neighborhoodinfodc.org/wards/Nbr_prof_wrd8.html [Accessed 2020-05-02].

[36] Rittel HWJ & Webber MM. Dilemmas in a General Theory of Planning. Policy Sciences. 1973;4(2): 155-169. DOI: 10.1007/bf01405730.

[37] Hacker K. Community-based participatory research. Sage Publications; 2013.

[38] Pavlish C & Pharris MD. Community-based collaborative action research. Jones & Bartlett Publishers; 2011.

[39] Byrd K, Palmarin I, McNeish R, Walker-Egea C, Ali Y, Beleche M, Boynton-Jarrett R. An Action Research Collaboration to Promote Mental Wellbeing Among Men of Color. Global Journal of Community Psychology Practice. 2019;10(3), 1-12.

[40] Bjørnsen HN, Espnes GA, Eilertsen MEB, Ringdal R, Moksnes UK. The Relationship Between Positive Mental Health Literacy and Mental Well-Being Among Adolescents: Implications for School Health Services. Journal of School Nursing. 2019;35(2): 107-116. doi: 10.1177/1059840517732125

[41] Kutcher S, Wei Y, Coniglio C. Mental Health Literacy: Past, Present, and Future. Canadian Journal of Psychiatry. 2016; 61(3):154-158. doi: 10.1177/0706743715616609

[42] Kusan S. Dialectics of mind, body, and place: Groundwork for a theory of mental health literacy. Sage Open. 2013;3(4), 1-16. http://dx.doi.org/10.1177/2158244013512131

[43] Wei Y, McGrath PJ, Hayden J, Kutcher S. Measurement properties of mental health literacy tools measuring help-seeking: a systematic review. Journal of Mental Health. 2017;26(6):543-555. doi: 10.1080/09638237.2016.1276532.

[44] Johns Hopkins University. Volunteer Summit 2010: At Home in the City: Forging a New Partnership with Baltimore [Internet]. 2010. Available from http://web.jhu.edu/administration/provost/_archive_052012/speeches%20and%20writings/101022%20Vol%20Summit/At%20Home%20in%20the%20City.pdf

[45] Porter ME. Anchor Institutions and Urban Economic Development: From Community Benefit to Shared Value [Internet]. 2010. Available from https://www.hbs.edu/ris/Publication%20Files/2010-1026 _ICEF_ANCHORS_MEP_13ec3cb4-bc71-4d2a-8832-e8880bced5f3.pdf

[46] Rutheiser C. The Promise and Prospects of Anchor Institutions: Some Thoughts on an Emerging Field [Internet]. N.d. Available from: https://www.huduser.gov/portal/pdredge/pdr_edge_hudpartrpt_062211.html.

[47] Ravenell J. How barbershops can keep men healthy. TED Talk [Internet]. 2016. Available from https://www.ted.com/talks/joseph_ravenell_how_barbershops_can_keep_men_healthy

[48] Nesbitt SD. Management of Hypertension in African Americans. US Cardiology. 2009;6(2):59-62.

[49] Center for Disease Control and Prevention. CDC Fact Sheet: HIV Among African Americans [Internet]. 2017. Available from https://www.cdc.gov/nchhstp/newsroom/docs/factsheets/cdc-hiv-aa508.pdf. Accessed 4-27-2018.

[50] Bhardwaj A, Srivastava S, Khan M, et al. Racial disparities in prostate cancer a molecular perspective. Frontiers in Bioscience. 2017;22(5):772-82.

[51] Frencher SK, Sharma AK, Teklehaimanot S, et al. PEP Talk: Prostate Education Program, "Cutting Through the Uncertainty of Prostate Cancer for Black Men Using Decision Support Instruments in Barbershops." Journal of Cancer Education 2015;31(3):506-513.

[52] Hess PL, Reingold JS, Jones J, et al. Barbershops as Hypertension Detection, Referral, and Follow-Up Centers for Black Men. Hypertension 2007;(530):1040-6.

[53] Luque JS, Rivers BM, Gwede CK, Kambon M, Green BL, Meade CD. Barbershop Communications on Prostate Cancer Screening Using Barber Health Advisers. American Journal of Mens Health 2010;5(2):129-139.

[54] Odedina F, Oluwayemisi AO, Pressey S, et al. Development and assessment of an evidence-based prostate cancer intervention programme for black men: the W.O.R.D. on prostate cancer video. ecancermedicalscience 2014;8(460).

[55] Victor RG, Lynch K, Li N, et al. A Cluster-Randomized Trial of Blood-Pressure Reduction in Black Barbershops. New England Journal of Medicine 2018;(378):1291– 1301.

[56] de Jong J, Stuart G, Kaboolian L. Embedded Education: An Innovation in Governance. Harvard Kennedy School Ash Center for Democratic Governance and Innovation [Internet]. 2015. Available from https://www.innovations.harvard.edu/embedded-education-innovation-governance.

[57] Embedded Education [Internet]. 2020. Available from http://www.embededu.org.

[58] The Confess Project [Internet]. 2020. Available from https://www.theconfessproject.com.

[59] Zak PJ. Why your brain loves good storytelling. Harvard Business Review [Internet]. 2014. Available from https://hbr.org/2014/10/why-your-brain-loves-good-storytelling

[60] Wilson D, Kaboolian L, de Jong J, Stuart G. Barbershops and Preventative Health: A Case of Embedded Education. Harvard Kennedy School Ash Center for Democratic Governance and Innovation [Internet]. 2017. Available from https://ash.harvard.edu/files/ash/files/case_study_barbershop.pdf.

[61] Kirkpatrick DL. & Kirkpatrick J. Evaluating Training Programs: The Four Levels (3rd ed.). San Francisco: Berrett-Koehler Publishers, Inc; 2006.

Chapter 13

Somewhere to Go: Implementing Medication-Based Treatment for Opioid Use Disorders in Rural Maryland and beyond

Seth Himelhoch, Marion Currens, Jewell Benford and Eric Weintraub

Abstract

Treatment for opioid use disorders is highly effective yet unavailable in many rural areas. "Somewhere to Go: Ensuring Access to Medication-Assisted Treatment in Rural Maryland" is a Robert Wood Johnson Funded Clinical Scholars project intended to expand the use of tele-health medication-based treatment for opioid use disorders services directly to rural areas in need. We demonstrated that a University-based substance use treatment team can successfully collaborate with a geographically distant rural substance use treatment clinic to provide medication-based treatment for opioid use disorders using a HIPPA compliant telehealth strategy. We provide an overview of the implementation strategies our team used to expand overall access in different locales throughout the State of Maryland and beyond. We describe implementation results of a tele-health medication-based treatment program for opioid use disorders that focuses on implementation successes and how to identify and overcome implementation challenges and barriers. Implementation of a telemedicine approach can be challenging, but careful consideration and forethought can map a successful path to program development, operation and sustainability.

Keywords: Medication assisted treatment MAT, Medication based treatment, Opioid Use Disorder OUD, rural, telemedicine, telehealth, video conferencing

1. Introduction

Rural America is impacted disproportionately by illicit and prescription opioid misuse [1–3]. Opioids include heroin and prescription opioid drugs such as oxycodone, hydrocodone, hydromorphone, methadone, tramadol, codeine and fentanyl. Prior to the 1990s, opioid misuse was predominantly an urban phenomenon centered on the use of heroin. A collective push in the mid-1990's encouraged an increase in the prescribing of opioids for the treatment of non-malignant pain. This included the American Pain Society endorsement of the subjective pain score as the "fifth vital sign" [4]. Furthermore, patient advocacy groups and pain specialists highlighted the need to aggressively "treat an epidemic" of undertreated pain.

Concomitantly, pharmaceutical companies initiated extensive marketing campaigns advocating for the use of long acting opioids such as OxyContin (Purdue Pharma, Stamford, CT) to treat chronic non-malignant pain. These campaigns specifically targeted primary care physicians, the most frequent prescribers of opioid pain medications. As a result, opioid prescribing in the United States skyrocketed with a 300 percent increase in opioid prescriptions between 1991 and 2009 [5]. By 2012, clinicians wrote 259 million opioid prescriptions, enough to distribute one bottle of opiates to each adult in the USA [6]. A direct correlation between the quantities of opioids prescribed and the morbidity and mortality associated with these medications is clear [7]. Since 1999, overdose deaths from opioids have quadrupled [8].

The devastating consequences of opioid misuse is particularly evident in rural communities. For example, the per capita overdose rates have been higher in rural areas, as compared to urban areas, since 2006 [9]. Factors hypothesized to contribute to the rise in opioid misuse in rural areas include: (1) an older population with more chronic pain; (2) increased occupational injury from heavy labor jobs; (3) cultural acceptance of the use of opioids to keep individuals working in heavy-labor occupations; (4) lack of economic opportunity resulting in unemployment and financial hardship; and (5) more extensive social and family networks which are the predominant networks for the distribution of prescription opioids [1, 10].

Treatment for opioid use disorders is highly effective [11, 12]. Medication-based treatment for opioid use disorders is the term used to describe a series of evidence-based treatments for opioid use disorders (OUD), which includes treatment with regulated opiate medication in combination with psychosocial interventions. Two of the medications approved by the FDA for the treatment of opioid use disorder are methadone and buprenorphine. Both medications have demonstrated greater efficacy than counseling alone in decreasing opioid use, increasing retention in substance abuse treatment, and significantly decreasing the risk of overdose and death [13–15]. A recent meta-analysis confirmed that patients on methadone maintenance therapy for opioid use disorder had a significantly decreased risk of death during treatment than after cessation; the same analysis suggested buprenorphine is similarly effective [16].

There are numerous barriers to accessing medication-based treatment for opioid use disorders in rural areas. For example, methadone maintenance clinics are overwhelmingly located in urban areas, are highly regulated by the federal government, and require daily attendance during the early phases of treatment [17, 18]. Clearly, residents in rural areas with opioid use disorders may lack the means of transportation to consistently attend methadone maintenance programs. Although buprenorphine treatment can be delivered in a less regulated way, which may overcome some of the access issues historically associated with methadone treatment, 60 percent of all rural counties lack a waivered provider and only two percent of buprenorphine-waivered physicians in the US practice in small and remote rural counties [19, 20].

2. Wicked problem impact project (WPIP) description

Rural communities in America are disproportionately affected by the opioid epidemic, a situation reflected in the state of Maryland. From 2010 to 2015, deaths related to prescription and non-prescription opiate overdose in the state nearly tripled, with substantial increases occurring in rural communities in Western Maryland and the Eastern Shore in particular. Although Medication-Assisted Treatment (MAT), which includes the use of medications (e.g. Methadone or Buprenorphine) with psychosocial interventions, is a lifesaving, evidence-based treatment for opioid use disorders, there are numerous barriers to accessing MAT in rural areas of Maryland. Factors affecting the rural population mirror those listed above for the larger body of the USA.

Our central project goal is to increase access to medication-assisted treatment to rural communities in Maryland using the telehealth model piloted in an existing treatment program (Wells House) located in Western Maryland. In order to advance this central goal, a small, diverse, multi-disciplinary, clinical team (Team JEMS) was created. Our primary team is comprised of a clinical social worker, nurse practitioner, and two addiction psychiatrists possessing a wealth of experience working in multi-disciplinary substance use settings. As our team and project have evolved, so has the necessity of cultivating relationships with both internal and external program stakeholders to help champion the cause of expanding access to medication-assisted treatment.

Providing increased access to evidenced-based, telehealth services to address the opioid crisis saves lives. "Somewhere to Go: Ensuring Access to Medication Assisted Treatment in Rural Maryland" is a Robert Wood Johnson Foundation-funded Clinical Scholars project intended to expand the use of telehealth medication-based treatment for opioid use disorders services directly to rural areas in need. Previous pilot data demonstrated that a University-based substance use treatment team can successfully collaborate with a geographically distant rural substance use treatment clinic to provide medication-based treatment for opioid use disorders using a HIPPA-compliant telehealth strategy. A chart review of over 150 people receiving substance abuse services demonstrated that approximately 60% were still in treatment at 3 months with 94% of them being free of opioid use [21]. The goal of the "Somewhere to Go" project was to address the significant health disparities in a rural Maryland community by initiating telemedicine-based opiate addiction treatment services in an area that had never previously engaged in telemedicine-based treatment.

3. Methods

Prior to 2015, the retirement of a rural waivered medical provider resulted in the loss of patient access to medication-based treatment for opioid use disorders across an entire region. In 2015, the University of Maryland School of Medicine's Division of Addiction Research and Treatment agreed to establish a pilot program to provide medication-based treatment for opioid use disorders using a telemedicine format for a rural Western Maryland Intensive Outpatient Treatment Program (IOP). A series of virtual and in-person meetings that included the leadership from both the Division of Addiction Treatment and Research and the rural, Western Maryland IOP occurred. The early meetings focused on ensuring organizational compatibility and establishing the telemedicine programmatic policies and procedures. These meetings resulted in formalized Standard Operating Procedures (SOP) that addressed the following areas: 1) informed consent, 2) privacy/HIPAA compliance, 3) video conferencing security, 4) initiation of telemedicine consults, 5) patient scheduling, 6) urine toxicology testing, and 7) medical records. Establishment of the agreement allowed for the forming of the new clinic to treat rural patients struggling with addiction disorders.

Program coordinators at both the University of Maryland and IOP sites began regular meetings to facilitate communication, arrange clinical schedules, and solve implementation problems efficiently. The program coordinators created two blocks of two hours for direct patient care appointments (i.e., 45-minute time slots for new evaluations and 20-minute follow-up appointments). At the initial telehealth visit, a full diagnostic patient evaluation occurred. Based on this assessment, the University of Maryland physician provided a differential diagnosis and treatment plan for the patient including the use of buprenorphine when indicated. At the end of each appointment, the physician entered clinical documentation on the University of Maryland electronic medical record that was electronically transferred to the IOP site.

The IOP coordinator made all follow-up appointments. The IOP program coordinator screened patients, coordinated the appointment schedules and forwarded appropriate clinical information (e.g., clinical notes and results of urine toxicology screens) to the University of Maryland program coordinator prior to each telehealth clinical encounter. An evaluation plan consisting of in-depth interviews with key stakeholders focusing on barriers and challenges occurred after about one year of implementation. Meetings with stakeholders are held approximately twice a year with the IOP program staff to discuss program operational and clinical issues.

The team also pursued additional funding to support and advance our telemedicine-based intervention and expand the number of rural patients who could be served.

4. Results

Since the inception of the telehealth program in August 2015, over 500 patients have been treated at the initial Western Maryland IOP site and at any one time, approximately 100 patients are in active treatment. At the time of the writing of this manuscript the telehealth program had been in operation for 4 ½ years. A chart review of the first 175 patients treated in the program demonstrated an over 50 percent retention rate at 3 months. Of those patients retained in the program for three months only 6 percent were actively using illicit opioids. While the IOP program incurred a small financial shortfall in supporting physician costs for the medication-based tele initiative, it made up for it by being able to recruit and retain patients in their IOP counseling program.

In 2018, our team was fortunate enough to secure additional funding of $210,000 via the CareFirst grant to expand the telehealth model to two underserved rural counties (Talbot, Dorchester) on the mid-shore of Maryland.

4.1 Stakeholder interviews: barriers and challenges to implementation

Stakeholder interviews provided insights into implementation challenges. Challenges fell into four broad categories: documentation, acceptance of medication-based treatment for opioid use disorders by IOP staff, and billing and regulatory issues. As each site contracted with different electronic medical record vendors, the primary technologic challenge was the de-novo need to design and create functional documentation at each site. Although this challenge was easy to overcome, there was an unexpected opportunity and financial cost for each site. In addition, integration of the two electronic medical records with the goal of improving communication between the two clinical staffs is an ongoing process. A more pressing challenge was the opposition of some IOP staff to use medication-based treatment for opioid use disorders as a “first-line” treatment approach. Many of the counselors in the program were trained and adhered to an abstinence model of care where the use of opioid agonist medication is viewed as replacing one addiction for another. To overcome this challenge, clinicians from the University of Maryland conducted several in-service trainings for the IOP staff. The IOP staff were also encouraged by their leadership to attend continuing education classes focused on medication-based treatment for opioid use disorders. Over time, these interventions lead to a "normalization" of the use of medication-assisted treatment at the IOP site. Billing for the services was another challenge. Although a formal business plan was not agreed to at the beginning of the implementation process, over time the two sites came together to create a "workable" billing arrangement. The result was for the IOP program to contract with the University for physician services and then the University independently billed insurance and collected revenue that was remitted to the IOP to cover costs. Finally, regulatory concerns associated with the Ryan Haight Act were an early implementation concern. The 2008 law, named after a California teenager who overdosed on opioids bought online without being formally evaluated by a physician, may in theory limit opportunities for providers to provide telemedicine for medication-based treatment for opioid use disorders. Engagement with the DEA in Maryland resulted in approval for a DEA level of care at the IOP site that allowed for patients to be seen via a telehealth interface and prescribed buprenorphine without a face-to-face encounter.

5. Discussion

5.1 Recommendations for success for other rural telemedicine initiatives

Through our experience we have found that nine areas are crucial to address when forming distance-based partnerships to provide care for addiction treatment using a telemedicine-based approach. These nine areas requiring forethought and planning include: creating the team; lead with values; be responsive and responsible; pilot policies and procedures; develop appointment structures; establish the role of substance use counselor; establish the role of the medication-based treatment for opioid use disorders prescribing clinician; ensure medication prescription is safe, reliable and compliant; and create monitoring and evaluation systems.

5.1.1 Creating the team

Developing a nimble leadership structure with the capacity to rapidly assimilate and share information is critical to successful implementation. This is even more important when two or more organizations who may be geographically quite distant are engaging in partnership. Taking the time to build a culture of leadership that is responsible, responsive, and value-based is essential for success.

5.1.2 Lead with values

Implementation of any new project rests on a foundation of shared goals and values. In our experience, taking the time to describe these shared set of values is essential to a successful project implementation. This is especially true when implementing a tele-health medication-assisted treatment program where two or more organizations may be working together for the first time. For example, "teamwork" is often a shared value that is fundamental to getting a project off the ground. Yet, if there is no consensus about the definition of "teamwork," unintended misunderstanding based on differing organizational cultures can quickly undermine the implementation effort. To remedy this, we recommend organizational leadership discuss their organizations' shared set of values with each other prior to project implementation. Values such as Teamwork; Excellence; Compassion; Integrity and Professionalism are good places to start.

5.1.3 Be responsive and responsible

Using shared values can assist in shaping and defining key leadership roles and responsibilities. Defining these roles early in the implementation process can significantly reduce miscommunication and allow for more rapid organizational integration. Additionally, creating a culture of shared responsibility that prioritizes responsiveness is extremely important. Accountability is key. Regular meetings, whether in-person or virtual, that are task oriented, agenda-driven, and based on shared values can guide and drive the implementation process.

5.1.4 Pilot policies and procedures

Prior to the initiation of clinical operations, the team's primary goal is to establish programmatic policies and procedures. Formalized Standard Operating Procedures (SOP) need to address the following areas: 1) informed consent, 2) privacy/HIPAA compliance, 3) video conferencing security, 4) initiation of telemedicine consults, 5) patient scheduling, 6) urine toxicology testing, and 7) medical records. Standardized templates for documentation of the initial evaluation and follow-up visits is highly recommended.

5.1.5 Develop appointment structures

In our experience, appointment structures are often organizationally dependent. However, we recommend starting with two blocks of two-hour appointments. These appointment slots are allocated for direct patient care, with 45-minute time slots for new evaluations and 20-minute follow-up appointments.

5.1.6 Establish the role of substance use Counselor

Substance use counselors at the distant clinic are the fulcrum of the intervention. Their job is to refer people who meet criteria for opioid use disorder and who demonstrate interest in medication-based treatment for opioid use disorders. They are responsible for scheduling appointments with the off-site medication-based treatment for opioid use disorders prescribing clinician. They are also the on-site provider responsible for ensuring evidence-based substance use counseling is in place and ensuring that data regarding substance use treatment outcomes (i.e., urine toxicological screening) are appropriately maintained and documented.

5.1.7 Establish the role of the medication-based treatment for opioid use disorders prescribing clinician

The role of the medication-based treatment for opioid use disorders prescribing clinician is to complete a full diagnostic patient evaluation including medical, psychiatric and substance abuse histories. Using information obtained through this meeting and the intake notes from onsite counselors, the clinician creates a differential diagnosis and treatment plan for the patient including the use of buprenorphine when indicated. Notes and updated medication logs from each encounter are placed in charts at both the originating and distant site. The prescribing clinician continues treatment through follow-up appointments for each patient.

5.1.8 Ensure medication prescription is safe, reliable and compliant

Each site will need to be compliant with state and federal regulations. We strongly advise meeting with officers from the local DEA office as well as State authorities prior to implementation. These agencies can provide critical advice regarding prescribing of regulated medication, use of HIPPA compliant technologies and ensuring that all providers are legally able to provide substance use care.

5.1.9 Create monitoring and evaluation systems

It is important to create an evaluation plan that is consistent with the goals of the implementation. One strategy is to use both chart review and informant interviews of clinicians, patients, and their families to provide a complementary approach to understanding the challenges and success of the goals of the project.

The effectiveness of telemedicine treatment approaches among diverse populations and clinical contexts, including rural populations, is well established. Expanding addiction treatment for rural patients via telemedicine is an important next step to ensure provision of accessible, evidence-based treatments where they are most in need. During the last 2 years, the University of Maryland School of Medicine's Division of Addiction Research and Treatment used the lessons learned from our original pilot program to implement several additional telemedicine sites throughout the State of Maryland. These programs are servicing several rural areas throughout the State of Maryland with good outcomes. Although issues pertaining to the implementation of a telemedicine program are extremely important and were the focus of this chapter, there are equally important issues pertaining to sustainability. The viability of our telemedicine program is primarily attributable to the State of Maryland Medicaid program's decision to allow both sites to be eligible for reimbursement. In our case, the University of Maryland School of Medicine's Division of Addiction Research and Treatment took on responsibility for physician billing and passed collections onto the remote site. Another sustainability challenge that we encountered was transitioning patients to the community once stabilized on medication-based treatment for opioid use disorders. In keeping with the hub-and-spoke model of medication-based treatment for opioid use disorders administration, we collaborated with the rural county's local health department leadership to identify providers in the community willing to continue prescriptions for patients already stabilized. This approach proved highly successful.

6. Conclusion

Our findings suggest that treatment with buprenorphine delivered by telemedicine to patients with opioid use disorders in a rural drug treatment program is effective. Implementation of a telemedicine approach can be challenging, but careful consideration and forethought can map a successful path to program development, operation and sustainability. Nevertheless, initiating a new clinic and addressing areas of health disparity where there are no other treatment options exist requires thoughtful planning and careful implementation on the part of the healthcare team. Despite the fact that an onsite clinic had previously served the rural area, the new policies and procedures for the telemedicine-based treatment plan still encountered obstacles that needed to be addressed, including local staff acceptance of new protocols. Given the importance of the issue of treating addictive disorders in some of the hardest hit and underserved areas, it is vital to address barriers that exist even at the policy level, such as with the Ryan Haight Act and working with the DEA for policy change and program approval. With collaboration and a team-based approach challenges such as these are manageable and should not deter a committed group from engaging in a similar venture to ameliorate health disparities in rural areas. Below are additional gems of insight the JEMS team discovered as they implemented their “Somewhere to Go” project for the Clinical Scholars National Leadership Institute.

7. Leader learning in the clinical scholars program

The JEMS team faced a significant set of challenges during their Fellowship experience and in the implementation of their Wicked Problem Impact Project. First, the relocation of a team member required the team to negotiate a tangible change which had direct impacts on team dynamics. Early investing in team commitment and functioning established a sense of cohesiveness and commitment to the project, which contributed to team success despite this difficulty. Second, for all team members, managing work/life balance presented challenges given the demands of the Clinical Scholars program, the requirements of implementing a successful Wicked Problem Impact Project, and the ongoing demands of both work and family obligations. Managing this balance has required a sustained commitment and investment in one’s project, team, and family. Our team members found it essential to realize value and purpose beyond the funding or even the project, and to recognize the potential application of our learning across the many dimensions of life. It was not necessarily easy to balance all of these goals and commitments, but each team member found it to be worthwhile just the same.

The third challenge represents the thorniest and most complex challenge of all. A strict interpretation of the Ryan Haight Act of 2008 had the potential to derail our project by casting the intervention as non-compliant with Federal rules. Given that opiate addiction is a politically charged topic, team members had to navigate some complexity with the press, who unfortunately cast the efforts in a stilted and dramatic light seemingly to create an enticing headline. While this unwanted publicity created unanticipated consequences, stakeholders who shared the vision of linking individuals and families to needed care in their communities were engaged. Through meetings with DEA representatives, the interpretation of the rules allowed for this project, and other similar telemedicine-based interventions across the country, to be successfully implemented.

7.1 Successes

Having our team and Wicked Problem selected by the Robert Wood Johnson Foundation was a critical and important initial success. The experience not only resulted in securing funding for our project, but also provided training, support, and guidance on how to grow individually as Clinical Scholars but also identify ways to refine and improve our project. Our team was fortunate enough to secure additional funding via the CareFirst grant to expand the telehealth model, which was a major coup and yielded several positive outcomes, including: 1) supporting our projects ability to expand the telehealth, Suboxone model to five additional sites within the State of Maryland; 2) increasing the number of physicians providing telehealth direct care and consultation and supervision to other providers; and 3) providing an opportunity to reduce some of the stigma associated with medication-assisted treatment.

The third major success has involved the opportunity to interact, network and meet with a diverse group of people in the RWJF universe. Learning about the vast array of wicked problems being addressed by other teams and their efforts to tackle and impact those problems has enriched our own perspective on the issues we face as a team and as individuals. Engagement in this process has facilitated personal and professional growth which transcends our wicked problem.

7.2 Lessons learned

Creating a team founded in shared values, informed by nimble leadership with the capacity to assimilate and share information rapidly, is critical for implementation. We highly recommend ongoing stakeholder meetings to facilitate communication, remedy potential problems and enhance evaluation of outcomes. We believe cultural sensitivity and community engagement is crucial for successful sustainability in rural communities. Our team learned that community leadership works best when shared and allows for the voices of multiple stakeholders to be heard. Community leadership requires listening that evolves to greater understanding of the perspective of others. Community leadership requires involvement of the community in order to cultivate a shared vision, shared responsibilities and shared roles in addressing the problems at hand.

Working within a community context is fraught with both landmines and inroads, risk and benefits. In Clinical Scholars we learned from our colleagues at Community-Campus Partnerships for Health (CCPH) that following the principle of "developing partnerships that balance power and share resources equitably among partners" is a good place to start. The CCPH principle referenced is the antithesis of the maxim "He who has the gold makes the rules" and hopefully helps guard against stepping on some of the potential landmines by promoting thought diversity and inclusiveness, and avoiding the dangers or disruptions associated with group think. In order to truly balance power and share resources equitably requires active communication and engagement to be successful.

8. Toolkit

A comprehensive toolkit can be found at https://clinicalscholarsnli.org/community-impact.

Author details

Seth Himelhoch[1*], Marion Currens[2], Jewell Benford[3] and Eric Weintraub[3]

1 University of Kentucky College of Medicine, Kentucky, United States

2 University of Maryland Medical Center Center for Addiction Medicine, Maryland, United States

3 University of Maryland School of Medicine, Maryland, United States

*Address all correspondence to: seth.himelhoch@uky.edu

References

[1] Keyes KM, Cerdá M, Brady JE, Havens JR, Galea S. Understanding the rural–urban differences in nonmedical prescription opioid use and abuse in the united states. American Journal of Public Health. 2014;104(2):e52–e59.

[2] Corso C, Townley C. Intervention, treatment, and prevention strategies to address opioid use disorders in rural areas: A primer on opportunities for Medicaid-safety net collaborations. National Academy for State Health Policy. 2016. Available from: nashp.org/wp-content/uploads/2016/09/Rural-Opioid-Primer1.pdf. [Accessed 2018-09-27].

[3] Hancock C, Mennenga H, King N, et al. Treating the rural opioid epidemic. National Rural Health Association. 2017. Accessed from: www.ruralhealthweb.org/NRHA/media/Emerge_NRHA/Advocacy/Policy%20documents/Treating-the-Rural-Opioid-Epidemic_Feb-2017_NRHA-Policy-Paper.pdf Accessed 27 September 2018.

[4] Okie S. A flood of opioids, a rising tide of deaths. New England Journal of Medicine. 2010;363:1981-1985.

[5] Centers for Disease Control and Prevention. Vital signs: Overdoses of prescription opioid pain relievers—United States, 1999-2008.MMWR Morbidity Mortal Weekly Report. 2011;60:1487-1492.6.

[6] Paulozzi LJ, Mack KA, Hockenberry JM, et al. Vital signs: Variation among states in prescribing of opioid pain relievers and benzodiazepines—United States, 2012. MMWR Morbidity Mortal Weekly Report. 2014;63:563-568.

[7] Bohnert AS, Valenstein M, Bair MJ, et al. Association between opioid prescribing patterns and opioid overdose-related deaths. JAMA.2011;305:1315-1321.

[8] Ahmad F, Escobedo L, Rossen L, Spencer M, Warner M, Sutton P. Provisional drug overdose death counts [Internet]. National Center for Health Statistics, Centers for Disease Control and Prevention; 2019. Available from: https://www.cdc.gov/nchs/nvss/vsrr/drug-overdose-data.htm#source.

[9] Guy GP, Zhang K, Bohm MK, Losby J, Lewis B, Young R, Murphy LB, Dowell D. Vital Signs: Changes in Opioid Prescribing in the United States, 2006-2015. MMWR Morbidity Mortal Weekly Report. 2017;66(26):697-704.

[10] Rigg KK, Monnat SM. Urban vs. rural differences in prescription opioid misuse among adults in the United States: Informing region specific drug policies and interventions. Internal Journal of Drug Policy. 2015;26:484– 491.

[11] Mattick RP, Breen C, Kimber J, Davoli M. Methadone maintenance therapy versus no opioid replacement therapy for opioid dependence. Cochrane Drugs and Alcohol Group, editor. Cochrane Database Syst Rev [Internet]. 2009. Available from: http://doi.wiley.com/10.1002/14651858.CD002209.pub2. [Accessed 2019-03-11].

[12] Fiellin DA, Pantalon MV, Chawarski MC, Moore BA, Sullivan LE, O'Connor PG, Schottenfeld RS. Counseling plus Buprenorphine–Naloxone Maintenance Therapy for Opioid Dependence. New England Journal of Medicine. 2006;355(4):365-374.

[13] Volkow ND, Frieden TR, Hyde PS, et al. Medication-assisted therapies-tackling the opioid-overdose epidemic. New England Journal of Medicine. 2014;370:2063-2066.

[14] Bart G. Maintenance medication for opiate addiction: The foundation of

recovery. Journal of Addictive Diseases. 2012;31:207-225.

[15] Connery HS. Medication-assisted treatment of opioid use disorder: Review of the evidence and future directions. Harv Rev Psychiatry. 2015; **23**: 63– 75. DOI: https://dx.doi.org/10.1080%2F10550887.2012.694598.

[16] Sordo L, Barrio G, Bravo M, Iciar Indave B, Degenhardt L Scientia, Wiessing L, Ferri M, Pastor-Barriuso R, Mortality risk during and after opioid substitution treatment: systematic review and meta-analysis of cohort studies. British Medical Journal. 2017;357:j1550.

[17] Rosenblum A, Cleland CM, Fong C, Kayman DJ, Tempalski B, Parrino M. Distance Traveled and Cross-State Commuting to Opioid Treatment Programs in the United States. J Environ Public Health. 2011;2011:1-10.

[18] Sigmon SC. Access to treatment for opioid dependence in rural America: Challenges and future directions. JAMA Psychiatry. 2014;71:359– 360.

[19] Dick AW, Pacula RL, Gordon AJ, Sorbero M, Burns RM, Leslie D, Stein BD. Growth in buprenorphine waivers for physicians increased potential access to opioid agonist treatment, 2002-11. Health Affairs (Millwood). 2015;34(6):1028-103422.

[20] Andrilla CHA, Coulthard C, Larson EH. Barriers rural physicians face prescribing buprenorphine for opioid use disorder. Annals of Family Medicine. 2017;15: 359-362.

[21] Weintraub E, Greenblatt AD, Chang J, Himelhoch S, Welsh C. Expanding access to buprenorphine treatment in rural areas with the use of telemedicine: Buprenorphine in Rural Areas With Telemedicine. The American Journal on Addictions. 2018;27(8):612-617. https://doi.org/10.1111/ajad.12805.

Chapter 14

Transforming Opioid Addictions Care in New Mexico: Combining Medication Treatment with Patient Autonomy, Civic Engagement and Integrative Healing

Anjali Taneja and William Wagner

Abstract

Opioid addiction is a complex issue. New Mexico has historically experienced some of the highest rates of deaths from opioid overdose, and opioid addictions have affected generations of New Mexicans – starting many years before the more recent national crisis. Treatment approaches to opioid and other addictions are fraught with paternalism, stigma, surveillance, criminalization, shaming, racism, discrimination, and issues with access to care. Current treatment paradigms fail to take into account the social and economic factors of people, community, and context. New paradigms embracing a broader, more-just contextualization of addictions, along with evidence-based treatment approaches are needed to transform medicine's historic role in the "war on drugs". The Strong Roots/Raices Fuertes program was developed by two community clinics, Casa de Salud and Centro Sávila, in Albuquerque, New Mexico. The program evolved from a desire to to acknowledge and right historical harms that the medical-industrial complex has caused; to provide rapid access to dignified, life-saving, evidence-based holistic treatment for opioid addictions in a community setting; and to build a model of care that transforms the biomedical model into one of solidarity with community and collective care. Five key concepts underpin the program design: 1) Harm Reduction, Autonomy, and Agency; 2) Healing-Centered Engagement; 3) Language and Cultural Humility; 4) Transforming Health Systems Design; 5) Workforce Diversity and Pipeline Training. The program's core components include conventional approaches such as low-barrier access buprenorphine (suboxone®) to medication treatment, primary care, case management, syringe exchange, and counseling/therapy in addition to more community-rooted and integrative healing modalities such as healing circles, acupuncture, massage, reiki, ear acudetox, and civic engagement. In sharing the values, lessons learned, and tools from our work in the Strong Roots/Raices Fuertes program, we hope to inspire and encourage others wishing to develop new systems of care for people dealing with addiction issues.

IntechOpen

Keywords: addictions, opioids, harm reduction, cultural humility, autonomy, agency, drug war, healing-centered engagement, health system design, New Mexico, racism, medication-assisted treatment

1. Introduction

This chapter shares how two community-based clinics in Albuquerque, New Mexico, USA, are working together to reframe treatment for opioid addictions. Program aims are to: 1) undo harms that the medical-industrial complex, structural inequities, and racism have created, and 2) reframe approaches to treatment. Our mix of evidence-based medicine, relational care, integrative healing modalities, trust-building with community, and a look beyond the biomedical model into structural issues aims to support individuals and our community in addressing root causes of pain and dealing with opioid addictions. The five-person team participating in the Clinical Scholars Program consisted of a Family Physician (AT), a Clinical Social Worker and Medical Anthropologist (WW), a Physician Assistant, a Family Nurse Practitioner and Curandera, and a Doctor of Oriental Medicine. We hope our experiences will guide others wishing to develop alternative systems of care for those dealing with addiction issues and support a broader responsibility of healthcare organizations in their communities.

1.1 A legacy of contradictions

The history of opioid pain pill and heroin use in the United States is fraught with contradictions, politics, moralizing, profit, stigma, and racism [1–3]. Use of these drugs has surged in recent years, triggering public health calls for responses to the epidemic, which in New Mexico has been fueled by political, social, and economic processes operating at the local level for decades, and in many cases, centuries. Acknowledging social suffering as a root cause of the epidemic shifts etiological explanations of the problem from historical, individual, moralistic, and medical frameworks to ones that take into consideration the roles of power, discrimination, and injustice in creating and maintaining racial health disparities.

Overwhelming evidence points to the pharmaceutical industry and the medical prescribing community as having key roles in manufacturing the current epidemic [4, 5]. However, the stigma associated with drug addiction is perpetuated by community perceptions rooted in racist, classist, and moralistic beliefs, and ignores the deep psychological, economic, social, and political forces that lead people to use drugs. Existing care systems erect barriers that include shortages of healthcare providers and clinics in the very communities needing them most—communities with high overdose death rates. The *War on Drugs* disproportionately targets and criminalizes minority communities and perpetuates the social exclusion, racism, disenfranchisement, and poverty that contribute to drug use [6–11]. The dominant treatment culture individualizes, judges, shames, fears, and blames people caught in cycles of use, abstinence, and relapse [9, 10].

1.2 New Mexico's colonial past: laying the groundwork for generational traumas

New Mexico's colonial and settler legacy frames the local context that has contributed to drug addiction in Albuquerque's South Valley. The South Valley has endured historic waves of invasion, displacement, dispossession, and campaigns to exterminate, subjugate, and assimilate the people. Colonial and settler structures that assigned racial identities and corresponding rights and privileges contributed to the erasure of the majority native and mestizo inhabitants from Albuquerque's social, political, and economic landscape. These structures remain in place today, albeit contested, adding to the belief held by many Strong Roots/Raices Fuertes patients that existing civic institutions and structures are not intended for them.

The South Valley was built along the Turquoise Trail, a route that weaves along the Rio Grande Valley between Mexico City and Santa Fe and was traveled for millennia by the region's first indigenous inhabitants [12]. After Spanish settlement it became known as the *Camino Real* [12]. The Spanish colonial administration created *castas* (castes) that reinforced racial hierarchies privileging European whiteness [12, 13]. Shortly after the signing of the Treaty of Guadalupe Hidalgo in 1848 that ended the Mexican American War, the Gadsden Purchase annexed the greater part of the Southwest and California as a US territory [14, 15]. The federal government denied statehood until there were more English-speaking white inhabitants [14, 15]. More than 60 years passed before New Mexico was recognized as a state in 1912 [14, 15]. Economic and political pressure to ascribe to whiteness forced many to cover up their indigenous and mestizo roots [16]. The promised benefits of assimilation never materialized for most and fueled racial tensions still present today [13–16].

Generations of South Valley families relied on military service as a pathway to greater economic stability. Soldiers wounded in the line of duty and treated with morphine found heroin a more accessible and affordable way to manage physical and psychological pain on their return home [17]. Many of the patients in the Strong Roots/Raices Fuertes program are children and grandchildren of veterans from the Korean and Vietnam Wars who grew up watching their role models struggle with finding a way to cope with their pain.

1.3 New Mexico today

New Mexico suffers high rates of opioid overdose deaths. For almost two decades, New Mexico ranked #1 or #2 for per-capita overdose death rates from heroin or opioid pain pill use [18]. The drop in recent years is in part due to the escalation of rates in other states experiencing the effects of the nationwide opioid crisis. In Bernalillo County, opioid overdose death rates are 22.2 per 100,000 people – nearly double the national rates (13.3 per 100,000 people) [19]. From 2010 to 2014, overdose death rates in the South Valley of Albuquerque ranged from 37.1 to 41.1 per 100,000 [20].

Because of the high overdose death rates, New Mexico has pioneered innovative harm reduction and treatment work. The state was the first to train first responders on naloxone administration for opioid overdoses, the first to pass a Good Samaritan 911 law, and one of the first states with an opioid addiction treatment program within a county jail, providing methadone to inmates. The state's Department of Health has a robust program supporting and funding syringe exchange sites and naloxone distribution for opioid overdose prevention.

A toxic mix of concentration of poverty with a greater concentration of industry and environmental exposures leaves the South Valley of Albuquerque experiencing huge disparities in access to primary care and behavioral health, and in health outcomes [21]. Some parts of the South Valley have a 15-year decrease in life expectancy compared to other parts of Bernalillo County [22]. However, the South Valley also boasts a high rate of home ownership, a mix of families present for generations and recent immigrants from Mexico and Central America, and a farming culture given its semi rural landscape.

1.4 Adverse childhood effects and opioid addictions

The Adverse Childhood Effects (ACES) study looks at kinds of childhood exposure to various factors including but not limited to physical, psychological, or sexual abuse; growing up in a household with one or more parent who uses drugs; mental illness; domestic violence; and having an incarcerated household member [23]. Exposure to multiple types of trauma in childhood builds up "toxic stress" and has shown to have lifelong impacts for children, including addictions in adulthood [24].

Nationally, 34 million children have had at least one adverse childhood experience (ACE), but in New Mexico, nearly 30% of children have two or more, the fourth highest in the country [25]. An individual with five or more ACEs is ten times more likely to use IV drugs as someone with no adverse childhood effects [26]. Children with four or more ACES have 32.6 times greater likelihood to have learning or behavioral issues [27]. A direct link between exposure to adverse childhood effects and juvenile delinquency has been demonstrated. Among all teens held in juvenile detention in 2011 in New Mexico, 100% of the girls and 96% of the boys had two or more ACEs [28].

1.5 From biomedical model to greater responsibility

"Addiction rates are higher in poor people—not because they are less moral or have greater access to drugs, but because they are more likely to experience childhood trauma, chronic stress, high school dropout, mental illness and unemployment, all of which raise the odds of getting and staying hooked."

- Maia Szalavitz, journalist

"When I work with addictions, the first question I ask is not why the addiction but why the pain."

- Dr. Gabor Mate, physician and author of *In The Realm of Hungry Ghosts*

The National Institutes on Drug Abuse and leading physicians and scientists refer to opioid dependence as a "chronic, progressive, relapsing, brain disorder" that requires treatment instead of criminalization [29]. However, this approach individualizes and medicalizes an issue that has roots beyond chemical changes in the brain. It also places individuals into a "cage" of sorts – someone labeled as having a relapsing progressive disorder may feel trapped, as if they can never improve, and others may treat them as such, reinforcing the perception. As neuroscientist and author Dr. Carl Hart states, "... if the problem is a person's neurobiological state after exposure to a drug, then either the drug must be eradicated from society through law enforcement or an individual's brain must be treated. In such a myopic approach, the socioeconomic and societal factors that contribute to drug addiction are considered a footnote in research, clinical practices, and policy, despite their apparent importance [30]." More recently, the opioid epidemic has been framed as a public health issue, but few public health solutions have arisen from this paradigm.

1.6 Two community clinics team up

Casa de Salud and Centro Sávila are two organizations in the South Valley of Albuquerque, New Mexico. Both clinics emerged from a recognition of significant gaps in New Mexico's public health safety net that leave thousands of community members without access to dignified healthcare.

Casa de Salud was founded in 2004 by medical practitioners, volunteers, and the Kalpulli Izkalli traditional healing collective. The clinic serves primarily uninsured New Mexicans and people with Medicaid. Services include safe, accessible, holistic, and culturally humble primary care; a wide variety of integrative healing options; transgender care; a syringe exchange; addictions care; medical debt support, and community organizing/advocacy. The clinic offers a unique, immersive health apprentice program as a pipeline health workforce opportunity primarily for students of color.

Centro Sávila opened its doors in 2011 to address the need for culturally and linguistically appropriate behavioral health services in New Mexico. Clinic staff work to decrease racial health disparities in Bernalillo County by providing outpatient mental health services; case management; health insurance enrollment assistance; food security support; drug and alcohol counseling and recovery support; and supervision, training, and research opportunities for students and health professionals. Central to this effort is the need for New Mexico's behavioral health provider workforce to reflect the same diversity of the state.

Support from the Robert Wood Johnson Foundation Clinical Scholars program in 2016 allowed staff from the two clinics to participate in the first cohort of the Clinical Scholars Program, deepen their existing partnership, and expand both the scope and depth of their efforts to combat opioid pain pill and heroin addiction and its underlying causes. Naming the Wicked Problem Impact Project "Strong Roots/Raices Fuertes" reflects the team's desire to lift up the community's strong culture and resiliency, while looking to address root causes of addictions in New Mexico. The *raison d'être* of the Strong Roots/Raices Fuertes program is a drive toward recognizing the contradictions inherent in providing health care to address problems with social, economic, and political roots. The program's health care providers recognized the *wicked problem* of addiction is fueled by social injustice and trauma.

2. Methods

The five clinicians of the Clinical Scholars Strong Roots/Raices Fuertes team were motivated by a drive to promote social justice and health equity in developing and implementing the Strong Roots/Raices Fuertes program. Aims of the program are to 1) provide rapid access to dignified evidence-based holistic treatment for opioid addictions in a community-based setting, and 2) develop a model to focus on mind/body/soul as well as collective care, going beyond the biomedical model. The team wanted to build tools to transform the medical-industrial complex that historically medicalizes, shames, and exploits communities. Underlying this aim was a desire to work in solidarity with the community to empower them to create change at the individual and systems levels instead of maintaining a power differential that silences people who use drugs.

2.1 Key concepts

The approach of the Strong Roots/Raices Fuertes program focuses on addressing individual healing as well as the underlying causes of addiction. Five key concepts underpinning the program design and thinking are 1) harm reduction, autonomy, and agency 2) healing-centered engagement for mind/body/soul 3) language and cultural humility, 4) transforming health systems design, and 5) workforce diversity and pipeline training.

2.1.1 Harm reduction, autonomy, and agency

Harm reduction, autonomy, and agency as concepts comprise a set of interconnected practical strategies to reduce the negative effects of health behaviors without necessarily stopping the behaviors completely. Harm reduction is based in values of humanism, pragmatism, individualism, incrementalism, and accountability without termination [31]. Guiding principles are to:

- meet people where they are
- accept that drug use is part of our world
- center on the person seeking treatment
- support individuals in their decision-making and recovery choices instead of replicating patterns of shame, blame, or trauma
- affirm the individual as his or her primary agent of change, a critical element for success, recovery, trust, and sense of purpose

2.1.2 Healing-centered engagement for mind/body/soul

Trauma-informed care reframes "What is wrong with this person?" to "What has happened to this person?" The latter frame is important but can lead care providers to prioritize individual traumas over collective traumas or community-based needs. Healing-centered engagement goes beyond trauma-informed care and is culturally rooted, reflective, and incorporates spirituality, civic action, and collective healing. The cultural rootedness strengthens trust from participants to support healing. A key innovation of Strong Roots/Raices Fuertes is opt-in access to multiple integrative healing services (**Table 1**) to restore the connection with mind/body/soul healing, and to lift up approaches to care that are culturally safe, hands-on, and relevant. Patients are also accepted as leaders with strength and agency, working together on structural and community level change.

2.1.3 Language and cultural humility

The role of language is critical in addiction treatment. Finding appropriate ways to discuss addictions without falling into the trap of focusing on personal character flaws or poor choices requires a macro frame that guides intervention on the

Frontline Advocacy/Case Management
Factors not directly related to health (e.g., lack of housing, food insecurity, transportation challenges, and access to ID / documentation) impact peoples' success in the program and in their lives beyond treatment. Case workers actively support patients with specific needs and coordinate care with services outside the program (e.g., referrals to specialist physicians, communicating with parole or probation officers). Community health workers, peer support networks, and navigators/promotoras assist patients in getting other basic needs met.
Emotional and Psychological Support with Behavioral Intervention
Culturally humble, licensed clinicians provide individual and group counseling and psychotherapy. Empathic, non-judgmental, and patient-driven meetings help identify emotional, thought, and behavior patterns that trigger substance use. Clinicians create a safe and confidential setting to help build trust, increase patients' insight into the ways substance use has affected their lives, and practice alternative and healthier behaviors that more effectively regulate and manage psychological and physical suffering.

Table 1.
Supportive and behavioral care components.

individual and family levels. Cultural humility reflects a need to be humble about our understanding of our patients' values and beliefs, be aware of our own assumptions and prejudices, understand and shift the power inherent in the clinician-patient relationship to a co-learning relationship, and hold ourselves and our institutions accountable to this practice. Cultural humility requires dedication, organizational buy-in, and regular practice among all staff and team members [32].

2.1.4 Transforming health systems design

Health system transformation requires the desire and investment in resources to reflect on user experience, patient care flow, and barriers to care, and to iterate on positive changes using direct feedback from patients and community members. Transformation helps systems move away from common barriers, such as distant locations that feel intimidating, (e.g. large hospitals, or clinic designs that treat patients in an assembly-line fashion by curt and overworked employees). Fee-for-service pay structures can oblige providers to filter access to healthcare services based on patients' ability to pay and language barriers can leave patients confused over what they are paying for.

2.1.5 Workforce diversity and pipeline training

Racial health disparities are exacerbated by disparities in the healthcare workforce. The demographic diversity of New Mexico's healthcare provider workforce does not look like the racial diversity of the general population. This gap reflects financial, geographic, and racial barriers that have historically limited access to pathways for professional development. Health care institutions play a critical leadership role in recruiting, training and hiring people that want to work in the communities they are from. Research shows that trust and patient satisfaction are directly related to concordance of patient and clinician racial/ethnic background. Medical schools across the country have increased diversity in general in the last twenty years, but the number of underrepresented minorities in medical school classes around the country – Black, Latinx, or Native American medical students – have actually decreased per 100,000 US population [33]. There is also a critical lack of social workers and therapists of color in New Mexico, a state with an almost 50% Latinx/Hispanic population. Internships and apprenticeships are powerful opportunities for students to serve their communities, in ways that are culturally humble, sensitive, skilled, and that understand the reality of patients from impacted communities.

2.2 Core components

Strong Roots/Raices Fuertes incorporates multiple core components that reflect both traditional medical approaches and integrative medicine. Core components are divided into four primary types: program orientation and primary care/medication treatment (**Table 2**), supportive care and behavioral care (**Table 1**), integrative healing modalities (**Table 3**) and purpose and leadership (**Table 4**). All fit the key concepts that guide program design, most already existed in the clinics with years of positive feedback about their value, and all offer the patients and community a wide array of options to choose from to meet their individual healing needs. Patients in the Strong Roots/Raices Fuertes program additionally have access to the New Mexico Department of Health's robust syringe exchange services program – as Casa de

Description	Approach
Orientation to Program	
A session in which clinicians • Share information about program format • Explain values of harm reduction, autonomy, and agency • Discuss philosophy of mind/body/soul healing with integrative care • Describe what is available to patients at each of the two clinics	To help equalize power, patients sit in a circle with clinicians, passing around a talking stick. • Use language of patients as leaders • Talk about why treatments are free, why care is made accessible, and how trauma may be stored in the body • Patients who wish to, may receive hands-on healing engagement at orientation sessions
Primary Care	
Patients in the Strong Roots/Raices Fuertes program may not be receiving primary care elsewhere, and many have untreated Hepatitis C. Patients receive primary care in the patient's preferred language (English/Spanish) for the range of health concerns they may be experiencing.	A key evidence-informed dimension is the program's emphasis on care for the 'whole patient'. Many patients come with a history of negative experiences with conventional western medicine such as • Feeling stigmatized, or not comfortable discussing the range of issues with which they need support • Having been asked to identify one 'single problem' to address in a visit • Experiencing moralized judgments from clinicians, or systems with barriers to care
Medication Treatment	
Buprenorphine (suboxone) • Reduces overdose death risk by 50% • Provides short-term and long-term success for opioid use disorder • Increases quality of life • Can easily be prescribed in outpatient treatment programs or primary care settings	Strong Roots (Raices Fuertes) program • Uses a harm reduction approach – "come for the suboxone; stay for everything else we offer!" • Has no mandatory requirements for additional services • Does not cut patients cut off from suboxone for urine drug test results that could otherwise result in a therapeutic discussion • Does not withhold medicine for arbitrary reasons.

Table 2.
Orientation and primary care/medication treatment.

Salud runs the busiest syringe exchange and naloxone distribution program in the South Valley.

2.3 Popular education workshops

The EleValle Collaborative is a collective of South Valley organizations that work together to improve the health and quality of life for residents and their families. The Strong Roots/Raices Fuertes program and the EleValle Collaborative supported development of two workshops, one two hours in length and the other six hours. A clinician from the Strong Roots/Raices Fuertes program trained six patient leaders in facilitation skills. Patient leaders helped develop and implement four two-hour workshops on various issues specifically for others in the community who care for people struggling with addictions or who were struggling with addictions themselves. Workshops included content on the history of the drug war, resiliency, storytelling, and trauma. A subsequent six-hour event for the community was

Acupuncture
East Asian Medicine (EAM) is thousands of years old, and is a system of medicine that looks at the entire body as a whole and includes relationships of the body systems as well as relationships of people to the world. It takes into account how all systems affect health and longevity and employs many different tools including diet, exercise, meditation, herbal therapy, cupping, moxibustion, and acupuncture. Acupuncture uses fine needles to stimulate and enhance the body's ability to heal itself, through channels or meridians – and has been used to effectively approach issues of energy, digestion, stress, anxiety, emotional and physical pain, cravings, neurological issues, immune system issues, blood pressure, and more.
Massage
Massage therapists use the healing power of human touch to hold, press, rub or otherwise manipulate muscles and other soft tissues. Massage has proven effective in healing trauma, managing pain, and integrating emotional pain and somatic experience. Many patients' addictions began when they needed relief from a physical or emotional trauma. By paying attention to the ways in which the body holds the variety of lived experiences ranging from stress, trauma and isolation, to love, joy and connectedness, massage therapists help patients to feel whole.
Reiki
Reiki is a Japanese healing technique shown to be effective in managing pain, calming the nervous system, and decreasing stress. It is based on the premise that a reiki practitioner can channel energy into a patient and assist him/her to activate natural healing processes to promote relaxation and balance, and restore emotional well-being. Reiki can also be practiced on oneself. A session can be hands-on, where a practitioner applies light touch during the session, or hands-off where they hold their hands slightly above a patient's body.
Ear Acudetox
Ear acudetox is an evidence-based, standardized ear acupuncture protocol used for heroin, alcohol, and cocaine addictions treatment, as well as for sleep, anxiety reduction, and stress reduction [34]. Following the National Acupuncture Detoxification Association (NADA) protocol, five very small needles are placed in each ear. Ear acudetox has been used as supportive care for people struggling with addictions since it was developed in the 1970's at Lincoln Hospital in Bronx, NYC, through community activism and a self-help model. It is currently practiced around the world.
Healing Circles
Healing circles are based on the Native American talking circle in which each participant is passed the sacred feather and given time to speak. The Strong Roots/Raices Fuertes program offers healing circles in which patients share their stories and support each other. Each three-hour session is co-facilitated by two healers: a nurse practitioner who is also a curandera or traditional Mexican healer, and a reiki master, both of whom are ear acudetox specialists. After the talking circle, participants are offered ear acudetox, reiki, and a limpia (cleansing ceremony), in a group setting, to provide healing, calmness, and closure to the talking circle.

Table 3.
Integrative healing modalities.

Civic Engagement
Civic engagement focuses its efforts at understanding root causes of addiction and building movement toward systems change. The Strong Roots/Raices Fuertes Program provides opportunities for patients to become engaged in civic leadership. Civic engagement efforts include advocating for changes to the criminal justice system, increased access to treatment, and opportunities to talk with elected officials and decision-makers. Patients receive training in storytelling for public speaking and peer-to-peer support around addictions. Popular Education workshops are delivered by patient leaders who train in facilitation, to help community members educate each other, toward action. A deeper understanding of the leadership capacity of and leadership development desires of community members also offers the two clinics opportunities to develop resources alongside patients and community members.

Table 4.
Purpose and leadership.

Leadership Survey Questions
1. Give an example of a time in your life when you showed leadership.
2. Currently, what are some ways that you show leadership with your friends, family, co-workers, or community?
3. Currently, do you feel like you are a leader in your community? [(Likert scale response from 1 (not at all) to 10 (very much)]
4. Are you interested in becoming more of a leader in your community? [(Likert scale response from 1 (not at all) to10 (very much)]
5. What are some of the most pressing issues facing your community that require more leadership?
6. If we (Casa de Salud, Centro Sávila, or ACCESS) offered regular opportunities to get together with others to build leadership skills and knowledge, are you likely to participate?
7. What are some skills that you are interested in building (for example, public speaking, writing, healing therapies)?
8. What types of activities would you be interested in (for example, a book club, a social club)?
9. What issues affecting your community do you want to learn more about (for example, the history of war on drugs, current policies regarding treatment of people who use drugs, etc.)?
10. When you think about building leadership skills and knowledge, what are some fears or barriers that you face?

Table 5.
Leadership survey questions.

created, composed of content from the two-hour workshops plus overdose prevention training. The goal of this process was to lift up those most impacted by addictions in our community and develop peer-to-peer education workshops that could be used locally and beyond.

2.4 Inherent leadership survey

The Strong Roots/Raices Fuertes program and the EleValle Collaborative also worked with a local evaluator to develop a ten-question leadership survey. The purpose was to gather a sense of inherent leadership and desires for leadership training, among individuals struggling with addictions. The survey was administered to 1) people who use drugs and who actively utilize the syringe exchange, and 2) patients in the Strong Roots/Raices Fuertes opioid addiction treatment program. Most had not attended the Popular Education workshops described above. Survey questions are shown in **Table 5**.

3. Outcomes

3.1 Partnering to improve care

Casa de Salud and Centro Savila met weekly and for several day-long retreats, to develop and implement the Strong Roots/Raices Fuertes program. Regular meetings were key for iterating on processes, for ensuring alignment with values and goals and language of the program, and for troubleshooting issues. In addition, the team regularly met to discuss patients, and approached their care from a truly transdisciplinary process, learning from each other to best partner with our patients for care. The two clinics improved upon pre-existing modalities and services that the organizations offered, and built new joint services and projects together. Outcomes for patient care are detailed more in the Evaluation section.

3.2 Response to integrative healing services

A key innovation of Strong Roots/Raices Fuertes is opt-in access to a variety of integrative healing services to restore the connection with mind/body/soul healing described earlier. These low-cost, high-touch, non-pharmacological, relational therapies are key components in patients' paths to recovery. One patient shared: "In other programs, nobody ever wanted to touch me. Here we experience healing touch, and that means everything to my confidence and my connection with society." Others have shared the ways in which bodywork and energy work helped release trauma, or as ongoing tools for stress and anxiety reduction.

3.3 Popular education workshops

More than thirty participants attended each of the four two-hour workshops; most were active drug users or had immediate family members who were actively using drugs or were in treatment. The six-hour workshop that combined content from the two-hour sessions and added overdose prevention training had 80 attendees. Overall, more than 200 community members participated in workshops. Survey feedback from these events was overwhelmingly positive. A toolkit for broad use of these workshops was developed in this process. The response from the community and the leadership development of patient/client leaders who facilitated these workshops was very moving. Patient leaders built confidence while training in facilitation skills and through delivering workshops. They described the process as transformative and engaging. Two of the patient leaders (33%) subsequently pursued Certified Peer Support Worker (CPSW) certifications, with an interest in building careers in this area.

3.4 Inherent leadership survey

One hundred and one people completed the Leadership Survey. In response to the prompt, "give an example of a time in your life when you showed leadership", resulting themes from patient stories included being leaders on their high school sports teams and current workplaces, and having roles as parents and caregivers.

Responses to the self-assessment of their leadership question ranged widely. Participants were asked to rate themselves on a scale of one (not at all) to ten (very much) as to whether they identified as leaders in their communities. More than a third of patients rated themselves as low on the leadership scale (three or lower), roughly half rated themselves in the middle range (four to seven), and almost 20% of patients self-identified as currently "very much" a leader in their communities (eight to ten). When asked if they were interested in becoming more of a leader in their community, more than 80% responded with positive interest. Some cited barriers to developing their leadership such as lack of time due to family and community responsibilities and fear of failure. Participants noted specific fears around leadership, including being labeled as a "junkie" if they spoke out about their recovery journey, or internal fears around their self-esteem or anxiety regarding public speaking. About 40% stated they were somewhat interested in developing their leadership and $\sim$ 40% responded they were "very much" interested.

In response to the question, "what are some of the most pressing issues facing your community that require more leadership?", several clear themes emerged including homelessness, police, violent crime, loss of connection to cultural heritage, and public services. One syringe exchange participant wrote, "the police and homeless are issues we face. As a community we need to step up and try to get more help for the homeless population and especially the youth. The police are killing and shooting with no real reason, people are fearing and not trusting the police." Another person shared, "homelessness, violent crime, non-violent offense charges being too drastic." On the issue of loss of connection to cultural heritage another wrote, "my community needs leadership to keep our traditions and language alive." These results were incredibly informative for next steps in leadership development work in partnership with our community.

3.5 Practicing leadership

Strong Roots/Raices Fuertes staff and patients together presented to state legislators and public health officials as well as government leaders and community health care providers. These presentations helped raise awareness about opioid addictions and harm reduction, the need for community focused approaches, and also focused on structural issues, such as the disproportionate effect of criminal justice efforts on communities of color and the harmful effects of the war on drugs. Our organizations have a voice at the Bernalillo County Addiction Treatment Advisory Board, at the county's Criminal Justice Coordinating Committee, and with the City of Albuquerque, which is exploring a new Department of Community Safety as an alternative to police, and is looking to us, among other organizations, to build infrastructure to improve support services for a community approach to addictions.

4. Evaluation

4.1 Framework and process

The Strong Roots/Raices Fuertes team aimed to build and analyze data that was meaningful to our clinics and to our patients. This was a topic of great discussion among team members of both clinics during regular team meetings. The values and key concepts of the program, including harm reduction and autonomy, meant that conventional indicators such as how many "relapses" patients experienced; length of stay in the program; positive urine drug screens for illicit substances; were not of primary interest.

Instead, the team aimed to learn about what barriers to care existed (from program design or external factors), and how transforming system design could improve patient care and engagement; what recovery journeys patients would choose within an opt-in program that valued autonomy and choice over prescriptive structured programming; how we could avail patients of naloxone and other tools more systematically; and how we could re-engage patients who stopped interacting with care.

With the help of an independent evaluator, we developed an Engagement and Registry system, populated using code that pulls data from Casa de Salud's electronic medical record (EMR), OpenEMR, an open source system with powerful and flexible reporting abilities. We also developed an external data process that captured information on anybody who expressed interest in the program – interest by phone, through the syringe exchange, through case management – who were not yet patients in the electronic medical record.

4.2 Data

Initial data show that over the course of two years after the program redesign, 68% of people who expressed any interest at all in the program – initial interest by phone, through primary care, or through the syringe exchange – followed through to starting buprenorphine medication, orientation, and engagement in optional healing modalities. Before the program components were redesigned to decrease the number of mandatory steps present in the first few weeks – despite the profound healing nature of the mandatory modalities – less than 40% of people who expressed interest in treatment and healing successfully completed orientations, healing circles and achieved medication treatment.

Data on days from interest in the program to starting medication treatment, before the program was redesigned, is limited and variable, given time cycles of mandatory components (orientation and healing circles) before start of medication treatment. However, from the limited prior data, it appears program redesign reduced average wait times to start medication from two weeks down to one week or less, in an already accessible program.

In addition, with a fully opt-in program for many components and services, 45% of patients engaged in opt-in components of the program, including acupuncture, massage, reiki, healing circles, counseling, coaching, case management, and more. Many patients engaged in multiple components of the program.

Each month, former patients also returned to the program after dropping off in communication and treatment – and they were welcomed back without judgment or hurdles to jump through. Over time, the clinics also proactively reached out to patients who dropped off, with the help of coding within the EMR that flagged staff when two to three months had lapsed since last communication with a patient.

Trainings on naloxone (Narcan®) as an overdose prevention tool were systematically incorporated into the program. At orientations, patients shared stories of saving others' lives with Narcan®, or receiving life saving treatment from others – and through story sharing they were lifted up as leaders. Patients encouraged friends in their peer networks to utilize the syringe exchange in order to use drugs more safely, if they were not ready to quit. Of the Narcan® units that Casa de Salud distributed to community members (within and outside of the treatment program), fully one-third of units were reported to be used to save community members' lives outside of any healthcare setting. And initial data collected by Casa de Salud a few months into the COVID-19 pandemic showed that more than 50% of units of Narcan® distributed were reported to be used on others in the community, which correlates to national data around an uptick of opioid overdoses in the U.S. during the initial few months of the pandemic [35].

The dynamic iterative model of changes in the program made the measurement of some outcomes challenging, and the opt-in model that meant that any single patient could engage in a unique set and frequency of programming available to them. However, an overwhelming number of patients reflect that healing touch improved their self-confidence and accelerated their healing process; that the program allowed them to connect mind–body-soul and reconnect to their bodies in new ways; that skilled counseling/therapy done at their own pace instead of starting from day one, allowed them to move through healing in their body first until they were ready to talk, and allowed for necessary trust building. Lastly, the ability to navigate warm handoffs and treatment among interdisciplinary providers allowed for interruptions in patients' triggers that curbed relapse risk (see link at the end of this chapter for a video of acupuncturist at Casa de Salud speaking to the power of a warm handoff and transdisciplinary care in a specific patient situation). We are building "practice-based evidence" alongside evidence-based practice.

The multiplier effect of the health apprentices program at Casa de Salud – future clinicians and healthcare leaders – and the social work interns at Centro Sávila – future therapists and advocates – is palpable as students enter institutions of higher education with community based practice knowledge gained in either institution, and then go on to practice healthcare, impact patients and communities, and mentor other future healthcare leaders.

Casa de Salud developed a unique immersive health apprenticeship program that provides more than 500 hours of immersive experience, primarily to students of color interested in healthcare careers and who want to work, live, and invest in their communities. Apprentices learn medical assistant skills such as phlebotomy, greet patients, support clinicians with procedures, staff the syringe exchange, and understand the administration of nonprofit integrative care. The apprentice program trains a future workforce that is culturally humble, bilingual, sensitive, skilled, and that understands the realities of patients from impacted communities. Apprentices deepen their understanding of how to provide care with dignity to communities, help close provider-client demographic gaps, and demonstrate what culturally-rooted and responsive care looks like. Apprentices at Casa de Salud share stories of transformation in their own attitudes in working with active drug users and people seeking treatment, and their impact on shifting attitudes among family members and friends. The effects of humanization, compassion, and passion for supporting drug users and people in recovery will be multiplied many times during the careers of these future clinicians and healthcare leaders.

In a survey of health apprentices conducted during the Clinical Scholars fellowship time period, 94% reported increased awareness of issues in the community during their apprenticeship, and 84% reported improved clinical skills. A total of 87% of apprentices were between the ages of 16 and 24 years of age and 84% of the apprentice team during this time period identified as women, and over 90% of apprentices identified as Latinx or Hispanic. About 60% of apprentices reported the highest parental level of education of either parent as a high school diploma or below. Each year, 20–30 students complete rigorous immersive apprenticeships at Casa de Salud. Over the course of the health apprenticeship program's history, upwards of 40% of former apprentices who Casa de Salud is in touch with are enrolled in or have completed health professional schooling, public health school, allied health fields, and other areas of education, and are working as clinicians and other professionals.

By investing in the human capital of apprentices and interns, Centro Sávila and Casa de Salud have begun to train a new generation whose commitment to local community will ease the recruitment and retention in healthcare provider shortage areas.

5. Discussion

> "So the opposite of addiction is not sobriety. It is human connection... You can build a system that is designed to help drug addicts to reconnect with the world — and so leave behind their addictions."

• Johann Hari, author of *Chasing the Scream.*

The Strong Roots/Raices Fuertes program has made important contributions to the South Valley community, residents of Bernalillo County, and the State of New Mexico. Through a three-year process that engaged staff and patients, the program evolved greatly. Access to low-cost, life-saving naloxone and buprenorphine has saved many lives - buprenorphine has been shown to reduce all cause mortality by a staggering 50%, and naloxone delivered by community members is estimated to have saved around 27,000 lives over an 18 year time period [36, 37]. The program's array of holistic services to support the recovery process is unique in that it prioritizes culturally-rooted practices and recognizes cultural, social, and historical factors that contribute to the opioid epidemic. The program earned the trust and respect of local community members and succeeded in recruiting and retaining patients. During one orientation, a patient shared she had learned about the program from her drug dealer, who respected her desire for treatment instead of drugs.

By far, the most popular service in the program was the low-to-no-cost medication treatment with buprenorphine. The importance of supporting patients with lifesaving evidence-based medicine, in the window of time they are ready, with dignity and without barriers or shame, is critical. Apprentices and staff sometimes "ghost call" other clinics, as patients, to explore barriers in the community such as wait times and hurdles to starting treatment. Often there are wait times of several weeks to several months, or many mandatory requirements in order to start medication treatment – which many programs do not even offer. Same-day or next-day buprenorphine start for people seeking treatment, is a goal for the Strong Roots/Raices Fuertes program.

Patients often reflect on their ability and power to choose their path and programming for their own recovery goals. Many of our patients have experienced overbearing surveillance from the criminal justice system and from the medical-industrial complex of clinics and for-profit treatment programs. Healthcare systems would benefit greatly from reworking treatment and recovery options to provide less surveillance and more autonomy.

Low-cost, relational, high-touch, healing modalities should be incorporated into treatment programs. Many of our patients reflected greater calm, decreased pain (previously a trigger for relapse), fewer withdrawal symptoms, more grounded nervous systems, improved sleep, and decreased anger and reactivity after receiving massage, reiki, acupuncture, ear acudetox, or participating in healing circles. Specific benefits from healing circles included building community, letting go of shame, connecting with others, not feeling alone, and reconnecting with their spirituality. Numerous patients reflected that high-touch healing modalities allowed them to connect to their bodies and feel human and cared for. Two patient leaders in the program were so transformed by massage, acupuncture, and reiki, that they pursued and completed Reiki certification courses, with Casa de Salud's reiki master. They utilized this training to practice reiki on themselves, for stress reduction and calming their nerves, and plan to continue certifications in this practice.

Healthcare must become anti-racist. A recent study showed that Black patients who tested positive for illicit drugs were discharged from treatment at a significantly higher rate than white patients [38]. Neighborhoods in need of healthcare and drug treatment options have systematically been denied appropriate treatment in part based on their racial and socioeconomic makeup. White Americans are almost 35 times more likely to have access to suboxone than Black Americans [39, 40].

Developing a unified approach to care and a common language requires time to iterate on the program and hold each other accountable. Clinicians and staff from both clinics meet regularly, for introspection, reflection, and improvement. Clinicians together shifted away from language of "addicts" and "clean vs dirty" urine samples, among other things. Feedback from patients provides valuable insights into ways to improve. The majority of our clinicians at both clinics, and all health apprentices/medical assistants are fully bilingual (English and Spanish) to support our community of patients, many of whom are monolingual Spanish speakers.

Casa de Salud and Centro Sávila are intentionally small clinics, in walking distance of each other, and rooted centrally in the South Valley community. The clinics are approachable, have a neighborhood appeal, are colorful and welcoming, and are non-clinical in feel. Many aspects of our clinical environments are designed to reflect our core principles, evident in the 'community' feel of clinical rooms, an inclusive front door setup shared by all patients and syringe exchange clients, and our reconceptualization of the 'front desk' as a space that welcomes rather than alienates or shames. Casa de Salud runs a syringe exchange program and has built trust with the drug using community through thousands of exchanges over the last 15 years.

In teaming up to improve support for patients seeking treatment and recovery for opioid addictions, we tried to put ourselves in our patients' shoes - patients who may be rejected by systems when seeking care, have internalized shame around barriers to care, and are finally ready to seek treatment and have a small window in which supporting them could go a long way. Significant introspection helped us identify barriers we were inadvertently creating with our orientation process or with prior mandatory requirements to start on treatment. Healthcare systems can incorporate shifts, small or large, to improve patient experience, flow, design, and accessibility to care. Clinicians in communities should engage with each other to reflect on their systems' inadvertent barriers to care and discuss ways to shift these in practice, on the ground level.

Both clinics recognize the critical financial barriers to care inherent in our healthcare system and magnified in the world of addictions treatment. Despite Medicaid expansion and the Affordable Care Act, more than 10% of the state's population is still uninsured, and undocumented patients have no meaningful way to access affordable health insurance. Many Strong Roots/Raices Fuertes patients are recently out of jail or prison and may not have Medicaid reinstated when starting treatment. The two weeks post-release from jail or prison have a several times elevation in overdose death risk for people struggling with opioid addiction [41–44]. Our clinics work hard to ensure patients had access to Medicaid or insurance on the health exchange, and for those who remained uninsured, we provide global care (as many visits for treatment, therapy, primary care, acupuncture, massage, reiki, and other services as patients needed), at a small monthly fee, which is subsidized or waived when financial barriers existed. Financial barriers cause avoidance of care or create a firm barrier to care; this is very apparent in treatment of addictions. We encourage clinicians to better understand their institutions' fees for care (especially for uninsured patients), collections policies, and any sliding scale options possible, and to advocate for positive change.

Fostering civic engagement that acknowledges the structural and systemic factors contributing to addiction engages new leaders to become the change they want to see in their communities. In the Strong Roots/Raices Fuertes program, we specifically include avenues for civic engagement for our patient population. We shift the language we use with patients; when they start in the program, we refer to them as leaders. We thank them for making this step in their recovery. We work on multiple approaches (e.g., patients co-designing and delivering community workshops, developing leadership skills) to support patients who were interested in doing something bigger than themselves, and/or speaking out for themselves and others.

One central aspect of the Strong Roots/Raices Fuertes Program is that our two organizations are small, community-rooted, non-profit startups that emerged out of a need to address gaps in New Mexico's public health safety net. The experience of "making the road by walking it" provided our program with a unique appreciation of the importance of community engagement and advocacy to address both the individual and systems levels of human suffering. In this time of the COVID-19 pandemic, clinicians around the country have united more than ever before, and discussions about healthcare workers organizing are inspiring, for greater long-term impact on systems change. Solidarity and partnerships with patients and our communities can result in sustainable building of power, with potential for immense policy change locally and nationally.

6. Toolkit

The Toolkit for our Wicked Problem Impact Project for Clinical Scholars can be found at www.ClinicalScholarsNLI.org/community-impact. Our Popular Education Workshop materials can be found in Appendix A (Spanish) and Appendix B (English). At the following link you can find a video of an acupuncturist talking about integrating our care for Strong Roots/Raices Fuertes patients (https://drive.google.com/file/d/1op5A_p_qGzJGFiVRTCkiP8NJsfFZLdGs/view).

Acknowledgements

We are grateful to the Robert Wood Johnson Foundation Clinical Scholars Program, and its program staff, for believing in the ideas of, and investing in the leadership development of and financial resources for, our Clinical Scholars team. We grew so much alongside our incredible national cohort of Clinical Scholars fellows from around the country. We dreamed and struggled and implemented together with our local Clinical Scholars team - thank you to Lorraine Cordova FNP, Dominic Villanueva DOM, and Kate Porterfield PA-C - in addition to numerous staff members at both Casa de Salud and Centro Savila, to build the Strong Roots/Raices Fuertes program. These staff members include clinicians and healers (Paula Terrero Reiki Master, Sarah Sidelko LMT, Alejandra Casarrubias RN, Leah Jo Carnine PA-C, Dina Bello DOM, Justin Remer-Thamert LMT, Laura Rifka Stern MD, Carlos Flores LMSW, Irini Georges LPCC, Carolina Verdezoto LCSW, Moriah Mahoney NP), Operations and Intake team staff (Elizabeth Boyce, Fizz Perkal, Sarah Sidelko), data/evaluation expertise (Judy Bartlett PhD), clinic flow coordinators (Phoenix León, Oscar Munoz, Tegan Whitney, Kenya Quiñonez, Denise Ornelas, Joe McDonald, and others), peer support/program staff (Robert Hoberg, Kristin Muniz LMSW), and all of our health apprentices. Every single patient leader we worked with in the Strong Roots/Raices Fuertes program humbles us and teaches us, and many contributed to the program's development. We stand by our patients as community leaders every day. We are also grateful to the EleValle South Valley Healthy Communities Collaborative for collaborative work in developing popular education workshops, and to artist Gabriela Hernandez/Joteria Undocumented for the design of the workshop materials. We thank the City of Albuquerque, especially Director of Equity and Inclusion Michelle Melendez; Bernalillo County; and the New Mexico Department of Health's Harm Reduction Division, for supporting our work.

In writing this chapter, we thank Dr. Nadine Ijaz PhD, for her coaching on the chapter development. We greatly thank the editorial team of Carol Lorenz, Edith Amponsah, and Lia Garman, and the Clinical Scholars Directors, for their generosity, patience, inspiration, and feedback on the writing.

A. Appendix

A.1 Popular Education Workshop Materials (Spanish)

- Causas fundamentales de la addicion
- Resilencia
- Guera contra las drogas
- Historias

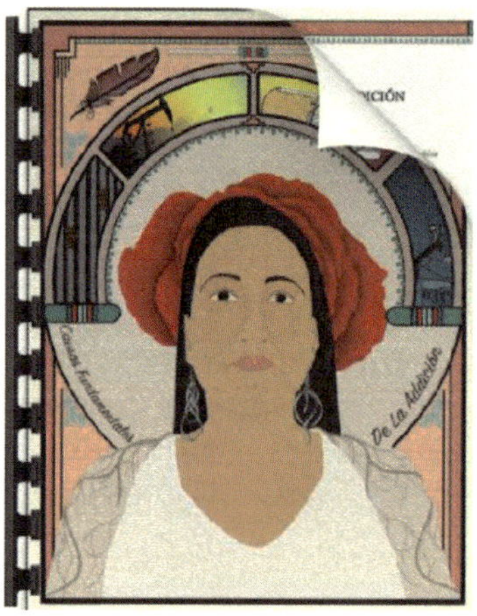

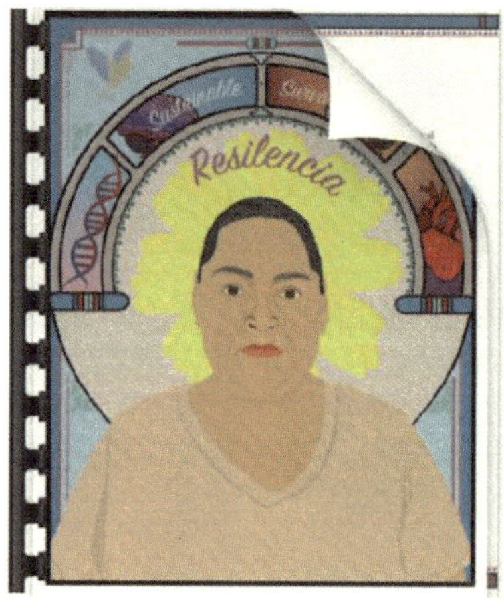

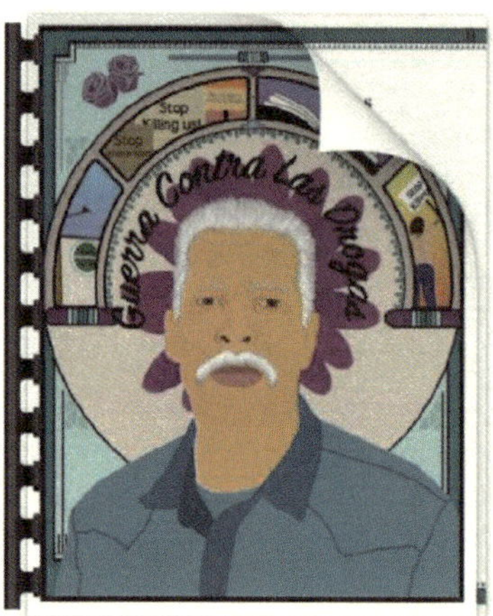

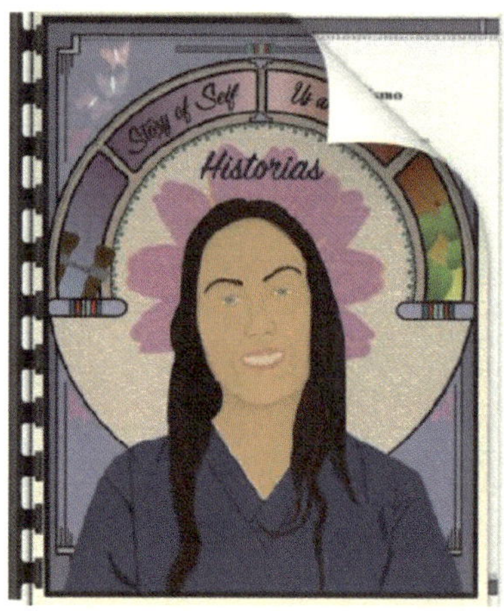

A.2 Popular Education Workshop Materials (English)

- Root causes of addictions
- Resilience
- The war on drugs
- Storytelling for social justice

DOI: http://dx.doi.org/10.5772/intechopen.98463

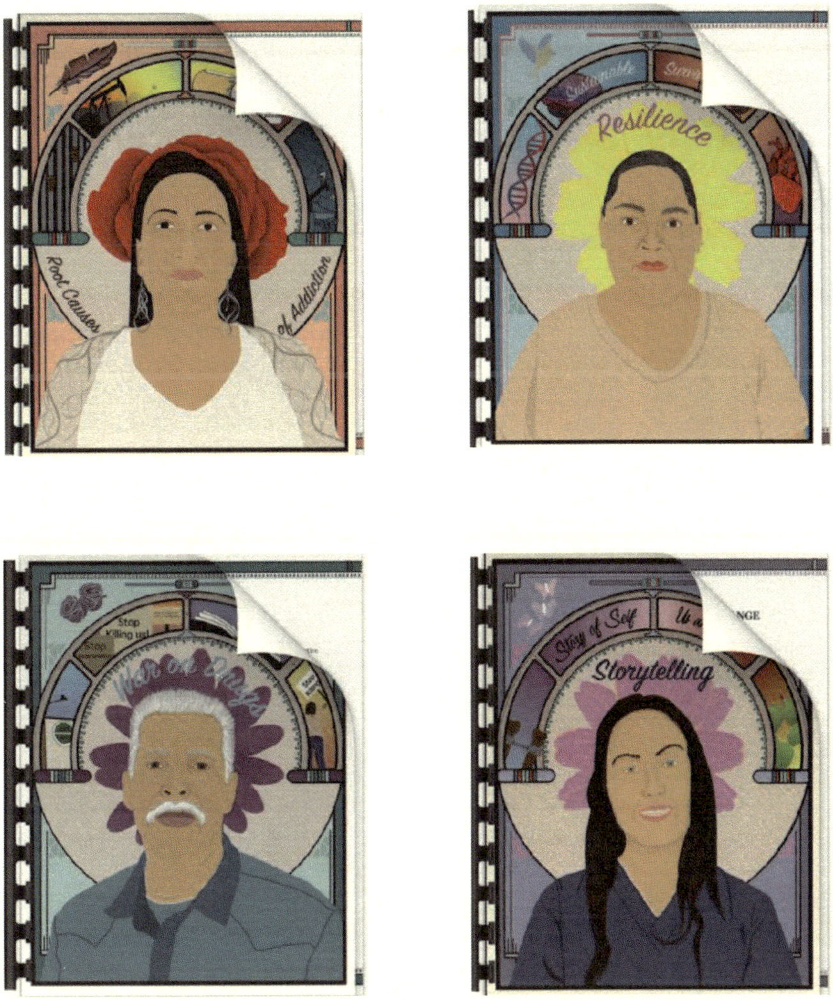

Author details

Anjali Taneja[1*] and William Wagner[2]

1 Casa de Salud, New Mexico, USA

2 Centro Sávila, New Mexico, USA

*Address all correspondence to: anjali@casadesaludnm.org

References

[1] Henninger A, Sung HE. History of substance abuse treatment. In: Bruinsma G, Weisburd D, editors. Encyclopedia Criminology and Criminal Justice. Springer: New York; 2014. DOI: 10.1007/978-1-4614-5690-2.

[2] Trickey E. Inside the Story of America's 19th-Century Opiate Addiction [Internet]. 2018. Available from: https://www.smithsonianmag.com/history/inside-story-americas-19th-century-opiate-addiction-180967673/ [Accessed: 2020-07-26].

[3] Nevius J. The Strange History of Opiates in America: From Morphine for Kids to Heroin for Soldiers [Internet]. 2016. Available from: https://www.theguardian.com/commentisfree/2016/mar/15/long-opiate-use-history-america-latest-epidemic [Accessed 2020-09-26].

[4] Hadland SE, Rivera-Aguirre A, Marshall BDL, Cerdá M. Association of pharmaceutical industry marketing of opioid products with mortality from opioid-related overdoses. JAMA Network Open. 2019;2(1):e186007. DOI:10.1001/jamanetworkopen.2018.6007.

[5] Jones MR, Viswanath O, Peck J, Kaye AD, Gill JS, Simopoulos TT. A brief history of the opioid epidemic and S \strategies for pain medicine. Pain and Therapy. 2018;7:13–21. DOI: 10.1007/s40122-018-0097-6.

[6] Coyne CJ, Hall AR. Four Decades and Counting: The Continued Failure of the War on Drugs [Internet]. 2017. Available from: https://www.cato.org/publications/policy-analysis/four-decades-counting-continued-failure-war-drugs [Accessed: 2020-07-14].

[7] Penal Reform INternational. The Unintended Negative Consequences of the 'War on Drugs': Mass Criminalisation and Punitive Sentencing Policies [Internet]. 2013. Available from: https://cdn.penalreform.org/wp-content/uploads/2013/05/PRI_war-on-drugs-briefing_March-2013.pdf [Accessed: 2020-07-14].

[8] Kain E. The War on Drugs Is a War on Minorities and the Poor [Internet]. 2011. Available from: https://www.forbes.com/sites/erikkain/2011/06/28/the-war-on-drugs-is-a-war-on-minorities-and-the-poor/#70f2cae6624c [Accessed: 2020-07-14].

[9] Drug Policy Alliance. Race and the Drug War [Internet]. Available from: https://www.drugpolicy.org/issues/race-and-drug-war [Accessed: 2020-07-14].

[10] Tsai AC, Kiang MV, Barnett ML, Beletsky L, Keyes KM, McGinty EE, Smith LR, Strathdee SA, Wakeman SE, Venkataramani AS. Stigma as a fundamental hindrance to the United States opioid overdose crisis response. PLoS Medicine. 2019;16(11):e1002969. DOI: 10.1371/journal.pmed.1002969.

[11] Boyd G. The Drug War Is the New Jim Crow [Internet]. 2001. Available from: https://www.aclu.org/other/drug-war-new-jim-crow [Accessed: 2020-07-14].

[12] Jackson HE. Following the Royal Road: A Guide to the Historic Camino Real de Tierra Adentro. University of New Mexico Press: New Mexico; 2006. 227 p.

[13] Carrera MM. Imagining Identity in New Spain: Race, Lineage, and the Colonial Body in Portraiture and Casta Paintings. 1st ed. University of Texas Press: Texas; 2003. 188 p.

[14] Gonzales M, Lamadrid ER, editors. Nación Genízara: Ethnogenesis, Place, and Identity in New Mexico. University of New Mexico Press: New Mexico; 2019. 376 p.

[15] Gómez LE. Manifest Destinies: The Making of the Mexican American Race. NYU Press: New York; 2018. 320 p. DOI: 10.2307/j.ctt1pwt9vn.

[16] Trujillo ML. Land of Disenchantment: Latina/o Identities and Transformations in Northern New Mexico. University of New Mexico Press: New Mexico; 2010. 288 p.

[17] Baca JS, Levertov D. Martín & Meditations on the South Valley. New Directions Publishing: New York; 1987. 104 p.

[18] Centers for Disease Control and Prevention. Drug Overdose Mortality by State [Internet]. 2020. Available from: https://www.cdc.gov/nchs/pressroom/sosmap/drug_poisoning_mortality/drug_poisoning.htm [Accessed: 2020-07-14].

[19] Opioid Accountability Initiative. Impact Report 2017-2018 [Internet]. 2018. Available from: http://www.bchealthcouncil.org/resources/Documents/OAI%20Impact%20Report%20-%202018.pdf [Accessed: 2020-07-14].

[20] New Mexico Department of Health. Complete Health Indicator Report of Drug Overdose Deaths [Internet]. 2019. Available from: https://ibis.health.state.nm.us/indicator/complete_profile/drugoverdosedth.html [Accessed: 2020-07-14].

[21] Joint Center for Political and Economic Studies. Place Matters for Health in Bernalillo County: Ensuring Opportunities for Good Health for All - A Report on Health Inequities in Bernalillo County, New Mexico [Internet]. 2012. Available from: http://www.bchealthcouncil.org/Resources/Documents/Place-Matters-for-Health-in-Bernalillo-County.pdf [Accessed: 2020-07-14].

[22] New Mexico Department of Health. Complete Health Indicator Report of Life Expectancy From Birth [Internet]. 2019. Available from: https://ibis.health.state.nm.us/indicator/complete_profile/LifeExpectBirth.html [Accessed: 2020-07-14].

[23] Felitti VJ, Anda RF, Nordenberg D, Williamson DF, Spitz AM, Edwards V, Marks JS. Relationship of childhood abuse and household dysfunction to many of the leading causes of death in adults: The adverse childhood experiences (ACE) study. American Journal of Preventive Medicine. 1998;14 (4):245-258.

[24] Centers for Disease Control and Prevention. Adverse Childhood Experiences (ACEs): Preventing Early Trauma to Improve Adult Health. 2019. Available from: https://www.cdc.gov/vitalsigns/aces/index.html [Accessed: 2020-07-14].

[25] Bethell, CD, Davis, MB, Gombojav, N, Stumbo, S, Powers, K. Issue Brief: A National and across State Profile on Adverse Childhood Experiences among Children and Possibilities to Heal and Thrive. Baltimore, MD: Johns Hopkins University School of Public Health; 2017. Available from: http://www.cahmi.org/projects/adverse-childhood-experiences-aces/

[26] Dube SR, Felitti VJ, Dong M, Chapman DP, Giles WH, Anda RF. Childhood abuse, neglect, and household dysfunction and the risk of illicit drug use: The adverse childhood experiences study. Pediatrics. 2003;111 (3):564-572. DOI:10.1542/peds.111.3.564.

[27] Burke NJ, Hellman JL, Scott BG, Weems CF, Carrion VG. The impact of adverse childhood experiences on an urban pediatric population. Child Abuse & Neglect. 2011;35(6):408-413. DOI: 10.1016/j.chiabu.2011.02.006.

[28] Cannon Y, Davis G, Hsi A, Bochte A. Adverse Childhood Experiences in

the New Mexico Juvenile Justice Population. 206. Available from: https://nmsc.unm.edu/reports/2016/adverse-childhood-experiences-in-the-new-mexico-juvenile-justice-population.pdf.

[29] National Institute on Drug Abuse. The Science of Drug Use and Addiction: The Basics [Internet]. 2018. Available from: https://www.drugabuse.gov/publications/media-guide/science-drug-use-addiction-basics#:~:text=Addiction%20is%20defined%20as%20a,disorder%20and%20a%20mental%20illness [Accessed: 2020-07-14].

[30] Grifell M, Hart CL. Is Drug Addiction a Brain Disease? [Internet]. 2018. Available from: https://www.americanscientist.org/article/is-drug-addiction-a-brain-disease [Accessd: 2020-07-14].

[31] Hawk M, Coulter RW, Egan JE, Fisk S, Friedman MR, Tula M, Kinsky S. Harm reduction principles for healthcare settings. Harm Reduction Journal. 2017;14(1):70. DOI: 10.1186/s12954-017-0196-4.

[32] Tervalon M, Murray-Garcia J. Cultural humility versus cultural competence: A critical distinction in defining physician training outcomes in multicultural education. Journal of Health Care for the Poor and Underserved. 1998;9(2):117-125. DOI: 10.1353/hpu.2010.0233.

[33] Stuyt EB, Voyles CA. The National Acupuncture Detoxification Association protocol, auricular acupuncture to support patients with substance abuse and behavioral health disorders: Current perspectives. Subst Abuse Rehabil. 2016;7:169-180. DOI: 10.2147/SAR.S99161.

[34] Talamantes, Efrain & Henderson, Mark & Fancher, Tonya & Mullan, Fitzhugh. (2019). Closing the Gap - Making Medical School Admissions More Equitable. The New England journal of medicine. 380. 803-805. 10.1056/NEJMp1808582.

[35] Alter A, Yeager C. The Consequences of COVID-19 on the Overdose Epidemic: Overdoses are Increasing [Internet]. Available from: https://files.constantcontact.com/a923b952701/dbf0b5a5-f730-4a6f-a786-47097f1eea78.pdf.

[36] Wheeler E, Jones TS, Gilbert MK, Davidson PJ. Opioid overdose prevention programs providing naloxone to laypersons—United States, 2014. Morbidity and Mortality Weekly Report. 2015;64(23):631.

[37] Larochelle MR, Bernson D, Land T, Stopka TJ, Wang N, Xuan Z, Bagley SM, Liebschutz JM, Walley AY. Medication for opioid use disorder after nonfatal opioid overdose and association with mortality: A cohort study. Annals of Internal Medicine. 2018;169(3):137-145. DOI: 10.7326/M17-3107.

[38] Gaither JR, Gordon K, Crystal S, Edelman EJ, Kerns RD, Justice AC, Fiellin DA, Becker WC. Racial disparities in discontinuation of long-term opioid therapy following illicit drug use among black and white patients. Drug and Alcohol Dependence. 2018;192:371-376. DOI: 10.1016/j.drugalcdep.2018.05.033.

[39] Lagisetty PA, Ross R, Bohnert A, Clay M, Maust DT. Buprenorphine treatment divide by race/ethnicity and payment. JAMA Psychiatry. 2019;76(9):979-981. DOI:10.1001/jamapsychiatry.2019.0876.

[40] Bebinger M. Opioid Addiction Drug Going Mostly to Whites, Even As Black Death Rate Rises [Internet]. 2019. Available from: https://www.npr.org/sections/health-shots/2019/05/08/721447601/addiction-medicine-mostly-prescribed-to-whites-even-as-opioid-deaths-rose-in-bla.

[41] Merrall EL, Kariminia A, Binswanger IA, Hobbs MS, Farrell M, Marsden J, Hutchinson SJ, Bird SM. Meta-analysis of drug-related deaths soon after release from prison. Addiction. 2010;105(9):1545-1554. DOI: 10.1111/j.1360-0443.2010.02990.x.

[42] Binswanger IA, Stern MF, Deyo RA, Heagerty PJ, Cheadle A, Elmore JG, Koepsell TD. Release from prison—A high risk of death for former inmates. New England Journal of Medicine. 2007; 356(2):157-165. DOI: 10.1056/NEJMsa064115.

[43] Joudrey PJ, Khan MR, Wang EA, Scheidell JD, Edelman EJ, McInnes DK, Fox AD. A conceptual model for understanding post-release opioid-related overdose risk. Addiction science & clinical practice. 2019;14(1):1-4. DOI: 10.1186/s13722-019-0145-5.

[44] Ranapurwala SI, Shanahan ME, Alexandridis AA, Proescholdbell SK, Naumann RB, Edwards Jr D, Marshall SW. Opioid overdose mortality among former North Carolina inmates: 2000–2015. American journal of public health. 2018;108(9):1207-1213. DOI: 10.2105/AJPH.2018.304514.

Chapter 15

Beautiful Ruin: Creating Healthfields

Laurel Berman

Abstract

Multiple programs promote redevelopment of land reuse sites, which are environmentally impacted or potentially contaminated sites. Historically, such programs have focused primarily on economic development. However, public health is an important consideration to address not only sustainable redevelopment but also health inequity and disparities. The Agency for Toxic Substances and Disease Registry's (ATSDR) Land Reuse Health Program is a special program to promote broad public health improvements through safe land reuse and redevelopment. Land reuse sites are virtually in every community in the U.S. and are a global problem. Brownfields are the greatest number of land reuse sites. With estimates of over 450,000 land reuse sites across the U.S., most communities suffer the burden of blight and contamination associated with these sites. ATSDR promotes and practices **Healthfields Redevelopment**: The safe reuse of environmentally distressed land to reduce exposures to contaminants and to improve overall health in the community. In this chapter, I highlight Navajo Nation Healthfields activities using ATSDR's **5-step Land Reuse Strategy to Safely Reuse Land and Improve Health (5-step Land Reuse Model)** and describe some of ATSDR's Healthfields projects and related tools and resources for communities to create their own Healthfields practice.

Keywords: Brownfields, land reuse, community revitalization, Healthfields, redevelopment, health outcomes, ATSDR

1. Introduction

Land reuse is the redevelopment of environmentally impacted sites. While there are many types of land reuse sites, brownfields—potentially contaminated, underused, or vacant properties—are the most numerous of these sites. Brownfields may have less serious contamination than other types of land reuse sites, such as Superfund sites, which are hazardous waste sites that are on the National Priorities List for remediation [1, 2]. Land reuse sites like brownfields exist all over the country and include old gas stations, abandoned manufacturing and commercial/industrial facilities, residential buildings, and incompatibly located or under-utilized sites [3].

Contaminated sites are routinely reused and redeveloped in the U.S. and throughout the world. In the U.S., multiple programs are in place to promote redevelopment. Two well-known programs are the U.S. Environmental Protection Agency's (EPA's) Brownfields Program [4] and Superfund Program [5]. Many federal and state programs promote economic development aspects of land reuse and redevelopment. However, land reuse and redevelopment is also an opportunity to reduce health inequity and disparities by redesigning communities to improve overall health.

The Agency for Toxic Substances and Disease Registry (ATSDR) in Atlanta, Georgia, is a federal public health agency of the **U.S. Department of Health and Human Services**. ATSDR protects communities from harmful health effects related to exposure to natural and man-made hazardous substances. We respond to environmental health emergencies; investigate emerging environmental health threats; conduct research on the health impacts of hazardous waste sites; and build the capabilities of and provide actionable guidance to state and local health partners. Our Land Reuse Health Program is a special program to promote broad public health improvements through safe land reuse and redevelopment. This includes economic development, as it is integrally tied to other health improvements, such as the ability to afford healthful food, participate in recreation, and clean up distressed environments.

Since the mid-1990s, ATSDR's Land Reuse Health Program has built skills and knowledge of communities and state, local, tribal, and territorial partners to integrate a public health focus in land reuse and redevelopment.

Some land reuse sites can pose significant harm to the health of people and ecosystems. People who live near or access land reuse sites often experience disproportionate exposure to environmental pollution, which can result in poor health outcomes, including higher rates of chronic disease; toxic exposures such as from mercury or lead based paint that result in adverse health effects; and cancer [6–8]. Children and other vulnerable populations, such as the elderly or pregnant women, may suffer even greater levels of adverse health impacts from exposure to environmental pollution. In their analysis of environmental threats to child health, Wigle, Arbuckle, and Walker, et al. [9] highlighted common environmental contaminants that included lead, methylmercury, polychlorinated biphenyls (PCBs), dioxin, polycyclic aromatic hydrocarbons (PAHs), pesticides, environmental tobacco smoke, air toxins (e.g. particulate matter and ozone), and many other contaminants that can harm children. Many of these contaminants and factors are commonly associated with land reuse sites and can be very toxic.

To illustrate typical contaminants of concern associated with land reuse sites such as brownfields, ATSDR's Land Reuse Team summarized EPA's Cleanups in My Community (CIMC) data from 2013 to 2017 [10]. We generated a list of U.S. entities that received EPA brownfields assessment or cleanup funding. We selected the measure of cities and counties in states that received the most funding as a proxy measure for states with the highest numbers of brownfields. In all there were 11 states with the highest number of brownfields. We selected 10 of the 11 states that also currently have ATSDR cooperative agreement funding to conduct public health assessments. In a subsequent analysis, we compared the 2013–2017 brownfields listings to brownfields on which public health assessments had been completed. As shown in **Figure 1**, we reviewed the "Top 10" states for suspected or confirmed contaminants of concern at brownfields. The majority of sites listed in the CIMC data base were undergoing site assessments. Very few were undergoing cleanup. The primary contaminants, from most to least common, ranged from metals (other metals and lead), volatile organic compounds (VOCs), petroleum, PAHs, asbestos, arsenic, chromium, cadmium, mercury, "other" [contaminants], semi-volatile organic compounds (SVOCs), selenium, copper, PCBs, nickel, iron, and pesticides. These contaminants can be highly toxic and can cause neurological effects (e.g. lead, mercury, and pesticides) or cancer (e.g. VOCs and chromium), among other adverse health effects.

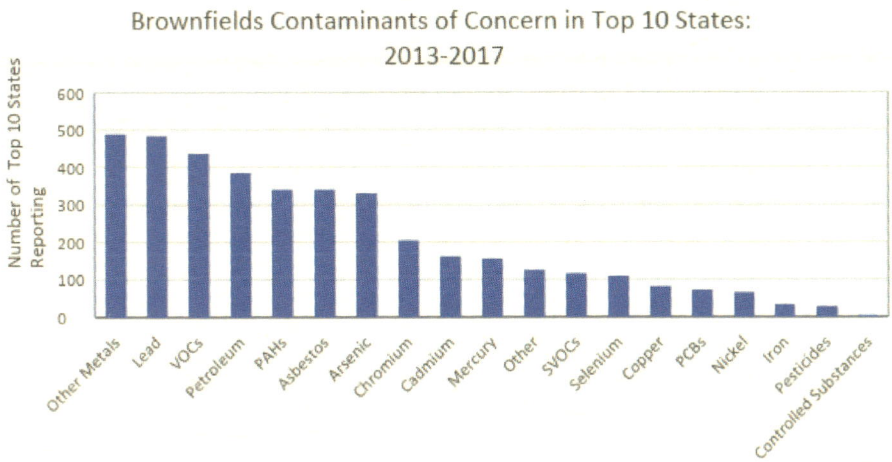

Figure 1.
Brownfields contaminants in "top 10" states that received the Most brownfields funding and are in cooperative agreements with ATSDR. Source: Berman, L. Agency for Toxic Substances and Disease Registry. Brownfields contaminants in "top 10" states that received the Most brownfields funding and are in cooperative agreements with ATSDR. Atlanta: Agency for Toxic Substances and Disease Registry; 2020.

2. The extent of the land reuse problem

Apart from potentially harmful chemical exposures, the blighted nature of land reuse sites alone can drag down communities. While blighted properties that are residential may have contamination issues, such as lead based paint or asbestos, at the same time they can be nuisances that attract youth, squatters, and vandals. According to the U.S. Government Accountability Office (2011), vacant and unattended residential properties can attract crime, cause blight, and pose a threat to public safety. The number of vacant residential properties increased 51 percent (%) from 2000 to 2010, from nearly 7 million to 10 million [11]. In their report, *Urban Blight and Public Health: Addressing the Impact of Substandard Housing, Abandoned Buildings, and Vacant Lots* (2017), de Leon and Shilling summarize literature that quantifies the impact of blight on health. They emphasize that exposure to substandard housing disproportionately impacts people of color and people of lower income, particularly in urban areas. In addition, neighborhoods with persistent blight can attract crime and vermin. The impacts on residents include mental distress; higher rates of chronic illness and sexually transmitted diseases; stunted brain and physical development in children; and limited opportunities for exercise [12].

Land reuse is no small problem. Land reuse sites are virtually in every community in the U.S. and are a problem worldwide. Brownfields are a majority component of land reuse sites. As mentioned above, there are estimates of 450,000 brownfields sites across the United States. In the map below, the gray circles represent over 22,000 brownfields sites that have been entered in the EPA's Assessment, Cleanup and Redevelopment Exchange System (ACRES) database by federal EPA Brownfields grantees. The sites designated by colored circles are communities with brownfields sites where ATSDR has implemented a community health project, provided technical assistance, performed a health assessment, launched a special initiative (e.g. a residential soil sampling event known as "SoilSHOP"), or provided other services to address concerns about contamination.

The map shown in **Figure 2** illustrates that land reuse sites such as brownfields exist everywhere throughout the U.S., particularly in the "rust belt" and former

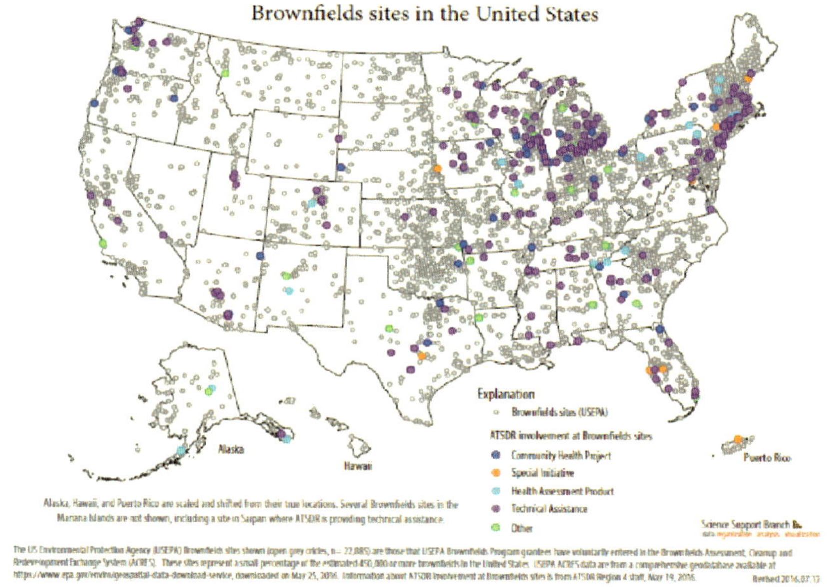

Figure 2.
ATSDR involvement at brownfields sites in the United States. Source: Science support branch. Agency for Toxic Substances and Disease Registry. Brownfields sites in the United States. Atlanta: Agency for Toxic Substances and Disease Registry; 2016.

industrial areas in the Eastern United States[1]. However, the sites represented in this map are only the known sites, meaning they are only a fraction of the total number of sites. The world of land reuse sites may continuously expand as more sites are created through bankruptcies, foreclosures, or abandonment. The 51% increase in vacant residential properties is one factor that can increase land reuse sites. Other factors include sites that were contaminated in the past and may be discovered during land expansion and development projects or when people become sick, smell odors, or suspect previous contamination.

The map in **Figure 2** shows that there are known land reuse/brownfields sites in Navajo Nation (Northern Arizona and New Mexico). Over 156,000 Navajo live within Navajo Nation, and over 33,000 live on the borders of or outside the Nation (e.g., Flagstaff, Holbrook, and Winslow) [13]. Over 50% of the population is below age 29. Navajo is rural and has low population density. The median household income for the Navajo Nation is $27,389, which is approximately half that of the State of Arizona ($51,310) overall. One-third (32%) of all households on the Navajo Nation have incomes of less the $15,000 when compared to the State of Arizona (17%) [14]. Many Navajo live without electricity (32% of the population), plumbing (31% of the population), water services (38% of the population), natural gas (86% of the population), and telephone services (60% of the population) [15].

The Division of Health and the Navajo Epidemiology Center (2013) report that Navajo people are burdened with many health issues such as alcoholism, diabetes, and cancer. They believe that from an epidemiologic perspective, many of these health issues may be related to socio-economic status and social behavior (see Ref. [13]).

Except for former uranium mining sites and associated health issues of exposure to uranium, it is not known whether health issues in Navajo Nation are related to the presence of land reuse sites. However, Navajo Nation, known for the Painted Desert, Canyon de Chelly, Monument Valley, and many other places of cultural

[1] ATSDR Region 4 staff provided the location data for ATSDR brownfields activities shown on the map.

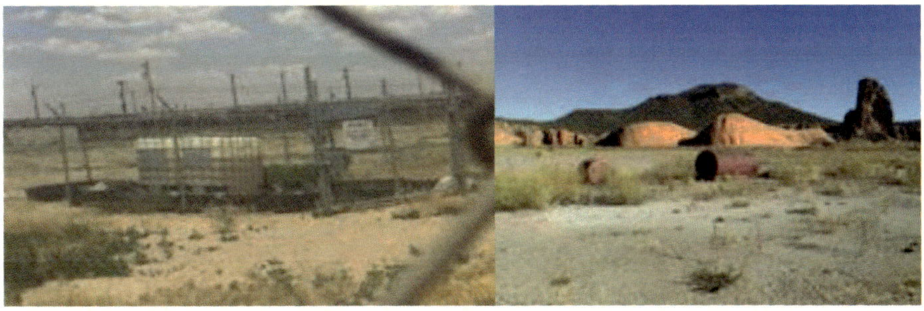

Figure 3.
Images of a petroleum spill remediation site in Chinle AZ (left) and the former Navajo Forest products industries site in red Lake NM. Source: Berman, L. Agency for Toxic Substances and Disease Registry. Brownfields images in Navajo nation. Atlanta: Agency for Toxic Substances and Disease Registry; 2017.

significance and beauty, is littered with land reuse sites and contamination. In Chinle, vacant former fast food restaurants, two sites with active petroleum spills, and other vacant land reuse sites are present. In a conversation with Navajo planner T. Begay (June 6, 2016) during a field visit to a petroleum spill site, he stated that one petroleum plume is currently being remediated and one petroleum plume may have migrated under a multi-unit apartment building, which can impact residents who live there. In Red Lake, the former Navajo Forest Products Industries (NFPI) site sits vacant, with waste left in place until 2019 (right photo of **Figure 3**, below). The site is reported to be over 100 acres [16]. The woodchip fill from the site has caught on fire more than once and when it does, it smolders for days, potentially exposing nearby residents and children at a nearby Head Start and a charter middle school to particulates (i.e., smoke) that may be toxic (interviews with US EPA representative (October 2016) and Navajo Nation EPA representative (June 2019). The images below highlight two land reuse sites in Chinle and Red Lake (**Figure 3**).

2.1 Healthfields redevelopment

ATSDR conducts public health assessments to determine whether exposure to hazardous substances associated with a hazardous waste site (i.e. a contaminated site) may be harmful. Of over 2700 public health assessments completed by ATSDR as of 2017, 274 were specifically on brownfields, and 42% of the time these assessments indicated a public health hazard. This emphasizes how important community health can be as a driver for redevelopment plans that reduce health inequity and disparities often associated with distressed environments.

ATSDR calls health-focused redevelopment **"Healthfields" Redevelopment**: The safe reuse of environmentally distressed land to reduce exposures to contaminants and to improve overall health in the community. Healthfields are integral to a Culture of Health. The Culture of Health Leaders (CoHL) is a program developed by the Robert Wood Johnson Foundation (RWJF) that supports and trains leaders working to improve health inequity and disparities in communities across the United States.

3. Methods used: the 5-step land reuse model to promote Healthfields

To address health risks and exposures related to land reuse sites, ATSDR integrates a public health model in land reuse and redevelopment, the **5-step Land Reuse Strategy to Safely Reuse Land and Improve Health (5-step Land Reuse Model)**. The steps of this model, shown in **Figure 4**, are steps to achieve

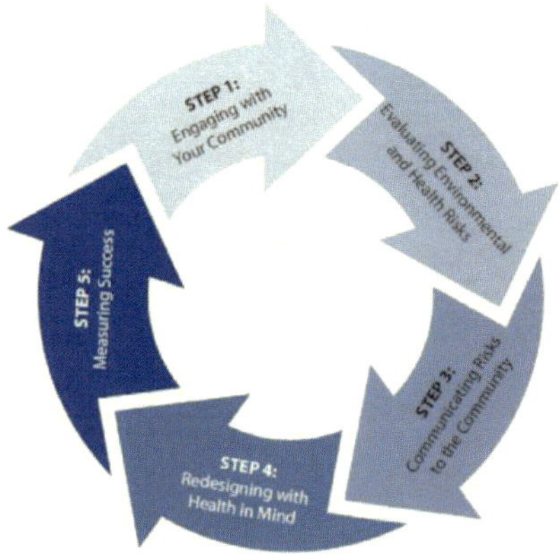

Figure 4.
ATSDR 5-step land reuse model. Source: Agency for Toxic Substances and Disease Registry. ATSDR 5-step land reuse model [image on internet]. Atlanta: Agency for Toxic Substances and Disease Registry; 2019–0904. Available from: https://www.atsdr.cdc.gov/sites/brownfields/land_reuse_toolkits.html#.

Healthfields and highlight activities that community revitalization partners can take to ensure that community health outcomes are at the forefront of redevelopment planning. ATSDR's goal is to promote Healthfields as a national effort effected at the local level.

In 2016, RWJF launched the first cohort in their CoHL Program. Forty individuals were selected to participate in this three-year program grounded in equity, diversity, and inclusion. ATSDR was able to leverage RWJF funding into ATSDR's 5-step Land Reuse Model Healthfields initiatives across the country, primarily through Community Partnerships projects and Land Reuse Toolkit Pilots, described below. Ultimately, ATSDR was able to focus intensively on Healthfields as a redevelopment option in our largest Community Partnership: Navajo Nation.

3.1 The 5-step land reuse model steps

Communities interested in renewing and reusing land reuse sites can follow the 5-step Land Reuse Model steps shown in **Figure 4** [17]. These steps can be followed sequentially or individually. For example, if a community is already engaged and contamination has been assessed, the Development Community may opt to start with Step 4 to redesign with health in mind.

Step 1: Engage the Development Community.

The Development Community includes stakeholders with an interest in redevelopment, including residents, nonprofits, officials, planners, environmental or health professionals, developers, and any others with an interest in health-focused community revitalization.

Step 2: Evaluate Environment and Health Issues.

Evaluating environment and health issues at the beginning of the project can help ensure a safer project and a plan to protect and improve public health.

Step 3: Communicate Risks or Health Issues to the Development Community.

Describing risks of contaminants or hazards associated with land reuse sites can help community members learn more about how revitalization projects can address health and environmental issues.

Step 4: Redesign the Community with Health in Mind.

It is important to ask questions to build a healthier community (i.e., what are the benefits?). Redevelopment can be planned to promote healthier places to live and work for the long term, helping to ensure a sustainable, community-driven plan.

Step 5: Measure Success: Environment and Health Change.

Select metrics that correspond to health factors that affect the community, such as assessing the number of sites that are slated for redevelopment, counting the number of grocery stores, or mapping sites with known contamination that are close to residential properties. Tracking these indicators can measure changes in environment and health over the course of redevelopment.

A strong Development Community can work together to assess, clean, and re-envision land reuse sites. Through the diverse partnerships and collaborations that Development Communities offer, public health and planning can lead the effort to reshape America, recycling and improving land and serving as a resource for creating Healthfields.

3.2 Community partnerships

To promote Healthfields, a team of volunteer, multi-sector community engagement and redevelopment experts, the Brownfields & Opportunity Working Network (BROWN), provided free consultative assistance to land reuse communities through ATSDR's Community Partnerships pilot projects. BROWN includes federal, state, and local environmental, housing, development, and health agency representatives; private sector planners and consultants; academics with expertise in community-based research; filmmakers who document land reuse sites and community conditions; and several others who are proponents of Healthfields.

During the 2014–2016 pilot period, BROWN collaboratively provided assistance to seven Community Partnerships in the U.S. and one partnership in Romania. The U.S. partnerships included Healthfields projects in Whitewright, Texas; K.I. Sawyer, Michigan (formerly K.I. Sawyer Air Force Base); Jacksonville, Florida; Howardville, Missouri; Baker City, Oregon; the Arizona Healthfields Initiative focused on creating Healthfields throughout the state; and the Navajo Nation (primarily Chinle and Red Lake). In each Community Partnership, BROWN provided consultative assistance that essentially reflected Steps 1 through 5 of the 5-step Land Reuse Model. We are beginning to quantify outcomes that measure changes in overall community health resulting from these projects. ATSDR is currently highlighting our initial pilot projects and BROWN resources as models for rapid assistance to new partnership communities. ATSDR welcomed two new Community Partnerships in 2018 (Atlanta GA and Andrews University in Berrien County MI). The Navajo Nation Community Partnership is the partnership of focus in this chapter, and it is the partnership that is geographically the largest.

3.3 Land reuse and redevelopment (Healthfields) toolkits

In 2017, ATSDR's Land Reuse Team created the Land Reuse and Redevelopment Toolkits (Land Reuse Toolkits/Healthfields Toolkits). The Land Reuse Toolkits provide guidance to communities to implement the 5 steps of the 5-step Land Reuse Model to create Healthfields. The Toolkits are synchronized and serve as a resource for the typical roles represented in a Development Community: the **Community Champion, Community Planner, Developer, Environmental or Health Professional,** and the **Municipal Agency** (**Figure 5**). The Land Reuse Toolkits are available at: (available at: https://www.atsdr.cdc.gov/sites/brownfields/land_reuse_toolkits.html.

In early 2018, ATSDR leveraged RWJF CoHL funding to provide in-person technical assistance to seven Land Reuse Toolkit Pilots. One of the pilots was an expansion of the Navajo Nation Community Partnership. Each pilot focused on at least one step of the 5-step Land Reuse Model. The Navajo Nation Land Reuse

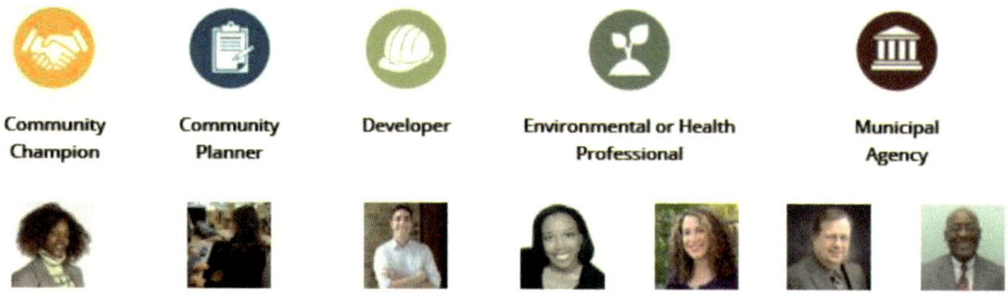

Figure 5.
Screen capture of the land reuse toolkit personas, who provided input into the toolkits. Source: Agency for Toxic Substances and Disease Registry. Land reuse toolkits (Healthfields toolkits) [image on internet]. Atlanta: Agency for Toxic Substances and Disease Registry; 2019–0904. Available from: https://www.atsdr.cdc.gov/sites/brownfields/land_reuse_toolkits.html#.

Toolkit Pilot initially focused on community engagement (step 1) and redesigning the community with health in mind (step 4). Navajo Nation completed intensive community engagement and visioning sessions, as well as a full rendering and plan for a vendor crafts village, and ultimately obtained funding to move towards the development phase of this project. During the summer of 2019, the Navajo Nation Land Reuse Toolkit Pilot began to implement the evaluation of environmental and health risks (step 2) by completing a Phase 1 Environmental Site Assessment at a site in Chinle and conducting stakeholder meetings about the former Navajo Forest Products Industries Site in Red Lake.

3.4 A culture of Healthfields in Navajo nation

Navajo Nation is vast. It extends over 27,000 square miles, through Arizona, Utah, and New Mexico (**Figure 6**). Navajo Nation is comprised of five governing Agencies (Tuba City, Chinle, Shiprock, Fort Defiance, and Crownpoint/Eastern) that are subdivided into 110 Chapters [18].

ATSDR leveraged RWJF CoHL funding into expanding the Navajo Nation Community Partnership into a strategic initiative focused primarily in Chinle, Red Lake, and Tsalie (Diné College) Chapters. The strategic initiative focuses on finding resources to clean up and redevelop properties in Chinle and Red Lake; and to provide a curriculum in Healthfields for Diné (Navajo) College students and for tribal environmental professionals in general.

Navajo Nation stakeholders include Navajo Department of Tourism, individual Chapters and Chapter members, Navajo natural resources and environmental agencies, National Park Service (NPS), BROWN members, and many others. We formed the Healthfields Redevelopment Coalition (HRC) as a sustainable entity to apply for redevelopment funding and to address community environmental health concerns. Key members include a planning contractor, an environmental consultant who is also a Culture of Health colleague, Navajo Department of Tourism, Navajo Nation EPA, Diné College, and Chinle and Red Lake Chapters.

The HRC is focusing on numerous sites throughout Navajo Nation. Currently, the HRC is advancing a Healthfields project on a vacant parcel of land in Chinle slated to be a vendor crafts village. Years of outreach and visioning have culminated in a plan for "Vendor Village" that will feature Navajo arts, culture, and a community recreation and cultural history amenity. To supplement the visioning process, we facilitated the use of ATSDR's Brownfields/Land Reuse Action Model (Action Model) (see: https://www.atsdr.cdc.gov/sites/brownfields/ model.html) to ensure that multiple stakeholders had equal opportunities to contribute to a health-focused redevelopment plan. During the Action Model process, stakeholders created metrics

DOI: http://dx.doi.org/10.5772/intechopen.98464

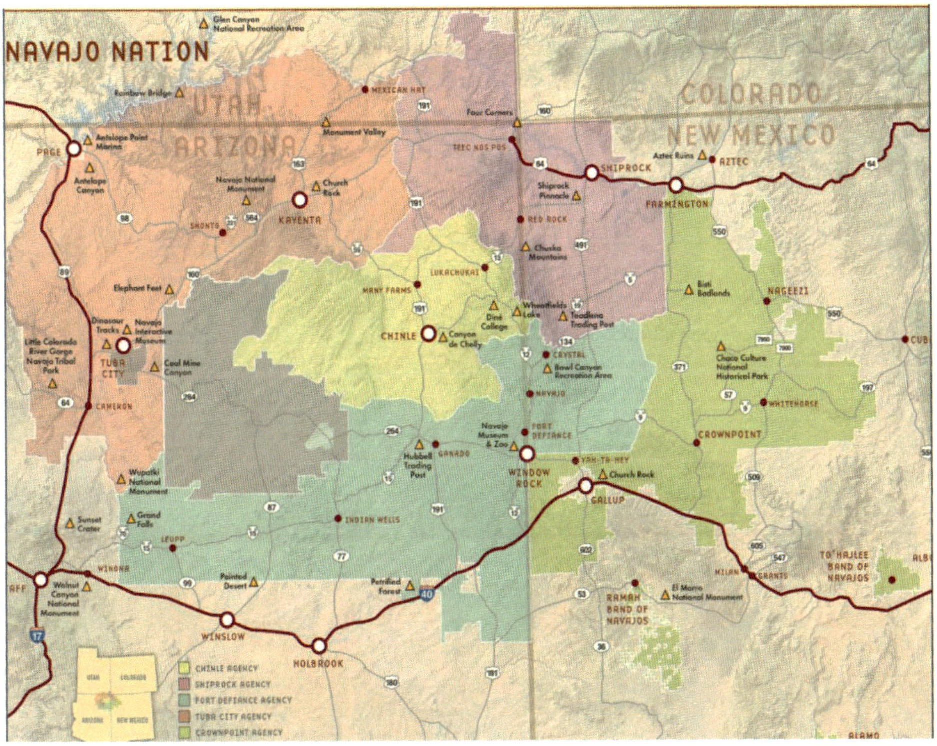

Figure 6.

Map of Navajo nation (Navajo nation tourism department, n.d.). Source: Navajo nation tourism department. Map of Navajo nation [image on internet]. Window rock, AZ: Navajo nation tourism department; 2019–0904. Available from: https://www.discovernavajo.com/hard-map.pdf.

to measure environment and health change over the course of redevelopment. In addition, the Land Reuse Team trained Chinle, Navajo, and other Chapter representatives on the ATSDR Land Reuse Site Tool, a tool that enables rapid inventorying of land reuse sites, site contamination, and environmental and health risks associated with land reuse sites.

To focus on advancing Healthfields, as well as education about Healthfields, ATSDR partnered with Diné College faculty who run a special Summer Institute for science, technology, engineering, and math students; the HRC; a Summer Institute mentor; and other partners to provide a Healthfields curriculum. HRC members and the Diné College Summer Institute mentor highlighted field activities for two Summer Institute students. ATSDR also created an EHLR Classroom Training Certificate course to ensure that environmental professionals have opportunities to engage in Healthfields practice.

4. Outcomes/results

The RWJF Culture of Health funding enhanced technical assistance through a $60,000 allocation to the Centers for Disease Control and Prevention (CDC) through the CDC Gift Foundation and a $35,000 separate allocation to Navajo partners for Healthfields-related projects. The RWJF funding supported ATSDR Land Reuse Team travel and technical assistance to several communities within Navajo Nation and in other projects focused on Healthfields. The RWJF funding also supported ATSDR's development of educational materials and resources, attendance at conferences and trainings, general strategic planning around Healthfields, and activities related to editing and production of the BROWN co-authored book, *Land Reuse and Redevelopment: Creating Healthy Communities*, which ATSDR intends to publish in 2020.

4.1 A culture of Healthfields in Navajo nation

The Navajo Community Partnership is incorporating history, education, and redevelopment success to drive small wins and long-term changes. The HRC will build on successful projects, incorporate culture, maximize positive health outcomes, and increase capacity to obtain resources.

Specific activities in the Navajo Nation Healthfields project included the development of community-driven indicators in Chinle to measure changes in environment and health over the course of redevelopment; funding for Healthfields projects; and environmental health (Healthfields) education (**Figure 7**).

Navajo Nation was one of 40 different communities across the U.S. that contributed to the development of a robust data set of public health indicators associated with land reuse and redevelopment. These were derived using the ATSDR Action Model (available at: https://www.atsdr.cdc.gov/sites/brownfields/model.html). Among the many Navajo indicators, those specifically related to Healthfields are provided in **Table 1**.

The Navajo Nation Healthfields project covers many different Chapters and community areas. By collaborating with another CoH leader, ATSDR cumulatively leveraged at least $105,000 in RWJF funds into Navajo Nation Healthfields projects. In addition, a lead HRC member was awarded over $400,000 in federal funding to finalize the Vendor Village plan (see **Figure 8**). Using CoH funding, in June 2019 a CoH colleague who is also an HRC member, performed the Phase 1 Environmental Site Assessment for the proposed Vendor Village site. Two Diné College Summer Institute students, HRC members, and the Chinle Chapter president observed and participated in the assessment. The site assessment saved the Chinle Chapter $5,000. After assessing two parcels, the HRC determined that the larger of the two parcels had few environmental issues of concern, and the smaller parcel had two older housing structures (pre-1970 or even earlier) and a small exterior burn pit that require further assessment to rule out the presence of asbestos containing material or lead based paint, which are routine findings of site assessments of properties with similar older structures.

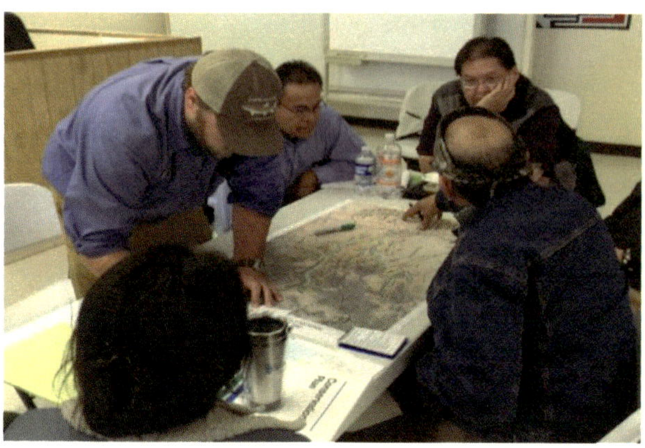

Figure 7.
Planning and visioning session in Navajo nation. Source: Berman, L. Agency for Toxic Substances and Disease Registry. Planning and visioning session in Navajo nation. Atlanta: Agency for Toxic Substances and Disease Registry; 2017.

Public health theme	Indicator
Environment/Land Reuse Agriculture and Land Reuse	Improved land management system Improved water efficiency/conservation Recognition of land uses by agencies Farming returns to residents
Community Development Watershed Health Interpretation/education of visitors Create a Navajo Narrative	Reduced 900 acres of tamarisk (an invasive species) Improved signage Cultural and other exhibits Community input training for guides Additional research and publications about Navajo culture and Healthfields Navajo language to be included in interpretative signs and exhibits
Business/ Economy Vending/Tours Home-based Business No fees to enter Canyon de Chelly	Establishing Vendor Village Less reported conflicts over use of area Actual (amount of) sales for vendors Decrease in illegal businesses More cooperation

Table 1.
Excerpt of Navajo nation action model indicators for the Chinle Vendor Village project.

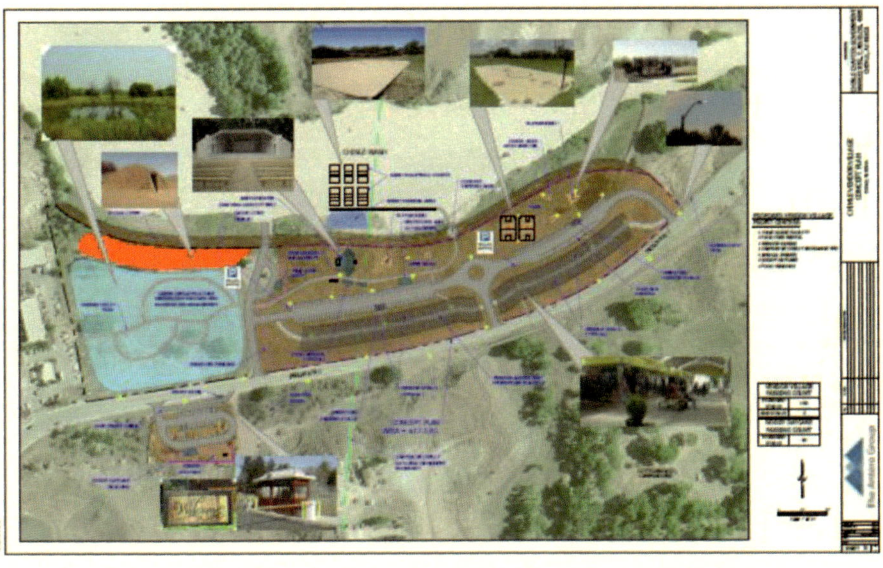

Figure 8.
Rendering of Vendor Village in Chinle, AZ. Source: Antero group. Economic development plan – Navajo nation. [image on internet]. Chicago: Antero group; 2019–0904. Available from: https://www.anterogroup.com/project/navajo-nation-economic-development/.

Through the partnership of Diné College in the HRC, two Diné students learned about and participated in the Phase 1 Environmental Site Assessment in Chinle and observed land reuse sites in Chinle, Red Lake, and Holbrook (see **Figures 9** and **10**). In July 2019, RWJF funds sponsored the two Diné students travel and expenses to extend their learning in Chicago for one week. They met federal partners and local experts engaged in land revitalization, environmental justice, public health, and development. I also immersed the students, along with four additional participants, in the pilot test of the EHLR Certificate Classroom Training course.

To promote Healthfields broadly, along with Land Reuse and HRC team members, ATSDR Land Reuse team members taught the EHLR Classroom

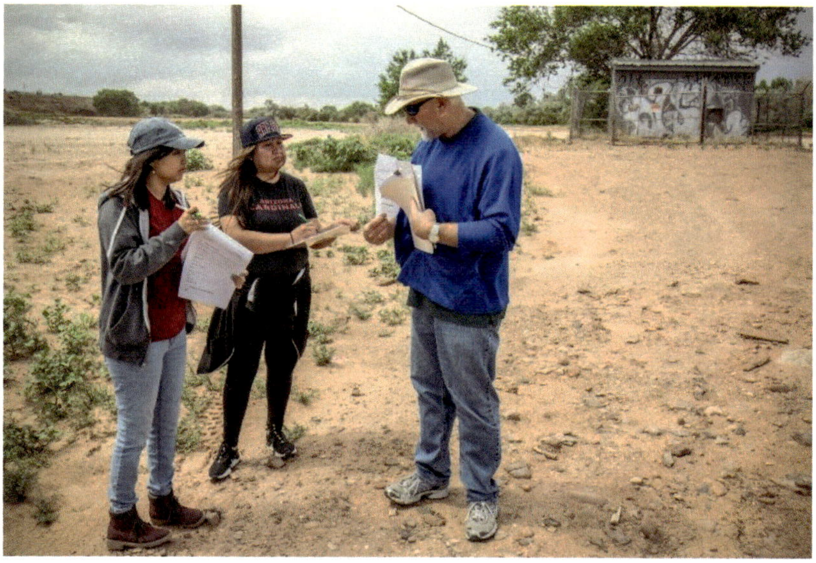

Figure 9.
Diné college students participating in a phase 1 environmental site assessment. Source: Lloyd DeGrane. Diné college students participating in a phase 1 environmental site assessment. Chicago: Lloyd DeGrane; 2019–0624.

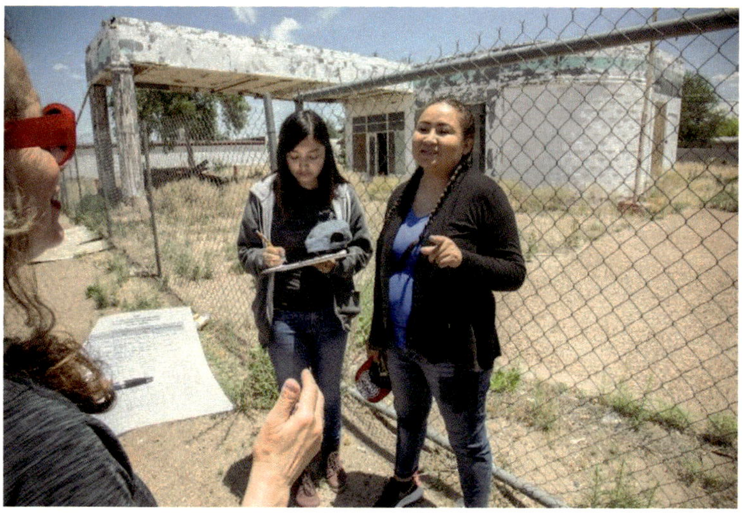

Figure 10.
Diné college students observing brownfields in Holbrook, AZ. Source: Lloyd DeGrane. Diné college students observing brownfields in Holbrook, AZ. Chicago: Lloyd DeGrane; 2019–0624.

Training Certificate course during the Institute for Tribal Environmental Professionals (ITEP) Tribal Environmental Lands Forum in August 2019. A total of 20 tribal environmental professionals participated in the course and successfully passed their course module tests. One of the environmental professionals serves Diné College, and we hope to jointly provide the training to Diné students in coming years. ATSDR will also host the EHLR Classroom Training Certificate as a free training on our land reuse website. Ultimately, the EHLR Classroom Training Certificate will remain available to future Diné College students, ITEP, tribal environmental professionals, and all environmental and planning professionals long into the future.

5. Discussion

Ultimately, Healthfields redevelopment in Navajo Nation can serve as a model for other regions of the country. ATSDR maintains the Healthfields tools and resources, such as the Action Model and Land Reuse Toolkits on our website, under "Healthfields Tools and Resources" at https://www.atsdr.cdc.gov/sites/brownfields/index.html. The real people engaged in Healthfields redevelopment who are the backbone of each Land Reuse Toolkit—community champions and planners, developers, environmental and health professionals, and municipal agencies—are change leaders who are models for others. Success stories about how pilot communities are using the toolkits to engage their communities, communicate risk, create Healthfields community designs, and many other purposes, can pave the way for Healthfields projects nationally.

To promote Healthfields, ATSDR and partners create manuscripts and commentaries about Healthfields and related resources. From 2018 to 2019, the *Journal of Environmental Health* featured a 3-part Healthfields series that focused on the development of the 5-step Land Reuse Model as a national resource; the capacity of local health departments to engage in health-focused land reuse and redevelopment; and community-driven public health indicators associated with land reuse and redevelopment. In addition, 49 BROWN members and their colleagues voluntarily created the book, *Land Reuse and Redevelopment: Creating Healthy Communities* that is slated to be published by ATSDR in 2020.

One exciting development in elevating Healthfields nationally has been connecting with other Culture of Health leaders. For example, a 2018 roundtable discussion during a RWJF CoHL convening blossomed into a new Healthfields project in Berrien County, Michigan. Key partners are faculty from Andrews University in Berrien Springs, Michigan. Andrews University is deeply committed to improving community health through education. Faculty partners are pursuing funding to become a Center for Excellence in Environmental Health. They have become one of ATSDR's newest Community Partnerships. Through this partnership, we are preparing our first publications that highlights the multi-media (land, air, and water) environmental landscape in Berrien County. In addition, Andrews University Environmental Health faculty intend to integrate the EHLR Certificate as a curriculum option for public health students.

The 5-step Land Reuse Model was formalized in the Land Reuse Toolkits and it is now the basis of the EHLR Certificate. The Certificate is geared to graduate students in public health, planning, and environmental science; environmental professionals; and planners. To ensure the training resources and Certificate are widely available, ATSDR will host the EHLR course materials indefinitely within our website at www.atsdr.cdc.gov/sites/brownfields. Soon, the EHLR Certificate will enable us to train thousands of environmental professionals, planners, and students, broadly promoting Healthfields.

As we gain traction promoting and featuring Healthfields projects, ATSDR can reflect on how much we accomplished with a small amount of funding. We hope that the successes, resources, and tools highlighted in this chapter will provide a roadmap and model for communities to implement in their own revitalization projects, helping to create sustainable health-focused land reuse programs across the country.

6. Leader learning

For leaders struggling with the problem of land reuse sites, blight, concerns about harmful contaminants and the associated health disparities and inequity in your communities, the 5-step Land Reuse Model approach to creating Healthfields can be adapted to your needs. The 5-step Land Reuse Model is fluid and does not always have to start with Step 1, Engaging with Your Community. However, unless your communities are already engaged and organized, I cannot emphasize enough how important meaningful community engagement (step 1) is to this process. It is like learning to crawl before you can walk. It takes practice, and it is a slow process. As leaders, you may make mistakes. It happens, you are human. Embracing your mistakes as opportunities to learn, and sharing this with your communities, helps with trust-building and is part of the process of community engagement.

It can take months to years to fully form an inclusive and engaged Development Community. As a leader, it is important to support your community's vision of what their end goal is in community revitalization. Keeping the vision in mind while building the coalition of the Development Community can ensure that everyone has a place at the table, everyone feels heard, and everyone is an expert. Once communities are fully engaged and collaborating, they are ready to take action to achieve equitable and just Healthfields revitalization.

7. Toolkits

If you live in or work with communities burdened by blight and land reuse sites, there are many resources available to walk you through the Healthfields process. These include:

ATSDR Land Reuse Toolkits (Healthfields Toolkits): https://www.atsdr.cdc.gov/sites/brownfields/land_reuse_toolkits.html#.
ATSDR Action Model: https://www.atsdr.cdc.gov/sites/brownfields/model.html
ATSDR Brownfields/Land Reuse Site Tool: https://www.atsdr.cdc.gov/sites/brownfields/site_inventory.html
ATSDR's Environmental Health and Land Reuse Classroom Training Certificate will be available within our website, along with a future online EHLR Certificate that we are developing with the National Environmental Health Association. Please check here to search for the Certificate: https://www.atsdr.cdc.gov/sites/brownfields/.

Additional resources, including a variety of federal agencies, tools, and information are provided on ATSDR's website: https://www.atsdr.cdc.gov/sites/brownfields/resources.html.

Acknowledgments

The RWJF funding helped to expand ATSDR's Community Partnership program in Navajo Nation and was used to partially support additional work in seven other Community Partnerships across the country. ATSDR's Land Reuse Team (Laurel Berman, Leann Bing, and Gary Perlman) benefitted greatly from the RWJF funding, which enabled face-to-face meetings with several of our Community Partnership partners. Many thanks are owed to ATSDR's Community Partnership partners, who diligently have incorporated our 5-step Land Reuse Model and a Healthfields focus in their redevelopment projects. Our Community Partnership communities have also "paid it forward" and helped each other, sharing best practices and successes as models for others. One of our Community Partnership partners, Dave Laney, is also an RWJF Culture of Health partner, who was an integral member of our Navajo Nation Community Partnership. I am most grateful for Dave's and BROWN member Eric Neagu's assistance in the Navajo Nation Community Partnership.

Author details

Laurel Berman
Agency for Toxic Substances and Disease Registry, Georgia, USA

*Address all correspondence to: laberman@cdc.gov

References

[1] United States Government Accountability Office. Economic Development Administration: Remediation Activities Account for a Small Percentage of Total Brownfield Grant Funding [Internet]. Washington, D.C.: United States Government Accountability Office; October 2005. 50 pp. Report No.: GAO-06-7. Available from: https://www.gao.gov/assets/250/248268.pdf

[2] United States Environmental Protection Agency (EPA). What is Superfund? 2018. Available from: https://www.epa.gov/superfund/what-superfund. [Accessed: 2019-0904]

[3] Agency for Toxic Substances and Disease Registry (ATSDR). ATSDR Land Reuse Health Program: What is a Brownfield or Land Reuse Site? 2017. Available from: https://www.atsdr.cdc.gov/sites/brownfields/. [Accessed: 2019-0904]

[4] EPA. Overview of EPA's Brownfields Program. Available at: https://www.epa.gov/brownfields/overview-epas-brownfields-program. 2018. [Accessed 2019-0904]

[5] EPA. Superfund. Available at: https://www.epa.gov/superfund. 2019. [Accessed 2019-0904]

[6] Massey, R. Environmental Justice: Income, Race, and Health. Medford, MA: Global Development and Environment Institute, Tufts University; 2004. 24 p.

[7] New Jersey Department of Health and Senior Services. Health Consultation: Mercury Exposure Investigation Using Serial Urine Testing and Medical Records Review. Atlanta: Agency for Toxic Substances and Disease Registry. 2007. 23 p.

[8] Litt, J.S., Tran, N.L., Burke, T.A. Examining Urban Brownfields through the Public Health "Macroscope". Environmental Health Perspectives. 2002, April; vol. 110, supplement 2: Community, Research, and Environmental Justice, pp. 183-193.

[9] Wigle, D.T., Arbuckle, T.E., Walker, M., Wade, M.G., Liu, S., Krewski, D. Environmental Hazards: Evidence for Effects on Child Health, Journal of Toxicology and Environmental Health, Part B: Critical Reviews [Internet]. 2007, Dec 10], 10:1-2: 3-39. Available from: http://dx.doi.org/10.1080/1093740060 1034563

[10] EPA. Cleanups in My Community. Available at: https://www.epa.gov/cleanups/cleanups-my-community. 2019. [Accessed 2019-0904]

[11] United States Government Accountability Office. Vacant Properties: Growing Number Increases Communities' Costs and Challenges. Washington, D.C.: United States Government Accountability Office; November 2011. 102 pp. Report No.: GAO-12-34.

[12] deLeon, E., Schilling, J. Urban Blight and Public Health: Addressing the Housing, Abandoned Buildings, and Vacant Lots [Internet]. The Urban Institute; 2017 Apr 11. 44 pp. Available from: https://www.urban.org/research/publication/urban-blight-and-public-health

[13] Navajo Nation Division of Health and Navajo Epidemiology Center. Navajo Population Profile 2010 U.S. Census. Window Rock, Arizona: Navajo Nation; December 2013. 53 pp. Available from: https://www.nec.navajo-nsn.gov/Portals/0/Reports/NN2010Population Profile.pdf

[14] Northern Arizona University. Demographic Analysis of the Navajo Nation Using 2010 Census and 2010

American Community Survey Estimates. Window Rock, Arizona: Not dated (post-2010). 68 pp. Available from: https://gotr.azgovernor.gov/sites/default/files/navajo_nation_0.pdf

[15] Landry, A. Not Alone In the Dark: Navajo Nation's Lack of Electricity Problem. Indian Country Today [Internet]. 2011 Feb 11 [cited 2019 Sept 04]; Archives. Available from: https://newsmaven.io/indiancountrytoday/archive/not-alone-in-the-dark-navajo-nation-s-lack-of-electricity-problem-yO5P4y3H6k6kuxF-U5FvvQ/

[16] Yurth, C. Lost logging legacy: Red Lake struggles to retrieve its former grandeur. Navajo Times [Internet]. 2014 Jan 2 [cited 2019 Sept 04]; Chapter Series. Available from: https://www.navajotimes.com/news/chapters/010214redlake.php.

[17] ATSDR. Redeveloping into a Healthy Community. Available from: https://www.atsdr.cdc.gov/sites/brownfields/. 2010. [Accessed 2019-0904]

[18] Navajo Nation Division of Community Development. Navajo Nation Chapters Information. Available from: https://www.navajochapters.org/About.aspx. N.d. [Accessed 2019-09040]